Veterinary Medicine: Prevention, Diagnosis and Treatment of Diseases in Animals

Veterinary Medicine: Prevention, Diagnosis and Treatment of Diseases in Animals

Edited by **Andrea Santoro**

SYRAWOOD
PUBLISHING HOUSE

New York

Published by Syrawood Publishing House,
750 Third Avenue, 9th Floor,
New York, NY 10017, USA
www.syrawoodpublishinghouse.com

Veterinary Medicine: Prevention, Diagnosis and Treatment of Diseases in Animals
Edited by Andrea Santoro

International Standard Book Number: 978-1-68286-117-2 (Hardback)

Contents

Preface

Diagnosis, treatment and prevention are the three core areas of veterinary medicine. This book is a compilation of chapters that discuss the most vital concepts like types of diseases, sources of infection, agents, techniques of diagnosis, etc. The objective of this text is to give a general view of the different areas of veterinary medicine. It will serve as a valuable source of reference for graduate and post graduate students of veterinary sciences and associated disciplines.

This book is the end result of constructive efforts and intensive research done by experts in this field. The aim of this book is to enlighten the readers with recent information in this area of research. The information provided in this profound book would serve as a valuable reference to students and researchers in this field.

At the end, I would like to thank all the authors for devoting their precious time and providing their valuable contributions to this book. I would also like to express my gratitude to my fellow colleagues who encouraged me throughout the process.

Editor

Differential modulation of immune response and cytokine profiles in the bursae and spleen of chickens infected with very virulent infectious bursal disease virus

Mehdi Rasoli[1], Swee Keong Yeap[1], Sheau Wei Tan[1], Kiarash Roohani[1], Ye Wen Kristeen-Teo[2], Noorjahan Banu Alitheen[1,2], Yasmin Abd Rahaman[1,3], Ideris Aini[1,3], Mohd Hair Bejo[1,3], Pete Kaiser[4] and Abdul Rahman Omar[1,3*]

Abstract

Background: Very virulent infectious bursal disease virus (vvIBDV) induces immunosuppression and inflammation in young birds, which subsequently leads to high mortality. In addition, infectious bursal disease (IBD) is one of the leading causes of vaccine failure on farms. Therefore, understanding the immunopathogenesis of IBDV in both the spleen and the bursae could help effective vaccine development. However, previous studies only profiled the differential expression of a limited number of cytokines, in either the spleen or the bursae of Fabricius of IBDV-infected chickens. Thus, this study aims to evaluate the *in vitro* and *in vivo* immunoregulatory effects of vvIBDV infection on macrophage-like cells, spleen and bursae of Fabricius.

Results: The viral load was increased during the progression of the *in vitro* infection in the HD11 macrophage cell line and *in vivo*, but no significant difference was observed between the spleen and the bursae tissue. vvIBDV infection induced the expression of pro-inflammatory and Th1 cytokines, and chemokines from HD11 cells in a time- and dosage-dependent manner. Furthermore, alterations in the lymphocyte populations, cytokine and chemokine expression, were observed in the vvIBDV-infected spleens and bursae. A drastic rise was detected in numbers of macrophages and pro-inflammatory cytokine expression in the spleen, as early as 2 days post-infection (dpi). On 4 dpi, macrophage and T lymphocyte infiltration, associated with the peak expression of pro-inflammatory cytokines in the bursae tissues of infected chickens were observed. The majority of the significantly regulated pro-inflammatory cytokines and chemokines, in vvIBDV-infected spleens and bursae, were also detected in vvIBDV-infected HD11 cells. This cellular infiltration subsequently resulted in a sharp rise in nitric oxide (NO) and lipid peroxidation levels.

Conclusion: This study suggests that macrophage may play an important role in regulating the early expression of pro-inflammatory cytokines, first in the spleen and then in the bursae, the latter tissue undergoing macrophage infiltration at 4 dpi.

Keywords: vvIBDV, Viral load, GeXP, Real-time PCR, Pro-inflammatory cytokines, Chemokines

* Correspondence: aro@upm.edu.my
[1]Institute of Bioscience, Universiti Putra Malaysia, Serdang 43400, Selangor, Malaysia
[3]Faculty of Veterinary Medicine, Universiti Putra Malaysia, Serdang 43400, Selangor, Malaysia
Full list of author information is available at the end of the article

Background

Infectious bursal disease is an important viral disease, resulting in an acute and contagious infection on poultry farms. The causative agent is infectious bursal disease virus (IBDV) which belongs to the *Birnaviridae* family. IBDV is categorised into different types based on virulence, and the very virulent (vv) strain is the most acute and lethal. Presently, vvIBDV outbreaks have been reported in various countries, causing severe economic losses in the poultry industry. This virus can overcome maternally derived antibodies (MDA) and can cause 80 to 100 percent mortality in susceptible chickens [1]. The main targets of IBDV are IgM-bearing B cells, found in the gut-associated lymphoid organs and the bursae of Fabricius. Following infection, depletion of B cells due to viral-induced apoptosis in B cell occurred, causing severe immunosuppression in young chickens [2]. The susceptibility of T cells to IBDV is not well characterised. However, T cells are a crucial component in the immunopathogenesis of IBDV, as infiltration of CD4$^+$ and CD8$^+$ cells was detected in the bursae between 1 to 10 dpi [3,4], without affecting the population of these cells in spleen and peripheral blood [5,6]. In addition, infection of one-day-old chicks results in a rapid decline in B cell numbers in the peripheral blood and spleen. Apart from B cells, macrophages can also be infected by IBDV *in vitro* [7].

Classical and vvIBDV induce differential host immune responses [8-10]. However, both virus strains upregulate the expression of Th1-like and pro-inflammatory cytokines, such as IL-12, IFN-γ, IL-1β, IL-6, iNOS, and IL-18, in bursae tissue, but vvIBDV-induced IFN-γ is expressed at greater magnitude, compared to classical IBDV. Modulation of IFN-γ gene expression that leads to subsequent production of nitric oxide by macrophages [11], probably associated with the bursae-infiltrating CD4$^+$ and CD8$^+$ cells [12]. Furthermore, Tippenhauer *et al.* [13] reported different strains of IBDV differentially regulated levels of types I and II IFN expression in infected spleens and bursae. However, the contribution of macrophages to the cytokines and chemokines induced following IBDV infection, *in vitro* or *in vivo*, is still unknown. In this study, the immunomodulatory effect of vvIBDV on the expression of selected cytokines, chemokines and other immune-related genes was evaluated, and correlated with viral load, in *in vitro* infection of the HD11 macrophage cell line, and *in vivo* infection, specifically in the spleens and bursae, of specific-pathogen-free (SPF) chickens.

Methods

Propagation of vvIBDV strain UPM0081 in SPF embryonated chicken eggs

The UPM0081 strain was first isolated during an IBD outbreak in 2000 in Kelantan, a northern state of peninsular Malaysia. Based on the virus pathogenicity and the VP2 sequence analysis (NCBI Acc. No. AY520910), it was characterised as a vvIBDV strain [14]. The virus was propagated using nine-day-old embryonated SPF chicken eggs and stored at -80°C. The median embryo infective dose of the virus (EID$_{50}$) was calculated using the Reed-Muench method [15].

In vitro vvIBDV infection of HD11 cells

The chicken monocyte macrophage cell line HD11 [16] was obtained from Dr. Delphine Beeckman (Ghent University, Belgium) and maintained in Dulbecco's modified Eagle's minimal essential medium (DMEM) (Sigma, USA), supplemented with 5% heat-inactivated foetal calf serum, 1% sodium pyruvate, 1% L-glutamine and 0.5% gentamicin (all products from Gibco, USA), at 41°C, 5% CO$_2$ and 90% humidity. The cells (10^6 cells/ml/well) were infected with vvIBDV strain UPM0081 at a multiplicity of infection (MOI) of 0.1 and 0.5 for 3 h at 41°C.

After incubation, the cells were washed, fresh complete medium was added, and further incubated for 3, 21 and 45 h. The uninfected control and the IBDV-infected cells were harvested and subjected to viral load detection using quantitative real-time polymerase chain reaction (qRT-PCR) and an immune-related gene expression study using the multiplex GeXP system.

Virus inoculation in SPF chickens

Nine-day-old SPF eggs were obtained from the Veterinary Research Institute, Ipoh, Perak, and hatched at the Laboratory of Vaccines and Immunotherapeutics, Institute of Bioscience, Universiti Putra Malaysia (UPM). The trial was conducted in the animal research facility at the Faculty of Veterinary Medicine, UPM. Three-week-old SPF chickens (n = 29) were randomly divided into three groups. The first group (n = 15) was subjected to oculonasal infection with 10^4 EID$_{50}$ of vvIBDV strain UPM0081, whilst the second group (n = 9) received phosphate-buffered saline (PBS), and were kept as the control. The third group, consisting of five UPM0081-infected chickens, was kept for clinical and mortality observations. Water and feed were provided *ad libitum*. Five birds from the infected group and three birds from the control group were killed and necropsied at 2, 4 and 5 dpi. The spleen and bursae were harvested, observed for lesions and cut into two pieces. One piece was submersed in RNAlater® solution (Ambion, USA) for ribonucleic acid (RNA) isolation and the remaining half was analysed with flow cytometry. The experimental trials were approved by the Animal Care and Use Committee, at the Faculty of Veterinary Medicine, UPM (reference number UPM/IACUC/AUP-R022/2014). Bursae was also fix in 10% formalin, embedded in paraffin, section and stained with Haematoxylin and Eosin (H&E) for histopathological examination. All bursae samples were assigned with the following lesion scoring where lesion scores of 1 representing no lesions; 2 representing mild reduction in overall follicle size, 3 representing moderate reduction in follicle size; 4 representing severe reduction in follicle size; and 5 representing necrosis and follicle atrophy [17].

Flow cytometry analysis of B cell, T cell, and macrophage populations, in the spleens and bursae of infected and uninfected SPF chickens

The spleens and bursae were harvested at 2, 4 and 5 dpi from both the control group and the infected chickens, and were washed using Hank's balanced salt solution. Afterwards, the samples were pressed through a 70 μm sterile wire mesh screen (SPL Life Sciences, China). The lymphocytes were isolated using Ficoll-Plaque Plus™ (Amersham Biosciences, USA) according to the recommended protocol by the manufacturer with slight modifications. Purified lymphocytes from each groups were separated into four different tubes and each of them were stained with 10 μg/ml of 10 μl FITC-labelled CD3, PE-labelled CD4, IgM and KUL01 and PerCP-labelled CD8 antibodies (Southern Biotech, USA), respectively, and analysed using a FACSCalibur™ flow cytometer with CellQuest™ Pro software (BD Bioscience, USA).

RNA extraction and cDNA synthesis

Total RNA from the HD11 cells, spleens and bursae was isolated using an RNeasy® Plus Mini Kit (Qiagen, Germany) according to the protocol provided by the supplier. The quality and quantity of the extracted RNA were determined using NanoDrop™ ND-1000 (Thermo Scientific, Wilmington, USA). SuperScript™ III reverse transcriptase (Invitrogen, USA), and oligo(dT)18 primer (Fermentas, Lithuania) were selected to synthesise the cDNA. Total RNA with the final concentration of 1 μg was used in the cDNA synthesis.

IBDV quantitative real-time RT-PCR

In order to detect the IBD viral load in infected HD11 cells, spleens and bursae, a forward primer of 5′-ATG CTC CAG ATG GGG TAC TTC-3′ and a reverse primer of 5′-TTG GAC CCG GTG TTC ACG-3′, targeting the VP2 gene of the IBDV, were designed and optimised using iQ™ SYBR® Green Supermix (Biorad, USA). The thermal cycling protocol of polymerase activation and DNA denaturation was 95°C for 3 min, followed by 40 cycles of denaturation of 15 s at 95°C, 30 s of annealing and extension at 58.7°C. The melt curve analysis was 65 to 95°C, at increments of 0.5°C every 5 s/step. No template control (NTC) was included to ensure no cross-contamination during sample preparation. To ensure the specific amplification from IBD viral RNA and not DNA contamination, no-RT control was used. Standard curve was generated in RT-qPCR with the tenfold serially diluted viral RNA ranged from 9 to 14 $\log_{10}$ copies number. The viral load in infected HD11 cells, spleens and bursae was quantify based on the generated standard curve.

Multiplex GeXP assay

GenomeLab™ GeXP assays were performed to measure 27 selected genes with immune function and glyceraldehyde-3-phosphate dehydrogenase (GAPDH) was used as the reference gene for normalisation according to the method previously reported [18]. Primers to amplify the target genes were designed using the GenomeLab eXpress Profiler software (Table 1), which produced fragment sizes ranging from 137 to 350 nucleotides. The gene expression data were normalised by dividing the peak area of each gene by the peak area of the GAPDH gene and the fold change of expression of each gene was calculated using the following formula: fold change = normalised data of the gene from treated samples/normalised data of the gene from untreated samples [18]. The data for each gene and technical replicate were averaged and calculated.

Quantitative real-time RT-PCR validation of GeXP data

The GeXP data for CXCLi2, IFN-γ, IL-12α and IL-18 gene expression in the spleen and bursae were validated via qRT-PCR, using the primers and probes described by Kaiser et al. [19] and Kogut et al. [20], with some modification of the PCR reaction protocols (Table 2). The amplification step was carried out in a 25 μl reaction by adding 4 μl of cDNA, 12.5 μl of iQ Supermix (100 mM KCl, 40 mM Tris–HCl, 1.6 mM dNTPs, iTaq DNA polymerase 50 units/ml, 6 mM MgCl$_2$, and stabilisers), 1 μl of 10 mM of each primer and 2 μl of 1 mM probe, topped up with sterile distilled water. Amplification and detection of specific products was carried out using CFX96™ Real-Time System (BioRad, USA) with the following cycle profile: 1 cycle at 95°C for 5 min, 40 cycles at 95°C for 20 s, and 58°C or 60°C for 30 s as indicated in Table 2 RNA extracted from HD11 and ConA-C1-Vick T cell lines was used to generate a standard curve by serial dilution (10^{-1} to 10^{-5}) [18]. For each qRT-PCR experiment, the test samples and the ten-fold serially diluted RNA were run in duplicate. A no template control was also included. No-template control and no-RT control were also included. Quantification was carried out according to the Pfaffl method with corrected efficiency for each primer set [21].

Nitric oxide and malondialdehyde assays

The uninfected and vvIBDV-infected spleens and bursae were homogenised, filtered through a 70 μm mesh, and

Table 1 GeXP primers sequence and amplicon sizes designed for quantification of chicken cytokines, chemokines and other immune-related genes

Gene	Accession number	Amplicon size (bp)	Forward primer sequence* (5′–3′)	Reverse primer sequence** (5′–3′)
Cytokines and chemokines				
CCL4	NM_204720	235	CTGCTCAAAGCCTGCCATC	GTGCAGCCATCCTGAAGC
CXCLi1	NM_205018	228	CCGATGCCAGTGCATAGAG	CCTTGTCCAGAATTGCCTTG
CXCLi2	NM_205498	165	CCTGGTTTCAGCTGCTCTGT	GCGTCAGCTTCACATCTTGA
GM-CSF	NM_001007078	242	TGAAAACAAATGGGACAGAGG	TTCTCCTCTGGGAGCACATC
IFN-γ	NM_205149	214	GAGCCATCACCAAGAAGATGA	TAGGTCCACCGTCAGCTACA
IL-1β	NM_204524	137	CCAGAAAGTGAGGCTCAACA	GTAGCCCTTGATGCCCAGT
IL-2	NM_204153	144	GTGGCTAACTAATCTGCTGTCCA	CCGTAGGGCTTACAGAAAGG
IL-4	NM_001007079	151	CGTCAAGATGAACGTGACAGA	AGGTTCTTGTGGCAGTGCT
IL-6	NM_204628	158	AGTTCACCGTGTGCGAGAAC	TTCGTCAGGCATTTCTCCTC
IL-10	NM_001004414	172	TAACATCCAACTGCTCAGCTC	TGATGACTGGTGCTGGTCTG
IL-12α	NM_213588	179	AAGGGACTCAACTGCTCCAG	TTGTGTTGCTCTGACTGTTGG
IL-15	NM_204571	193	ATTCCCGATCCAGATTCTGTT	ACAGTTGGTACTGGAGACAAATACT
IL-16	NM_204352	200	GCCTCACAAGAATCAACAACTG	TGCTTTGTTCCAACGAGGTC
IL-17 F	NM_204460	340	TCCATGGGATTACAGGATCG	AGGCAAGGCAGTTCTCCTG
IL-18	NM_204608	207	CGTCAATAGCCAGTTGCTTG	CTTCTACCTGGACGCTGAATG
IL-21	NM_001024835	186	TGTGGTGAAAGATAAGGATGTCG	CAGTTTTGGCGAATGTAGCA
IL-22	XM_416079	256	CAGCCCTACATCAGGAATCG	GAACTGTGCCACATCCTCAG
TGF-β3	NM_205454	347	AATCAGCATACACTGCCCTTG	TCGGAAGTCAATGTAAAGAGGAC
TNFSF13B	NM_204327	333	GGCAAGGTCTCCACTAGAGC	TCAGAAGCCAAGGGACAATG
Toll-like receptors				
TLR2-1	NM_204278	249	TCAGCTACACCAAAATGTTCAACC	CGTGATTTTGCCTGTGAGC
TLR3	NM_001011691	263	TGCATAAGAAGGAGCAGGAAG	CTGGCCAGTTCAAGATGCAG
TLR4	NM_001030693	270	CATCTCTGGAGTTCCTGCTG	AGGCTGCTAGACCCAGGTG
TLR5	NM_001024586	277	CACTCAGGTTCTCGGTATTCG	AATCCAGGTGCTTCAGCAAG
TLR7	NM_001011688	284	GAGTGAGTTATGCCACTCCTCTC	TCAAAGGCTTCCACATCAC
Others				
iNOS	NM_204961	221	TATGCTCTGCCTGCTGTTGC	ATGCAAGTTTGTTGCTTTCC
MHCI	NM_001044683	291	GGAAACCTGCGTGGAGTG	TGGTGACCCAGGTGTGGTA
MHCII	NM_001044679	298	AGTACGCGCACTTCGACA	AGAAGCCCGTCACGTAGC
GAPDH	NM_204305	312	CTGGCAAAGTCCAAGTGGTG	AGCACCACCCTTCAGATGAG
KAN^r***	-	325	ATCATCAGCATTGCATTCGATTCCTGTTTG	ATTCCGACTCGTCCAACATC

*Forward universal primer sequence (AGGTGACACTATAGAATA).
**Reverse universal primer sequence (GTACGACTCACTATAGGGA).
***Internal control.

pelleted at 500 xg for 10 min. Supernatants from both the spleen and bursae were subjected to quantification of nitric oxide and malondialdehyde levels. NO was quantified using the Griess assay, where 150 μl of the supernatant was added to 20 μl of Griess reagent (Invitrogen, USA) and 130 μl of deionised water, followed by 30 min incubation at room temperature. The sample's absorbance was read at 548 nm using a μQuant ELISA Reader (BioTek Instruments, USA).

For the malondialdehyde (MDA) determination, 200 μl of supernatant were added to 800 μl of PBS, 25 μl of butylated hydroxytoluene (Sigma, USA), and 500 μl of trichloroacetic acid and 2-thiobarbituric acid (Sigma, USA), followed by 2 h incubation on ice. The mixture was then pelleted at 500 xg for 15 min and 1 ml of the supernatant was collected and added to 75 μl of 0.1 M ethylene diamine tetraacetic acid and 250 μl of 0.05 M 2-thiobarbituric acid (Sigma, USA). Finally, the sample

Table 2 Real-time quantitative RT-PCR probes and primers

Target		Probe or primer sequence (5'–3')	Accession no.	Annealing temperature
CXCLi2	Probe	(FAM)-TCTTTACCAGCGTCCTACCTTGCGACA-(BHQ1)	AJ009800	60°C
	F	GCCCTCCTCCTGGTTTCAG		
	R	TGGCACCGCAGCTCATT		
GAPDH	Probe	(FAM[a])-CGCCATCACTATCTTCCAGG-(BHQ1)	NM_204305	58°C
	F[b]	GAACGGGAAACTTGTGAT		
	R[b]	GACTCCACAACATACTCA		
IFN-γ	Probe	(FAM)-TGGCCAAGCTCCCGATGAACGA-(BHQ1)	Y07922	58°C
	F	GTGAAGAAGGTGAAAGATATCATGGA		
	R	GCTTTGCGCTGGATTCTCA		
IL-1β	Probe	(FAM)-CCACACTGCAGCTGGAGGAAGCC-(BHQ1)	AJ245728	60°C
	F	GCTCTACATGTCGTGTGTGATGAG		
	R	TGTCGATGTCCCGCATGA		
IL-10	Probe	(FAM)-CGACGATTCGGCGCTGTCACC-(BHQ1)	AJ621614	58°C
	F	CATGCTGCTGGGCCTGAA		
	R	CGTCTCCTTGATCTGCTTGATG		
IL-12α	Probe	(FAM)-CCAGCGTCCTCTGCTTCTGCACCTT-(BHQ1)	AY262751	58°C
	F	TGGCCGCTGCAAACG		
	R	ACCTCTTCAAGGGTGCACTCA		
IL-18	Probe	(FAM)-CCGCGCCTTCAGCAGGGATG-(BHQ1)	AJ276026	60°C
	F	AGGTGAAATCTGGCAGTGGAAT		
	R	ACCTGGACGCTGAATGCAA		

[a]FAM, 6-carboxyfluorescein; BHQ1, Black Hole Quencher.
[b]F, forward primer; R, reverse primer.

was boiled for 15 min, cooled to room temperature, and the absorbance recorded at 548 nm by the μQuant ELISA Reader. A standard curve for MDA was prepared concurrently using thiobarbituric reactive substances (Sigma, USA).

Statistical analysis
The results from this study were subjected to one-way ANOVA analysis with Duncan's post-hoc test using SPSS version 21, where P < 0.05 is considered as significant.

Results
In vitro infection of HD11 cells with vvIBDV
IBDV in the infected cells was detected by quantitative real-time RT-PCR. As shown in Table 3, IBDV RNA was detected in HD11 cells as early as 6 h post-infection (hpi), with slight increased at 48 hpi.

vvIBDV-induced expression of cytokines, chemokines and other immune-related genes by HD11 cells
mRNA expression levels of the pro-inflammatory cytokine IL-1β, the pro-inflammatory chemokines CCL4, CXCLi1 and CXCLi2, and the Th1 cytokines IL-12α and IL-18 were all upregulated in vvIBDV-infected HD11

cells throughout the experiment (Table 4). At both MOI, mRNA expression levels of IL-1β, CCL4, CXCLi2, IL-12α and IL-18 peaked at 24 hpi, whereas those of CXCLi1 peaked at 6 hpi. In contrast, mRNA expression levels of the anti-inflammatory cytokine IL-10 were generally down-regulated.

Of the TLRs measured, only the mRNA expression levels of TLR3 were significantly altered post-infection, with levels increasing with time post-infection at both MOI. For MHC class I, mRNA expression levels were

Table 3 Detection of virus RNA in HD11 cells infected with vvIBDV strain UPM0081 by SYBR Green real-time qRT-PCR

Sample	Mean Cq		Viral copy number (log$_{10}$)	
	0.1 MOI	0.5 MOI	0.1 MOI	0.5 MOI
Uninfected	ND	ND	ND	ND
6 hours	18.89	18.42	14.16	14.29
24 hours	18.85	18.28	14.17	14.33
48 hours	18.05	17.30	14.40	14.61

Statistical differences between groups were assessed by one-way ANOVA followed by a Duncan post-hoc test.
ND = not detected.

Table 4 Relative fold changes in gene expression in HD11 cells infected with different MOI of vvIBDV strain UPM0081 at 6, 24 and 48 hpi

Gene	6 hpi		24 hpi		48 hpi	
	0.1 MOI	0.5 MOI	0.1 MOI	0.5 MOI	0.1 MOI	0.5 MOI
Pro-inflammatory cytokines and chemokines						
IL-1β	<2	2.33 ± 0.19^a	5.53 ± 0.37^b	6.74 ± 1.78^b	<2	2.92 ± 0.65^a
CCL4	$2.47 \pm 1.03^{a,b}$	$4.07 \pm 0.64^{a,b}$	3.89 ± 0.85^b	5.07 ± 1.17^a	2.69 ± 0.78^a	3.29 ± 0.90^a
CXCLi1	3.39 ± 0.45^a	4.34 ± 0.54^b	1.99 ± 0.35^c	2.32 ± 0.49^c	<2	<2
CXCLi2	2.24 ± 0.41^a	2.44 ± 0.27^a	6.44 ± 0.75^b	9.02 ± 0.45^c	3.84 ± 0.40^d	4.40 ± 1.14^d
Th1 cytokines						
IL-12α	2.10 ± 0.39^a	3.32 ± 0.78^b	3.43 ± 0.31^b	4.32 ± 1.2^b	<2	<2
IL-18	<2	3.05 ± 0.53^a	2.46 ± 0.23^b	3.34 ± 0.50^b	<2	<2
Treg cytokine						
IL-10	-2.44 ± 0.23^a	-4.17 ± 0.10^b	-2.00 ± 0.33^c	-2.86 ± 0.36^d	<2	$-2.22 \pm 0.13^{a,c}$
Toll-like receptors						
TLR2-1	<2	<2	<2	<2	<2	<2
TLR3	<2	$2.65 \pm 0.37^{a,b}$	2.00 ± 0.90^a	4.90 ± 0.44^c	3.22 ± 0.14^b	5.22 ± 0.45^c
TLR4	<2	<2	<2	<2	<2	<2
TLR5	<2	<2	<2	<2	<2	<2
TLR7	<2	<2	<2	<2	<2	<2
Others						
IL-15	<2	<2	<2	<2	<2	<2
IL-16	<2	<2	<2	-2.13 ± 0.15	<2	<2
iNOS	3.67 ± 0.53^a	$4.73 \pm 0.16^{b,c}$	$3.52 \pm 1.1^{a,b}$	7.51 ± 0.73^d	5.57 ± 0.61^c	5.68 ± 0.44^c
MHCI	<2	<2	<2	-2.22 ± 0.22^a	2.59 ± 1.18^b	3.13 ± 1.40^b
MHCII	-2.33 ± 0.08^a	-3.13 ± 0.08^b	<2	-4.55 ± 0.14^c	<2	-5.26 ± 0.09^d
TGF-β3	<2	<2	<2	<2	<2	<2

Statistical differences between groups were assessed by one-way ANOVA followed by a Duncan post-hoc test. Means labelled with different letters are significantly different, $p < 0.05$. <2: less than a 2-fold change.

upregulated at 48 hpi for both MOI, but downregulated at 24 hpi only for the MOI of 0.5. For MHC class II, at an MOI of 0.1 mRNA expression levels were downregulated only at 6 hpi, whereas with an MOI of 0.5, mRNA expression levels were increasingly downregulated with time. For iNOS, mRNA expression levels were upregulated at all time-points for both MOIs, with peak expression being at 48 hpi for an MOI of 0.1 and 24 hpi for an MOI of 0.5.

For the other genes measured, there was very little difference in mRNA expression levels, regardless of MOI or time-point.

qRT-PCR quantification of viral load in infected spleens and bursae

Clinical signs, including diarrhoea, depression, feather ruffling and loss of appetite, were observed in chickens infected with vvIBDV strain UPM0081, starting from 3 days post-infection (dpi), while 100 percent mortality was observed at 6 dpi. A mottled spleen and bursae

haemorrhages were observed in the infected chickens from 3 dpi onwards (Data not shown). Lesion scoring 4 and 5 were recorded in the histology of bursal from vvIBDV strain UPM0081 infected chicken at 4 and 5 dpi, respectively (Figure 1).

Virus in vvIBDV-infected spleens and bursae was detected as early as 2 dpi and peaked at 5 dpi for both spleen and bursae, with 13.49 $\log_{10}$ and 13.97 $\log_{10}$ copies number, respectively. Viral loads were generally higher in the bursae of Fabricius compared to the spleen, but the differences were not significant (Table 5).

Flow cytometry immunophenotyping of vvIBDV-infected spleens and bursae

In order to study changes in the percentage of T and B lymphocytes and macrophages isolated from the bursae and spleens, the cells harvested from bursae or spleen were counted and stained with antibodies against CD3$^+$/CD4$^+$, CD3$^+$/CD8$^+$, IgM$^+$ and KUL01$^+$ and analysed by flow cytometry. Overall, IBDV infection caused a

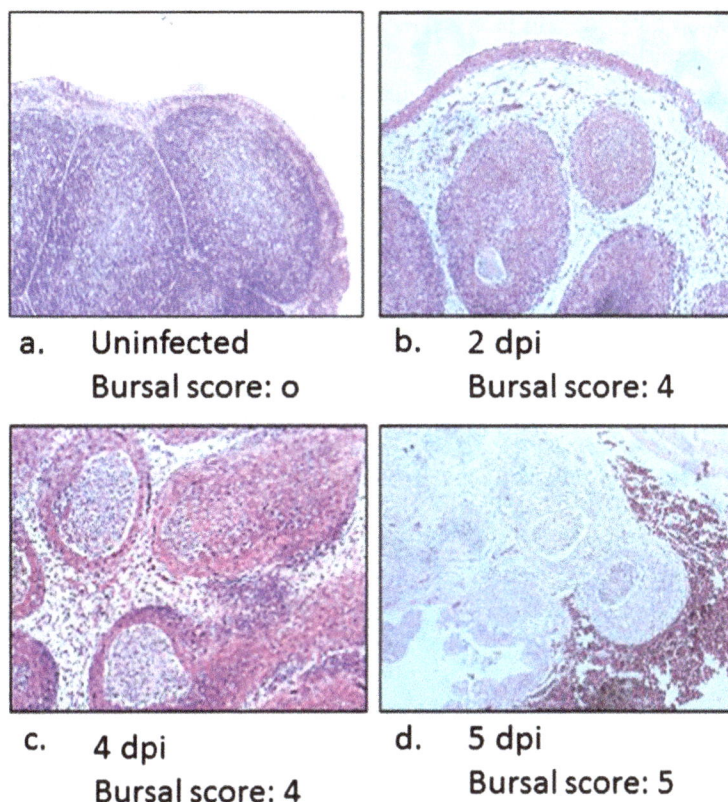

Figure 1 Bursal histopathology of (a) uninfected, (b) 2 day, (c) 4 day and (d) 5 day post vvIBDV strain UPM0081 infected chicken. Bursal was scored from 0-5 based on the lesion scoring. (100X).

significant increase in the percentage of KUL01$^+$ cells (macrophages), CD3$^+$/CD4$^+$ T cells and CD3$^+$/CD8$^+$ T cells in the bursae of Fabricius (Table 6).

In the bursa of chickens infected with vvIBDV strain UPM0081, the KUL01$^+$ macrophage population increased from ~9.90x10^6 cells in the control birds to 20.68x10^6 and 12.92x10^6 cells at 4 and 5 dpi, respectively (Table 6). However, there was no indication of an

Table 5 Detection of virus RNA in the spleens and bursae of chickens infected with vvIBDV strain UPM0081 by SYBR Green real-time qRT-PCR

Sample	Mean Cq		Viral copy number (log 10)	
	Spleen	Bursae	Spleen	Bursae
Uninfected	ND*	ND*	ND*	ND*
Day 2	30.42 ± 1.78^a	29.13 ± 2.48^{a,b}	10.93^a	11.29^{a,b}
Day 4	27.30 ± 0.84^{b,c}	25.92 ± 1.60^c	11.81^{b,c}	12.19^c
Day 5	21.29 ± 2.13^d	19.57 ± 0.21^d	13.49^d	13.97^d

Values are the mean percentages of total cells ± SD per tissue of 5 chickens, each with three technical repeats. Statistical differences between groups were assessed by one-way ANOVA followed by a Duncan post-hoc test. Means labelled with different superscript letters are significantly different (p < 0.05) between organs at different sampling days.
*ND = not detected.

increased macrophage population at 2 dpi in the infected bursae. In contrast, IBDV induced an increased in the KUL01$^+$ macrophage population in the spleen from 6.26x10^6 cells in the control to 18.54 x10^6 cells at 2 dpi. However, the splenic macrophage cell number in infected chickens decreased sharply at 4 and 5 dpi (Table 6).

An increased in CD3$^+$/CD4$^+$ and CD3$^+$/CD8$^+$ T cells was also detected in the infected bursae, reaching peaks of 4.25x10^6 and 3.52x10^6 cells, respectively, at 5 dpi (Table 6). However, the population of splenic CD4$^+$ and CD8$^+$ cells were initially high and reduced significantly at 5 dpi (Table 6). IgM$^+$ cells in the bursae of infected chickens reduced significantly from 189.83x10^6 cells in the control to 35.52x10^6 cells at 5 dpi. Similarly, the splenic IgM$^+$ cell number decreased from 57.36x10^6 cells in control birds, to 14.57x10^6 cells at 5 dpi (Table 6).

Expression profiles of immune-related genes in IBDV-infected spleens and bursae

A multiplex quantitative GeXP assay was used to quantify the mRNA expression levels of immune-related genes in the spleens and bursae of SPF chickens infected with vvIBDV strain UPM0081 at 2, 4 and 5 dpi. Of the

Table 6 The cell number of IgM$^+$ cells, KUL01$^+$ macrophages, CD3$^+$CD4$^+$ cells and CD3$^+$CD8$^+$ cells in bursae and spleens of 3-week-old chickens infected with vvIBDV strain UPM0081 at 2, 4 and 5 dpi

		Bursae (x10^{6}cell/bursae)	Spleen (x10^{6}cell/spleen)
Average number of cells	Day 0	230.00 ± 2.73^a	190.00 ± 3.41^a
	Day 2	173.00 ± 3.64^b	150.00 ± 2.76^b
	Day 4	116.00 ± 1.66^c	66.40 ± 2.31^c
	Day 5	54.00 ± 1.37^d	34.40 ± 2.32^d
IgM$^+$	Day 0	189.83 ± 0.83^a	57.36 ± 1.21^a
	Day 2	138.99 ± 0.50^b	44.35 ± 0.15^b
	Day 4	72.21 ± 0.55^c	23.27 ± 1.00^c
	Day 5	35.52 ± 3.07^d	14.57 ± 1.55^d
KUL-1$^+$	Day 0	9.90 ± 0.52^a	6.26 ± 0.13^a
	Day 2	8.76 ± 0.22^a	18.54 ± 0.93^b
	Day 4	20.68 ± 2.16^b	2.08 ± 0.31^c
	Day 5	12.92 ± 3.50^c	2.75 ± 0.49^c
CD3$^+$CD4$^+$	Day 0	1.73 ± 0.12^a	41.49 ± 0.80^a
	Day 2	1.67 ± 0.09^a	33.04 ± 1.51^b
	Day 4	3.82 ± 0.43^b	16.52 ± 2.12^c
	Day 5	4.25 ± 0.48^b	7.58 ± 0.53^d
CD3$^+$CD8$^+$	Day 0	1.67 ± 0.14^a	62.36 ± 0.61^a
	Day 2	1.86 ± 0.30^a	48.68 ± 0.98^b
	Day 4	3.05 ± 0.38^b	20.87 ± 0.66^c
	Day 5	3.52 ± 0.20^b	6.81 ± 0.38^d

The number of cell (mean ± SD) of the cell subsets were determined by trypan blue cell count and flow cytometry using a FACSCalibur with CellQuest Pro software (BD Bioscience, USA). Statistical differences between groups were assessed by one-way ANOVA followed by a Duncan post-hoc test. Means labelled with different superscript letters are significantly different (p < 0.05) between organs at different sampling days.

27 genes evaluated in this study, 20 genes were significantly regulated (>2-fold up or down) in the bursae and spleen post-infection (Table 7). In general, IBDV infection induced significant upregulation of pro-inflammatory cytokines and chemokines and Th1 cytokines in both tissues.

In the bursae of infected birds, the mRNA expression levels of the pro-inflammatory cytokine IL-1β were not statistically different from those in controls. All of the other pro-inflammatory cytokines and chemokines have increased mRNA expression levels, at least at some time-points post-infection, but with different patterns. IL-6 and CXCLi2 mRNA expression levels peaked at 4 dpi and were upregulated throughout the experiment. CCL4 and CXCLi1 mRNA expression levels were only upregulated from 4 dpi, but peaked at 5 and 4 dpi, respectively. Again, mRNA expression levels of the Th1 cytokines measured were upregulated compared to

controls at all time-points post-infection. IL-18 was consistently upregulated, whereas IFN-γ and IL-12α mRNA expression levels increased until 4 dpi but then plateaued. mRNA expression levels of the T cell proliferative cytokines IL-2 and IL-15, and the anti-inflammatory (Treg) cytokine IL-10 were essentially unaltered at most time-points from levels in the controls.

Expression levels of mRNA for the two TLRs measured were either downregulated (at 2 and 4 dpi for TLR7 and 4 dpi for TLR3) or unaltered compared to levels in controls. MHC class I and II mRNA expression levels were only upregulated at 4 dpi, and unaltered at the other time-points. iNOS mRNA levels showed a similar pattern of expression to those of IFN-γ and IL-12α.

Expression levels of the other molecules measured were varied. TGF-β3 mRNA expression levels were downregulated at 4 and 5 dpi, whereas those of the TNF superfamily member 13B were upregulated at the same time-points. IL-16 mRNA expression levels were slightly downregulated at 4 dpi, whereas those of IL-17F were unaltered compared to those in controls.

The spleen showed strong upregulation of the mRNA expression levels of pro-inflammatory cytokines and chemokines, Th1 cytokines and iNOS at all time-points, but there are few other changes compared to levels in controls. Upregulation of IL-1β mRNA expression levels appeared to be biphasic, higher at 2 and 5 dpi than at 4 dpi. IL-6 mRNA expression levels peaked at 2 dpi. The mRNA expression levels of the pro-inflammatory chemokines are consistently upregulated throughout the experiment but do not alter with time. Expression levels of mRNA for the three Th1 cytokines also peaked at 2 dpi. iNOS mRNA expression levels increased throughout the course of the experiment and peaked at 5 dpi.

Expression levels of the T cell proliferative and anti-inflammatory cytokines measured were largely unaltered in the spleen, as were levels of the TLRs measured, TGF-β3 and IL-17F. mRNA expression levels for MHC class I, MHC class II and TNFSF13B were all upregulated at 4 dpi (and at 5 dpi also for the latter), whereas IL-16 mRNA expression levels were downregulated at 4 dpi.

Validation of the GeXP gene expression profiles using qRT-PCR

In order to confirm the data obtained from the GeXP multiplex assay, qRT-PCR was performed to quantify the mRNA expression levels of selected cytokines, namely IFN-γ, IL-12α, IL-18 and CXCLi2 (Figure 2). Overall, qRT-PCR detected higher fold changes than the GeXP assay in all of the genes quantified, but confirmed the expression patterns previously detected by the GeXP assay (Table 7).

Table 7 Relative fold changes in gene expression in bursae and spleens of SPF chickens infected with vvIBDV strain UPM0081 at 2, 4 and 5 dpi, using a multiplex quantitative GeXP assay

	2 dpi		4 dpi		5dpi	
	Bursae	Spleen	Bursae	Spleen	Bursae	Spleen
Pro-inflammatory cytokines and chemokines						
IL-1β	<2	7.17 ± 2.17[b]	<2	3.26 ± 1.18[a]	<2	9.31 ± 2.59[b]
IL-6	2.22 ± 0.37[a]	6.51 ± 0.60[b,c]	10.96 ± 3.52[d]	3.35 ± 0.76[a,b]	9.74 ± 3.48[c,d]	2.28 ± 0.40[a]
CCL4	<2	2.61 ± 0.67[a,b]	4.93 ± 2.05[b,c]	2.29 ± 0.30[a]	5.69 ± 2.53[c]	2.19 ± 0.78[a]
CXCLi1	<2	2.16 ± 0.39[a]	4.24 ± 2.24[b]	2.45 ± 0.62[a,b]	2.23 ± 0.44[a]	2.59 ± 0.51[a,b]
CXCLi2	3.56 ± 1.54[a]	2.84 ± 0.95[a]	10.34 ± 3.64[b]	2.86 ± 1.20[a]	4.45 ± 1.95[a]	2.70 ± 1.18[a]
Th1 cytokines						
IFN-γ	9.55 ± 2.29[a]	12.30 ± 4.75[a]	26.20 ± 5.23[b]	9.29 ± 4.24[a]	26.22 ± 6.78[b]	9.87 ± 2.92[a]
IL-12α	4.76 ± 2.69[a]	23.95 ± 7.96[b]	10.63 ± 2.58[a]	15.52 ± 9.23[a,b]	11.62 ± 3.25[a]	8.06 ± 4.53[a]
IL-18	5.69 ± 1.92[a]	11.16 ± 2.04[b]	4.03 ± 1.03[a]	4.38 ± 1.59[a]	4.90 ± 3.01[a]	3.97 ± 1.35[a]
T cell proliferative cytokines						
IL-2	<2	<2	-3.57 ± 0.09	<2	<2	<2
IL-15	<2	<2	<2	<2	<2	2.39 ± 0.59
Treg cytokines						
IL-10	<2	<2	<2	<2	2.10 ± 0.13	<2
Toll-like receptors						
TLR3	<2	<2	-2.33 ± 0.18	<2	<2	<2
TLR7	-2.00 ± 0.11[a]	<2	-3.70 ± 0.09[b]	<2	<2	<2
Others						
iNOS	2.32 ± 0.50[a]	2.53 ± 0.52[a]	4.27 ± 0.70[b,c]	2.87 ± 0.91[a,b]	4.65 ± 1.29[c]	3.81 ± 0.72[a,b,c]
MHCI	<2	<2	2.14 ± 0.30[a]	2.24 ± 0.35[a]	<2	<2
MHCII	<2	<2	2.93 ± 1.01[a]	2.08 ± 0.49[a]	<2	<2
TGF-β3	<2	-2.00 ± 0.13[a]	-5.26 ± 0.07[b]	<2	-2.44 ± 0.10[a]	<2
TNFSF13B	<2	<2	2.83 ± 0.82[a]	2.46 ± 0.62[a]	3.30 ± 1.50[a]	3.11 ± 0.43[a]
IL-16	<2	<2	-2.04 ± 0.21[a]	-2.56 ± 0.10[a]	<2	<2
IL-17 F	<2	<2	<2	<2	<2	2.00 ± 0.22

Statistical differences between groups were assessed by one-way ANOVA followed by a Duncan post-hoc test. Means labelled with different superscript letters are significantly different ($p < 0.05$) between organs at different sampling days <2: less than a 2-fold change.

In the bursae of chickens infected with vvIBDV strain UPM0081, the Th1 cytokines IFN-γ and IL-12α were up-regulated as early as 2 dpi (Figure 2). The highest upregulation of IFN-γ mRNA levels was 113-fold at 5 dpi (Figure 2). IL-18 mRNA expression levels were upregulated from 2 dpi and remained unchanged until 5 dpi. CXCLi2 mRNA expression levels were up-regulated 9-fold as early as 2 dpi, peaked at 4 dpi at 40-fold, but decreased to 20-fold at 5 dpi (Figure 2).

In the spleens of chickens infected with vvIBDV strain UPM0081, IFN-γ mRNA expression levels were up-regulated 44-fold at 2 dpi and decreased thereafter (Figure 2). IL-12α mRNA expression levels were 106-fold up-regulated at 2 dpi, but decreased thereafter to 26-fold at 5 dpi. IL-18 mRNA expression levels were up-regulated moderately after infection, with a peak of

11-fold at 2 dpi. CXCLi2 mRNA expression levels were up-regulated at all time-points (up to 4-fold at 5 dpi).

NO and MDA levels in vvIBDV-infected spleen and bursae
Nitric oxide, which acts as a pro-inflammatory mediator and the production of which is often used as a measure of IFN-γ activity, was up-regulated in both the bursae and spleens of vvIBDV-infected chickens (Figure 3a). NO levels in the bursae increased more than those in the spleen and in both organs peaked at 5 dpi. Similarly, the lipid peroxidation rate in vvIBDV-infected spleens and bursae was measured using malondialdehyde as an oxidative stress marker. Similarly to NO, at 3 dpi MDA levels in the bursae increased throughout the experiment (Figure 3b), whilst levels in the spleen were also elevated but only at 4 and 5 dpi, with there being no significant

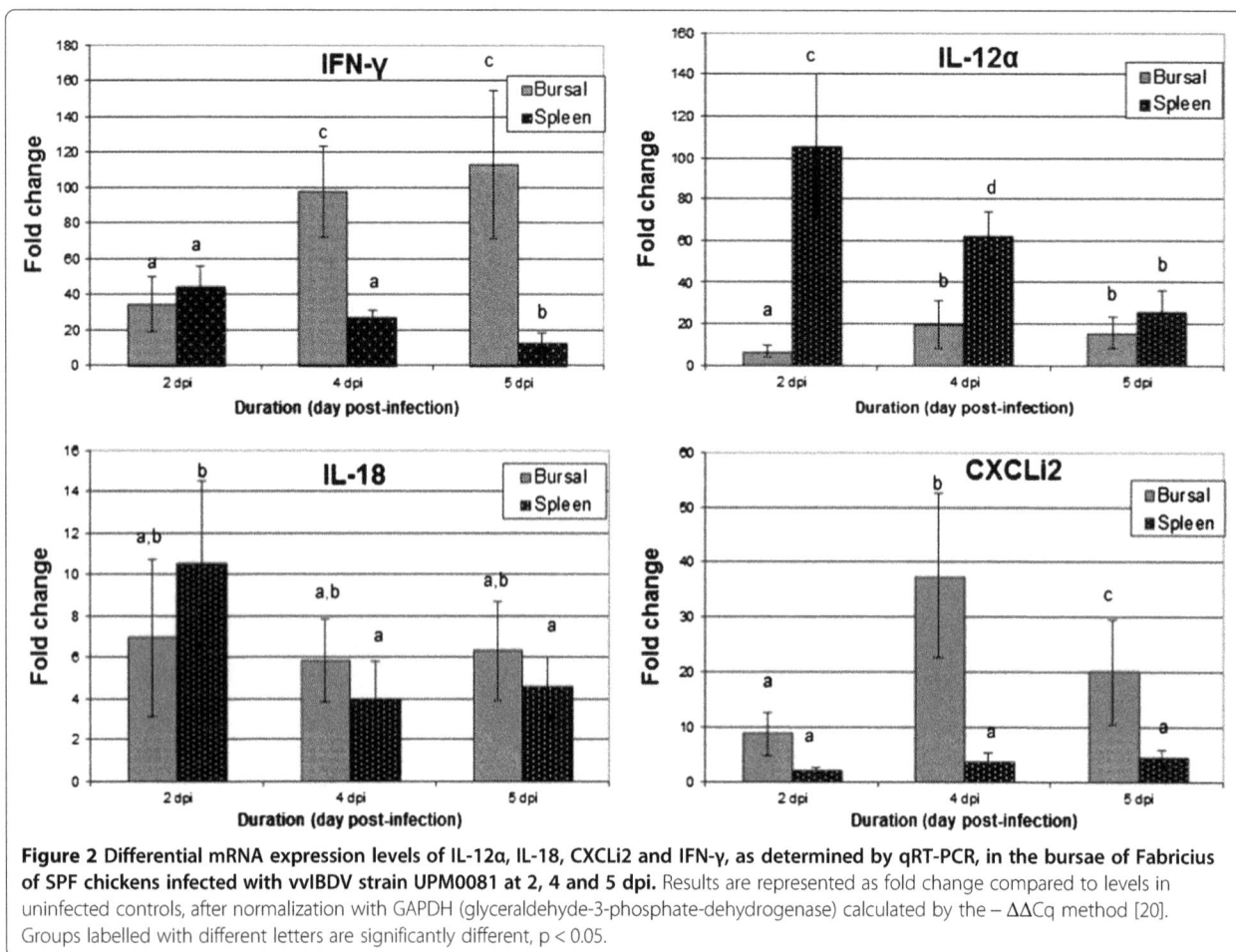

Figure 2 Differential mRNA expression levels of IL-12α, IL-18, CXCLi2 and IFN-γ, as determined by qRT-PCR, in the bursae of Fabricius of SPF chickens infected with vvIBDV strain UPM0081 at 2, 4 and 5 dpi. Results are represented as fold change compared to levels in uninfected controls, after normalization with GAPDH (glyceraldehyde-3-phosphate-dehydrogenase) calculated by the $-\Delta\Delta Cq$ method [20]. Groups labelled with different letters are significantly different, $p < 0.05$.

difference between levels at those latter two time-points (Figure 3b).

Discussion

IBDV infection is associated with up-regulation of pro-inflammatory cytokines and destruction of actively dividing IgM^+ B lymphocytes [8,10]. These previous studies looked at alterations of expression of a limited panel of cytokines, chemokines and TLRs following infection with classical and very virulent strains of IBDV [8,10]; we believe this is the most exhaustive study to date, and the first to compare responses to *in vitro* infection of macrophage-like cells (HD11 cell line) with those to *in vivo* infection in the spleen and bursae. Changes in the numbers of macrophages, T and B cells in the two tissues following infection were also quantified.

It has been proposed that macrophages play a critical role in spreading IBDV from the gut to the bursae [22]. This study illustrates that vvIBDV infection of HD11 cells can be detected as early as 6 h after adding virus to the cells, and that viral load was maximal at the end of the experiment, 48 hpi. After *in vivo* infection with

vvIBDV, virus was detected in both the spleen and bursae as early as 2 dpi using qRT-PCR, confirming an earlier study that detected the IBDV genome in the spleen and bursae as early as 3 dpi [10]. Increased viral load in both the spleen and bursae was associated with the progression of the disease and histological changes in the respective tissues (Figure 1). Although the load of IBDV was higher in the bursae than in the spleens, these results were not statistically significant (Table 5), indicating both spleen and bursae are equally susceptible to vvIBDV infection. This study also confirms a previous study by Rautenschlein *et al.* [23] that showed that infection with virulent strains of IBDV are associated with severe lesions in non-bursae organs, including the spleen.

IBDV infection is associated with activation of innate and adaptive antiviral immune responses, via proliferation of different effector cells, including macrophages and T cells [10]. Although similar viral loads were observed in the vvIBDV-infected spleens and bursae, kinetics of changes in macrophage numbers were different in the two organs (Table 6). In the infected spleens, there

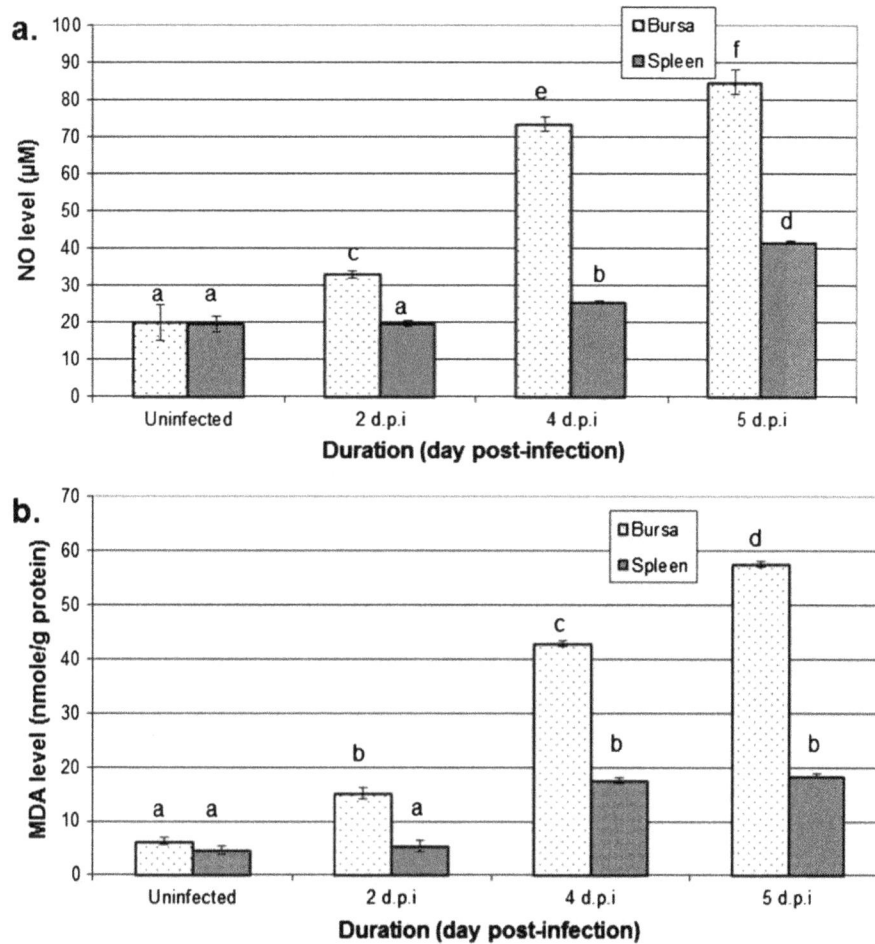

Figure 3 Level of inflammatory mediator (a) nitric oxide (NO) and lipid peroxidation reactive aldehydes (b) malondialdehyde (MDA) in the spleens and bursae of chickens infected with vvIBDV strain UPM0081 at 2, 4 and 5 dpi. Differences between control and treated groups were determined by one-way ANOVA (p < 0.05). Means labelled with different letters are significantly different, p < 0.05.

was a rapid increase in macrophage numbers at 2 dpi, followed by a marked reduction at 4 dpi back to levels in control spleens. In the infected bursae, macrophage numbers were increased at 4 and 5 dpi. This finding supports an earlier study, where bursae macrophage numbers increased significantly at 3 and 5 dpi [24]. The decreased in macrophage numbers in the spleen at 4 dpi could reflect migration of splenic macrophages to the bursae. Khatri and Sharma [25] reported that acute infection by IBDV was associated with lysis of macrophages that contributed to a reduction in innate immunity, followed by a rapid recovery of macrophage numbers and a revival of innate immunity. Changes in macrophage numbers in the infected tissues could consequently alter the expression levels of various cytokines and chemokines, which in turn could enhance the infiltration of heterophils, macrophages [25] and T cells [12] into the bursae. In this study, increasing numbers of CD4$^+$ and CD8$^+$ T cells, as similarly reported

by Kim *et al.* [12], were also observed in the bursae from 4 to 5 dpi. The CD4$^+$ T and CD8$^+$ T cells may have migrated from the spleen, as there was a significant decrease in numbers of these cells in the spleen at 5 dpi (Table 6). However, as has been previously suggested [26], it is still not clear whether the changes in cell numbers in the vvIBDV-infected bursae were the result of cell migration to/from other tissues or the periphery, or if there were expansions/contractions of the resident cell populations.

Expression of immune genes in response to *in vitro* infection of HD11 cells was remarkably similar to expression of immune genes in the bursae and spleen following *in vivo* infection, although the precise kinetics of expression sometimes differed slightly for the same gene between the different cells and tissues. In HD11 cells, spleens and bursae, infection with vvIBDV strain UPM0081 induced increased mRNA expression levels, in a dose-dependent manner, of pro-inflammatory cytokines and chemokines, Th1 cytokines, iNOS and MHC class I. This result is similar as previously reported [24,25] where IBDV infection promoted upregulation of proinflammatory cytokines including IL-1β, IL-6, IL-18 and iNOS of adherent putative macrophage cell isolated from bursae of IBDV challenged chicken. This is typical of the immune response to infection with a virus – an innate immune response is triggered, followed by a Th1 response leading to increased viral antigen presentation in the context of MHC class I, and the production of effector molecules, such as NO through the induction of iNOS.

Differences from this pattern were slight but the main ones will be discussed. In the in vitro HD11 cell infection model, mRNA expression levels of TLR3, which recognises dsRNA (IBDV is a dsRNA virus), were also upregulated. MHC class II mRNA expression levels were down-regulated, as were those of the anti-inflammatory cytokine IL-10, indicating that the macrophage-like cells were switched to a strong Th1-promoting anti-viral phenotype for the HD11 in vitro model. The tissues studied in the in vivo infection model are of course a complex mix of immune and non-immune cells. In the bursae, in contrast to infected HD11 cells, mRNA expression levels of both TLR3 (recognises double-stranded viral RNA) and TLR7 (recognises single-stranded viral RNA) were downregulated. Based on previous report by Rauf et al. [10], TLR3 reacted differently post-infected with different strains of IBDV where upregulation of TLR3 was recorded post-classical IBDV infection but in contrary downregulation was observed post-variant IBDV infection. Another study also indicated that response of TLR3 may play an important role in resistance of the indigenous chicken against vvIBDV infection [27]. mRNA expression levels of both MHC class I and II were upregulated, but only transiently, whereas IL-10 mRNA expression levels were unaltered from those in controls. In the spleens, mRNA expression levels of the TLRs were unaltered from those in controls, but levels of both MHC class I and II were upregulated. IBDV has been reported to inhibit immunoproliferation of spleen CD4 and CD8 T cell via non MHC-restricted interaction [28]. Furthermore, upregulation may delay the recovery of IBDV infected chicken since MHC-II was found to restrict T-cell dependent secondary antibody response against IBDV [29]. Different pattern of TLR 3 and IL10 responses maybe contributed by the complex interaction of immune and non-immune cell in both spleen and bursae. Although HD11 has been widely used as the chicken macrophages cell line model for cytokines study and has shown similar pattern in proinflammatory response post LPS stimulation, the nature of HD11 as a cell line transformed by avian myelocytomatosis virus (MC29) [16,30] may contribute to the slight differences in gene expression as noticed in this study.

Parallels can be drawn between this study and previous studies measuring the immune response to IBDV infection. In this study, IL-15 mRNA expression levels were unaltered, as previously reported [8]. Levels of expression of the mRNA for TLR3 and TLR7 were downregulated at 3 dpi, again as previously described [10]. IL-16 is a chemoattractant for CD4+ T cells, and is also involved in the development of B cells in the bursae [31]. IBDV infection is associated with down-regulation of IL-16 [27]. In this study, IL-16 was down-regulated at 4 dpi in infected spleens and bursae. Upregulation of IFN-γ expression in infected bursae and spleens was detected throughout the experiment, again consistent with previous studies [23,32], and as stated above suggesting the involvement of inflammatory and cell-mediated responses in the immune response to infection and possibly the associated tissue destruction/immunopathology seen in the bursae following IBDV infection. T cells infiltrate IBDV-infected bursae tissue to clear the virus [13]. However, this infiltration and induction of local inflammation may exacerbate bursae lesions and thus delay bursae recovery [11]. Previous report has stated the important of TLR3 in controlling the virus replication through coordinating stimulation of proinflammatory mediators (including proinflammatory cytokines and type II interferon) and antiviral mediators (such as type I interferon). Inhibition of TLR3-mediated antiviral response may subsequently lead to non-TLR3-mediated recognition that resulting in increased proinflammatory responses associated with increased virus replication [33] which is similar to the results in this study.

The substantial increase in the mRNA expression levels of pro-inflammatory cytokines presumably drove the increased iNOS mRNA expression levels and increased the levels of NO, which subsequently contributed to oxidative stress, as indicated by the levels of lipid peroxidation in the infected organs (Figure 3). As reported by Akaike and Maeda [34], oxidative stress and NO induce immune cell apoptosis. Therefore, our results suggest that oxidative stress may also play an important role in the impairment of the bursae and lymphocyte function during IBDV infection.

Understanding on the role of cytokines to the pathogenesis of vvIBDV offers the potential to design better vaccine against the prevention of disease. For example, this study has reported the importance of TLR3 in IBD progression similar to other previous findings [10,27]. Thus, it is possible to design a TLR3 ligands as a potential adjuvant to the current vaccine since previous study has reported the success of using TLR3 ligand poly-ICLC to enhance vaccine efficacy in mouse model [35]. Besides, enhancing other T cell proliferating cytokines such as IL-2, which was found downregulated, via preparing plasmid DNA vaccine adjuvant may help to improve the efficacy of vaccine to stimulate better cell-mediated immunity against vvIBDV infection [36].

Conclusion

In summary, this study indicated that cells of the macrophage-like cell line, HD11, infected with vvIBDV provide a good model to study the overall effects of *in vivo* vvIBDV infection, at least as occur in the bursae and spleen, suggesting that macrophages may play an important role in promoting inflammation and tissue damage in the vvIBDV-infected chicken. Future studies should elucidate the precise identities and roles of the cells producing the differentially expressed immune molecules described in this study and the relative contribution of macrophages in immunopathology of vvIBDV infection.

Competing interests
The authors declare that they have no competing interest.

Authors' contributions
MR, SKY, PK and ARO designed the experiment. MR, SKY, SWT and KR carried out the animal trials. MR and SWT propagated IBDV and performed the GeXP assays. MR, SKY and YWKT performed flow cytometry, NO and MDA assays. YAR performed histopathology study; MR, KR and SWT performed gene expression qRT-PCR. YWKT and SWT performed viral load qRT-PCR. MR, SKY, PK and ARO prepared the manuscript. NBA, AI, MHB, PK and ARO performed data analysis and proof-read the manuscript. All authors read and approved the final manuscript.

Acknowledgements
The study was supported by an Institute of Bioscience, Higher Institution Centre of Excellence (IBS HICoE) grant from the Ministry of Higher Education, Government of Malaysia. Mehdi Rasoli was funded by a Graduate Research Fellowship, Universiti Putra Malaysia. Pete Kaiser was supported by a Biotechnology and Biological Sciences Research Council Institute Strategic Programme Grant to The Roslin Institute. Authors would like to thanks Miss Amanda Teo Siak Mun for validation of viral load and immunophenotyping assays.

Author details
[1]Institute of Bioscience, Universiti Putra Malaysia, Serdang 43400, Selangor, Malaysia. [2]Faculty of Biotechnology and Biomolecular Sciences, Universiti Putra Malaysia, Serdang 43400, Selangor, Malaysia. [3]Faculty of Veterinary Medicine, Universiti Putra Malaysia, Serdang 43400, Selangor, Malaysia. [4]The Roslin Institute and R(D)SVS, University of Edinburgh, Easter Bush, Midlothian EH25 9RG, UK.

References
1. Van Den Berg TP. Acute infectious bursal disease in poultry: a review. Avian Pathol. 2000;29(3):175–94.
2. Withers DR, Young JR, Davison TF. Infectious bursal disease virus-induced immunosuppression in the chick is associated with the presence of undifferentiated follicles in the recovering bursa. Viral Immunol. 2005;18(1):127–37.
3. Sharma JM, Kim I-J, Rautenschlein S, Yeh H-Y. Infectious bursal disease virus of chickens: pathogenesis and immunosuppression. Dev Comp Immunol. 2000;24(2):223–35.
4. Vervelde L, Davison T. Comparison of the in situ changes in lymphoid cells during infection with infectious bursal disease virus in chickens of different ages. Avian Pathol. 1997;26(4):803–21.
5. Hirai K, Funakoshi T, Nakai T, Shimakura S. Sequential changes in the number of surface immunoglobulin-bearing B lymphocytes in infectious bursal disease virus-infected chickens. Avian Dis. 1981;25(2):484–96.
6. Rodenberg J, Sharma J, Belzer S, Nordgren R, Naqi S. Flow cytometric analysis of B cell and T cell subpopulations in specific-pathogen-free chickens infected with infectious bursal disease virus. Avian Dis. 1994;38(1):16–21.
7. Khatri M, Sharma JM. Infectious bursal disease virus infection induces macrophage activation via p38 MAPK and NF-κB pathways. Virus Res. 2006;118(1):70–7.
8. Eldaghayes I, Rothwell L, Williams A, Withers D, Balu S, Davison F, et al. Infectious bursal disease virus: strains that differ in virulence differentially modulate the innate immune response to infection in the chicken bursa. Viral Immunol. 2006;19(1):83–91.
9. Palmquist JM, Khatri M, Cha R, Goddeeris B, Walcheck B, Sharma J. In vivo activation of chicken macrophages by infectious bursal disease virus. Viral Immunol. 2006;19(2):305–15.
10. Rauf A, Khatri M, Murgia MV, Jung K, Saif YM. Differential modulation of cytokine, chemokine and Toll like receptor expression in chickens infected with classical and variant infectious bursal disease virus. Vet Res. 2011;42(1):85.
11. Kim I-J, Karaca K, Pertile TL, Erickson SA, Sharma JM. Enhanced expression of cytokine genes in spleen macrophages during acute infection with infectious bursal disease virus in chickens. Vet Immunol Immunopathol. 1998;61:331–41.
12. Kim I-J, You SK, Kim H, Yeh H-Y, Sharma JM. Characteristics of bursal T lymphocytes induced by infectious bursal disease virus. J Virol. 2000;74(19):8884–92.
13. Tippenhauer M, Heller DE, Weigend S, Rautenschlein S. The host genotype influences infectious bursal disease virus pathogenesis in chickens by modulation of T cells responses and cytokine gene expression. Dev Comp Immunol. 2013;40(1):1–10.
14. Tan D, Hair-Bejo M, Omar A, Aini I. Pathogenicity and molecular analysis of an infectious bursal disease virus isolated from Malaysian village chickens. Avian Dis. 2004;48(2):410–6.
15. Reed LJ, Muench H. A simple method of estimating fifty per cent endpoints. Am J Epidemiol. 1938;27(3):493–7.
16. Beug H, von Kirchbach A, Döderlein G, Conscience J-F, Graf T. Chicken hematopoietic cells transformed by seven strains of defective avian leukemia viruses display three distinct phenotypes of differentiation. Cell. 1979;18(2):375.
17. Hamoud MM, Villegas P, Williams SM. Detection of infectious bursal disease virus from formalin-fixed paraffin-embedded tissue by immunohistochemistry and real-time reverse transcription-polymerase chain reaction. J Vet Diagn Invest. 2007;19:35–42.
18. Rasoli M, Yeap SK, Tan SW, Moeini H, Ideris A, Bejo MH, et al. Alteration in lymphocyte responses, cytokine and chemokine profiles in chickens infected with genotype VII and VIII velogenic Newcastle disease virus. Comp Immunol Microbiol Infect Dis. 2014;37(1):11–21.
19. Kaiser P, Rothwell L, Galyov EE, Barrow PA, Burnside J, Wigley P. Differential cytokine expression in avian cells in response to invasion by Salmonella typhimurium, Salmonella enteritidis and Salmonella gallinarum. Microbiology. 2000;146(12):3217–26.
20. Kogut MH, Rothwell L, Kaiser P. Differential regulation of cytokine gene expression by avian heterophils during receptor-mediated phagocytosis of opsonized and nonopsonized Salmonella enteritidis. J Interf Cytok. 2003;23(6):319–27.
21. Pfaffl MW. A new mathematical model for relative quantification in real-time RT–PCR. Nucleic Acids Res. 2001;29(9):e45.
22. Käufer I, Weiss E. Electron-microscope studies on the pathogenesis of infectious bursal disease after intrabursal application of the causal virus. Avian Dis. 1976;20(3):483–95.
23. Rautenschlein S, Yeh H, Sharma J. Comparative immunopathogenesis of mild, intermediate, and virulent strains of classic infectious bursal disease virus. Avian Dis. 2003;47(1):66–78.
24. Khatri M, Palmquist JM, Cha RM, Sharma JM. Infection and activation of bursal macrophages by virulent infectious bursal disease virus. Virus Res. 2005;113(1):44–50.
25. Khatri M, Sharma J. Modulation of macrophages by infectious bursal disease virus. Cytogenet Genome Res. 2007;117(1–4):388–93.
26. Williams AE, Davison T. Enhanced immunopathology induced by very virulent infectious bursal disease virus. Avian Pathol. 2005;34(1):4–14.

27. Raj GD, Rajanathan TMC, Kumanan K, Elankumaran S. Changes in the cytokine and Toll-Like receptor gene expression following infection of indigenous and commercial chickens with infectious bursal disease virus. Indian J Virol. 2011;22(2):146–51.

28. Kim I-J, Sharma JM. IBDV-induced bursal T lymphocytes inhibit mitogenic response of normal splenocytes. Vet Immunol Immunopathol. 2000;74(1):47–57.

29. Dalgaard TS, Bumstead N, Jorgensen PH. Major histocompatibility complex-linked immune response of young chickens vaccinated with an attenuated live infectious bursal disease virus vaccine followed by an infection. Poult Sci. 2002;81:649–56.

30. Ciraci C, Tuggle CK, Wannemuehler M, Nettleton D, Lamont SJ. Unique genome-wide transcriptome profiles of chicken macrophages exposed to Salmonella-derived endotoxin. BMC Genomics. 2010;11:545.

31. Min W, Lillehoj HS. Identification and characterization of chicken interleukin-16 cDNA. Dev Comp Immunol. 2004;28(2):153–62.

32. Gelb J, Eidson C, Fletcher O, Kleven S. Studies on interferon induction by infectious bursal disease virus (IBDV). II. Interferon production in White Leghorn chickens infected with an attenuated or pathogenic isolates of IBDV. Avian Dis. 1979;23(3):634–45.

33. Hewson AC, Jardine A, Edwards MR, Laza-Stanca V, Johnston SL. Toll-like receptor 3 is induced by and mediates antiviral activity against Rhinovirus infection of human bronchial epithelial cells. J Virol. 2005;79:12273–9.

34. Akaike T, Maeda H. Nitric oxide and virus infection. Immunology. 2000;101(3):300–8.

35. Zhu X, Nishimura F, Sasaki K, Fujita M, Dusak JE, Eguchi J, et al. Toll like receptor-3 ligand poly-ICLC promotes the efficacy of peripheral vaccinations with tumor antigen-derived peptide epitopes in murine CNS tumor models. J Transl Med. 2007;5:10.

36. Park JH, Sung HW, Yoon BI, Kwon HM. Protection of chicken against very virulent IBDV provided by in ovo priming with DNA vaccine and boosting with killed vaccine and the adjuvant effects of plasmid-encoded chicken interleukin-2 and interferon-gamma. J Vet Sci. 2009;10:131–9.

2

Efficacy of multivalent, modified- live virus (MLV) vaccines administered to early weaned beef calves subsequently challenged with virulent *Bovine viral diarrhea virus* type 2

Manuel F Chamorro[1], Paul H Walz[2]*, Thomas Passler[1], Edzard van Santen[4], Julie Gard[1], Soren P Rodning[3], Kay P Riddell[2], Patricia K Galik[2] and Yijing Zhang[2]

Abstract

Background: Vaccination of young calves against *Bovine viral diarrhea virus* (BVDV) is desirable in dairy and beef operations to reduce clinical disease and prevent spread of the virus among cattle. Although protection from clinical disease by multivalent, modified-live virus (MLV) vaccines has been demonstrated, the ability of MLV vaccines to prevent viremia and viral shedding in young calves possessing passive immunity is not known. The purpose of this study was to compare the ability of three different MLV vaccines to prevent clinical disease, viremia, and virus shedding in early weaned beef calves possessing maternal immunity that were vaccinated once at 45 days prior to challenge with virulent BVDV 2.

Results: At 45 days following vaccination, calves that received vaccines B and C had significantly higher BVDV 1 and BVDV 2 serum antibody titers compared with control calves. Serum antibody titers for BVDV 1 and BVDV 2 were not significantly different between control calves and calves that received vaccine D. Following BVDV 2 challenge, a higher proportion of control calves and calves that received vaccine D presented viremia and shed virus compared with calves that received vaccines B and C. Rectal temperatures and clinical scores were not significantly different between groups at any time period. Calves that received vaccines B and C had significantly higher mean body weights at BVDV 2 challenge and at the end of the study compared with control calves.

Conclusions: Moderate to low maternally-derived BVDV antibody levels protected all calves against severe clinical disease after challenge with virulent BVDV 2. Vaccines B and C induced a greater antibody response to BVDV 1 and BVDV 2, and resulted in reduced viremia and virus shedding in vaccinated calves after challenge indicating a greater efficacy in preventing virus transmission and reducing negative effects of viremia.

Keywords: Early weaning, BVDV, MLV, Vaccine, Antibody titres, Virus, Isolation, Shedding

Background

Bovine viral diarrhea virus (BVDV) is an important cause of respiratory, enteric, and reproductive disease in cattle and has been associated with major economic losses in cattle operations worldwide [1]. Vaccination of young calves against BVDV reduces the number of acute infections in the herd and limits spread of virus among cattle populations [1,2]; however, effective vaccination of young calves against BVDV can be challenging due to the presence of maternally-derived BVDV antibodies at the time of vaccination [3]. Although maternally-derived BVDV antibodies can provide protection against acute BVDV infection and clinical disease, humoral immune responses to vaccination might be adversely affected [4]. Concentration of maternally-derived BVDV antibodies and age of calf at the time of vaccination are important factors in the induction of adequate immune responses following BVDV immunization [5-7]. Calves with moderate

* Correspondence: walzpau@auburn.edu
[2]Department of Pathobiology, College of Veterinary Medicine, Auburn University, Auburn, AL, USA
Full list of author information is available at the end of the article

to high maternally-derived BVDV antibody levels at vaccination do not usually respond with an increase in BVDV antibodies but are protected against clinical disease, have a slower decay rate of maternal immunity, and develop anamnestic antibody responses following BVDV challenge [8-10]. Calves with low maternally-derived BVDV antibody levels respond to vaccination by increasing BVDV antibody titers. The priming of naive B and T cells, the induction of specific cell mediated immune memory responses, and the induction of anamnestic antibody responses have been identified as the main source of protection of young calves vaccinated in the presence of maternally-derived antibodies and subsequently challenged with virulent BVDV [11-15].

Early weaned beef calves possess variable levels of maternally-derived BVDV antibodies at 2–4 months of age and therefore could benefit from vaccination prior to stress of weaning and shipment. A single dose of a multivalent, MLV BVDV vaccine was demonstrated to be effective in protecting young calves possessing different levels of maternal immunity against acute BVDV infection [16]. In addition to prevention of clinical disease, vaccination should limit the spread of BVDV by reducing virus shedding and horizontal transmission, a desirable outcome of vaccination in herds or units where populations of highly stressed cattle are commingled. However, experimental studies comparing different multivalent MLV vaccines containing BVDV in their ability to prevent viremia and viral shedding in young calves possessing maternally-derived immunity that subsequently undergo challenge with virulent BVDV are limited. The objective of this study was to evaluate the ability of three different commercially available, multivalent MLV vaccines containing BVDV to prevent clinical disease and reduce shedding of virus when administered to early weaned beef calves subsequently challenged with virulent BVDV 2 at 45 days after vaccination.

Results

Four groups of early weaned beef calves were vaccinated (B, C, and D) or received phosphate saline (A) at weaning at a median calf age of 72.2 days. The calves were born from cows that had been previously vaccinated at least once during the last 2 years with a MLV vaccine. The vaccine used in the cows during the previous 2 years was the same vaccine used in experimental calves from group D. Forty five days after weaning calves were challenged with BVDV 2 1373. Evaluation of clinical responses to challenge and sample collection was performed from day 0 (challenge day) until day 28.

Serum virus neutralization titers

Thirty days prior to vaccination (day –75) and at a median calf age of 44 days, the mean levels of maternally-derived BVDV 1 NADL and BVDV 2 125c serum antibodies were similar between groups (Table 1). At vaccination (day –45), a significant effect of time (day) was detected (P = 0.0001) as decay of maternally-derived antibodies for BVDV 1 NADL and BVDV 2 125c occurred in all groups; however, mean levels of BVDV 1 and BVDV 2 antibodies were not significantly different (P > 0.05) between groups. Forty-five days after vaccination, which corresponded to the time of BVDV 2 challenge (day 0), a significant effect of group and time (day) was detected (P = 0.0001 and P = 0.0001, respectively). Groups B and C calves had mean levels of serum BVDV 1 NADL antibodies significantly greater than controls (P = 0.0033 and P = 0.0002, respectively). Additionally, on day 0, mean levels of BVDV 1 NADL antibodies were similar between group D and the control group (P = 0.2641). With respect to BVDV 2 125c, group C calves had mean levels of antibodies significantly greater than the control group (P = 0.0368). Twenty eight days following challenge, a significant effect of time (day) was detected (p = 0.0001) with respect to the levels of BVDV 2 125c. The mean BVDV 2 125c serum antibody levels increased similarly in all groups (P > 0.05); in contrast, time (day) and group effects were significant (P = 0.0001 and P = 0.0001, respectively) for BVDV 1 NADL mean antibody levels as these were higher in group B and C calves compared to the control group (P < 0.00001). When antibodies to the challenge strain BVDV 2 1373 were examined at day 0, a significant effect of group and time (day) was detected (P = 0.0001 and P = 0.0001). Calves from groups B and C had greater levels of antibodies compared with control calves (P = 0.05 and P = 0.025, respectively). At day 28 after challenge, a significant (P = 0.0001) effect of time (day) was detected as all groups had increased and similar levels of antibodies to the challenge BVDV strain (P > 0.05).

Among vaccinated groups, seroconversion, as defined as a 4-fold or greater rise in antibody titers to BVDV 1 NADL after vaccination (at day 0) was observed in 16.6% of the calves from group B, 50% of the calves from group C, and 9% of the calves from group D. Similarly, seroconversion to BVDV 2 125c after vaccination was observed in 16.6% of the calves from group B, 8.3% of the calves from group C, and 9% of the calves from group D. None of the calves in group A (control) seroconverted to BVDV 1 NADL or BVDV 2 125c. The proportion of calves that seroconverted to BVDV 2 125c after vaccination was not significantly different between groups (P > 0.05); however, a higher proportion of calves from group C (50%) seroconverted to BVDV 1 NADL with a fourfold increase in antibody titers.

Virus isolation

Virus positive samples in serum and WBC samples were detected more frequently and for a longer time in the

Table 1 Geometric mean (95% CI) of virus neutralizing serum antibody titers to BVDV 1, BVDV 2, and BVDV 2 1373 from vaccinated (B, C, and D) and unvaccinated (A) calves at each time period

Virus	Group	Day of Study			
		−75	−45	0	28
BVDV 1 NADL	A	157.58 (31.12 − 831.74)	60.12 (14.52 − 250.73)	15.03 (5.93 − 38.05)	35.75 (17.38 − 74.02)
	B	135.29[NS] (28.64 − 639.14)	67.64[NS] (17.50 − 259.57)	**107.63*** (62.68 − 183.54)	**861.07*** (377.41 - 1951)
	C	222.86[NS] (67.64 − 765.36)	101.12[NS] (30.27 − 337.79)	**202.25*** (110.66 − 369.64)	**680.28*** (225.97 - 2048)
	D	194.01[NS] (45.56 − 903.88)	95.67[NS] (22.47 − 407.31)	36.25[NS] (12.04 − 108.38)	57.70[NS] (12.99 − 213.78)
BVDV 2 125c	A	107.63 (23.10 - 498)	47.83 (13.08 − 173.64)	14.22 (4.08 − 49.18)	608.87 (292.03 − 1260.69)
	B	101.12[NS] (23.26 − 439.58)	60.12[NS] (15.67 − 232.32)	42.52[NS] (22.47 − 80.44)	809[NS] (455.08 − 1438.15)
	C	128[NS] (38.85 − 418.76)	85.03[NS] (26.53 − 272.47)	**60.12*** (26.35 − 138.14)	1820.34[NS] (955.42 − 3468.26)
	D	128[NS] (40.78 − 398.93)	90.50[NS] (31.34 − 259.57)	29.85[NS] (15.24 − 58.89)	286.02[NS] (149.08 − 1541.37)
BVDV 2 1373	A	–	–	16.91 (5.02 − 56.44)	861.07 (424.61 − 1734.13)
	B	–	–	**76.10*** (47.50 − 121.09)	643.59[NS] (352.13 − 1176.26)
	C	–	–	**93.05*** (49.18 − 176.06)	1530.72[NS] (617.37 − 3795.30)
	D	–	–	56.10[NS] (28.44 − 11.43)	544.95[NS] (245.57 − 1200.98)

NS, *Means within BVDV strain and Day of Study are not significantly different (NS) from the control group A or are significantly different (*) based on Dunnett's test at $P = 0.05$.

control group compared with groups, B, C, and D (Figure 1). The total proportion of calves that tested positive to BVDV 2 in serum and WBC samples after challenge (days 0 to 28) was higher in the control group (90%) and group D (54.5%) compared with groups B (16%) and C (25%) (Table 2). A significant effect of group and time (day) was detected on days 6, 8, 10, and 14 after challenge with BVDV 2 1373 ($P = 0.0001$ and $P = 0.0001$, respectively). On day 6 post-challenge, the control group had a higher proportion of calves with positive BVDV samples (58.3%)

compared with groups B (8.3%) and C (8.3%) ($P < 0.05$) but not with group D (36.3%). Additionally, at days 8, 10, and 14 post-challenge, a higher proportion of calves in the control group had BVDV positive samples compared with calves in groups B, C, and D. The proportion of viremic calves (calves with positive serum or WBC samples) that shed virus after challenge (calves whose nasal swab samples tested positive to BVDV by virus isolation) was higher in the control group (72.7%) compared with groups B (0) and C (0) and D (33.3%) ($P < 0.05$).

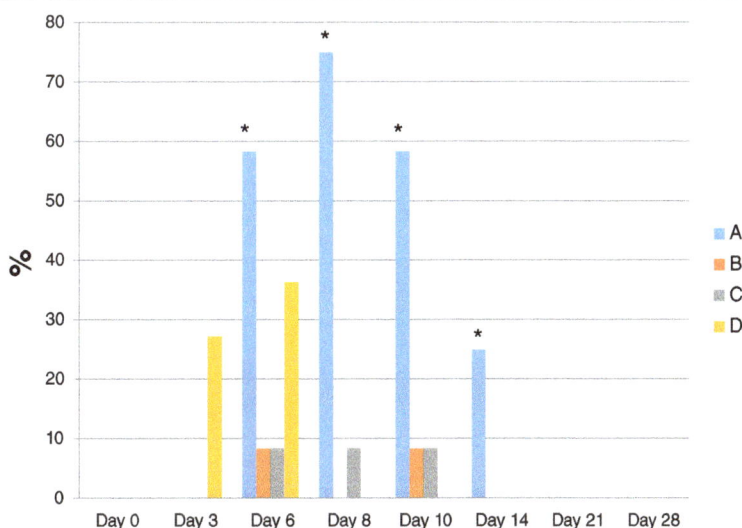

Figure 1 Total proportion of calves with a positive virus isolation result in WBC and serum samples at each time point after challenge with BVDV 2 1373. The proportion of vaccinated (B, C and D) and control (A) calves with positive virus isolation WBC or serum samples at each time point (day) after challenge with BVDV 2 1373 was higher and more frequent in the control group (A) compared with groups B and C and D. The star *sign refers to statistical significance ($P < 0.05$).

Table 2 Total number and proportion of calves (%) that became viremic and shed virus in nasal secretions after challenge (days 0 to 28) with BVDV 2 1373 in each group

Group	Number of viremic¥ calves (%)	Number of viremic calves that shed virus (%)
A	11 (90)*	8 (72.7)*
B	2 (16.6)	0
C	3 (25)	0
D	6 (54.5)*	2 (33.3)

¥, viremic calves = calves with a BVDV positive sample in WBC or serum. A higher proportion of control (A) and group D calves became viremic and shed virus after challenge compared with calves from groups B and C. The star *sign refers to statistical significance (P < 0.05).

Clinical scores and body weight

There were no detectable adverse vaccine reactions in any of the calves. One calf in group D was euthanized on the day prior to challenge with BVDV 2 1373 due to rectal prolapse. Vaccinated and control calves demonstrated clinical protection against challenge with virulent BVDV 2 1373 as only one calf in the control group developed mild diarrhea and anorexia on day 14 post-challenge. The proportion of calves with clinical scores of ≥ 2 for respiratory, diarrhea, and depression parameters was similar between groups (P > 0.05). A mild increase in body temperature, nasal secretion, and loose feces was observed in all calves after challenge independent of group designation. A significant effect of time (day) on rectal temperatures was observed (P < 0.00001). On day 8, the mean rectal temperatures of all groups were increased compared with other days post-challenge.

The average body weight at weaning (day −45) was not significantly different between groups (A = 206.56 +/− 3.53, B = 207.25 +/− 8.33, C = 214.08 +/− 9.25, D = 188.41 +/− 10.08); however, a significant effect of group and time (day)

was detected at day 0 and at the end of the study (P = 0.0001 and P = 0.0001, respectively). Calves from group B and C had significantly higher mean body weights at both time points compared with control calves (B = 257.5 +/− 13.14, C = 257.5 +/− 11.87 vs. A = 242.5 +/− 11.08 and B = 345 +/− 15.72, C = 333.75 +/− 12.17 vs. A = 267.91 +/− 12.63, respectively). At the same times (day 0 and end of the trial), the mean body weights of calves from group D were not significantly different compared with control calves (240 +/− 15.25 vs. 242.5 +/− 11.08 and 300.90 +/− 14.7 vs. 267.91 +/− 12.63, respectively) (P = 0.568 and P = 0.262, respectively).

Hematology

A significant effect of time (day) but not group was detected in the mean WBC counts, as mean WBC decreased in all groups from day 0 (challenge) until day 6 post-challenge (P = 0.0001); however, significant differences were not observed between groups (P > 0.05). On day 8 post-challenge, a significant effect of group and time (day) was detected. The mean WBC count from Group D calves was significantly higher compared with control calves (P = 0.007). At the same time, the mean WBC from calves in groups B and C were not significantly different compared to control calves (Figure 2). Effects of group and time (day) were not detected in platelet counts at any time point after challenge with BVDV 1373 (Figure 3).

Discussion

High levels of BVDV-specific antibodies from colostrum or vaccination effectively protect calves against severe clinical disease induced by challenge with virulent BVDV [3,9]; however, prevention of viremia and virus shedding are variable in cattle vaccinated with MLV vaccines and subsequently challenged with virulent BVDV [17-19]. In

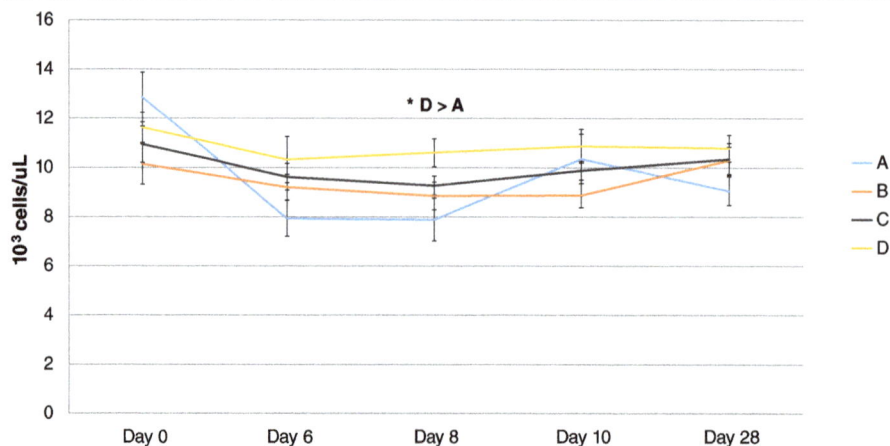

Figure 2 Mean white blood cell count (+/−SEM) after challenge with BVDV 2 1373. Mean WBC between vaccinated (B, C, and D) and control (A) calves after challenge. In all calves mean WBC decreased until day 6 after challenge. At day 8 after challenge calves from group D had higher mean WBC compared with the control group (P = 0.007).

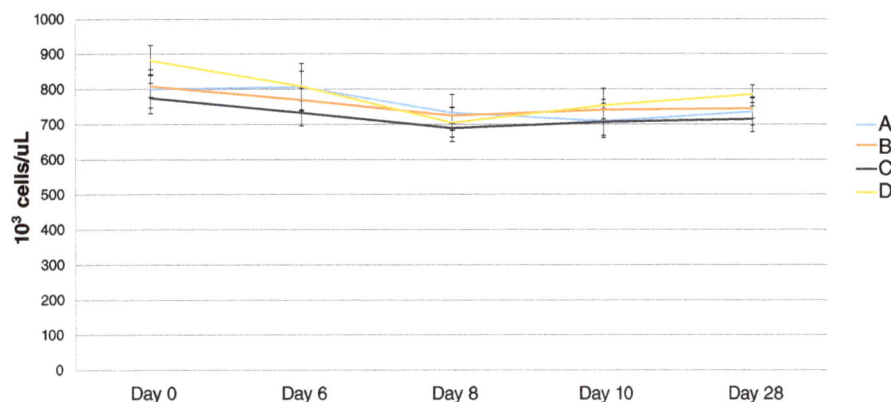

Figure 3 Mean platelet count (+/−SEM) after challenge with BVDV 2 1373. Mean platelet count after challenge with BVDV 2 1373 was not significantly different between vaccinated (B, C, and D) and control (A) calves.

the current study, calves from all groups had similar clinical scores and rectal temperatures, and mortality was not observed after challenge with virulent BVDV 2 1373. This could be associated with protection offered by maternally-derived BVDV antibodies in vaccinated and unvaccinated calves as has been previously reported [11], or could have resulted from lower virulence of the challenge virus than in previous reports [20]. Pestiviruses constantly undergo genetic change due to the poor proof-reading capability of the RNA-dependent RNA polymerase, resulting in variability of phenotypic characteristics such as host-cell tropism and virulence [21]. Repeated passage in cell culture was previously reported to result in attenuation of a BVDV isolate, and may have occurred with the BVDV 1373 used in this study [22].

Interestingly, only calves from group D had an increased white blood cell count compared with control calves at day 8 post-challenge. Prevention of leukopenia is one of several parameters used to evaluate response to vaccination after challenge with BVDV [9,11], and in this case the lack of a decrease in WBC counts observed in group D could have been related to the effects of vaccination or to the presence of high levels of specific maternal antibodies. Despite their ability to reduce clinical disease, maternally-derived BVDV antibodies were not as effective in preventing viremia and viral shedding in calves from the control group as 11/12 (90%) of the calves became viremic and of those 8/11 (72.2%) shed virus after challenge. For this study, we chose VI as our testing method in order to document clinically relevant shedding of live virus [23]. Prior to challenge, the geometric mean of serum BVDV 2 1373 antibody titers of control calves was significantly lower compared with titers from groups B and C (16.91 vs. 76.10 and 93.05, respectively). Low serum antibody titers prior to challenge with BVDV have been associated with an increased risk of viremia and clinical disease as demonstrated in

previous studies [3,4]. Other reports have indicated that calves with serum maternally-derived BVDV antibody titers < 64 before challenge with virulent BVDV have a higher risk of developing clinical disease and systemic spread of the virus compared to calves with greater antibody titers [3,8].

Antibody response to vaccination with MLV BVDV vaccines of young calves in the presence of maternally-derived BVDV antibodies has produced variable results. Previous studies have demonstrated that 40 to 90-day-old calves with maternally-derived antibody titers ≤ 32 against BVDV 1 and BVDV 2 prior to vaccination seroconvert after vaccination [5-7,10]; additionally, these calves can develop an anamnestic response when a second dose of vaccine is administered [5,10]. In contrast, similar studies have demonstrated that 3 to 56-day-old calves with BVDV 1 and BVDV 2 maternally-derived antibody titers ≥ 32 prior to vaccination usually do not seroconvert to vaccination and clinical protection against challenge with BVDV is variable [4,9,13]. In our study, a small proportion of calves vaccinated at weaning, at a median age of 72.2 days, seroconverted to BVDV 2 after vaccination. In contrast, 50% of calves from group C seroconverted to BVDV 1 suggesting a greater ability of the vaccine C to overcome maternal interference to BVDV 1. The higher levels of antibodies to BVDV 1 NADL and BVDV 2 1373 before challenge, the lower proportion of viremia, and the absence of viral shedding after challenge observed in calves from groups B and C suggests that vaccination with B and C may have primed B cell responses to increase specific antibody production or may have delayed the normal decay of maternal BVDV antibodies [6-8,10]. Additionally, the higher levels of antibodies at challenge could have reduced viremia and prevented viral shedding in calves from the same groups. The reduction of viremia and viral shedding is a highly desirable outcome of vaccination since this could prevent BVDV transmission in operations such as feedlots and stocker units where high numbers of cattle from multiple origins are commingled.

The higher proportion of calves with viremia and virus shedding observed in group D could have been a consequence of the presence of more specific maternal antibodies induced by previous vaccination of the dams with vaccine D. The presence of more specific BVDV antibodies induced by vaccine D on colostra from the dams could have exerted a more efficient blockage of humoral cell responses of calves vaccinated with D. Similar results were detected in a recent study in which lower antibody levels to BVDV 1a, BVDV 1b, and BVDV 2 and a higher proportion of viremia after BVDV 2 challenge were observed in calves 42 days after vaccination with D [19]. Protection against viremia and virus shedding after experimental challenge with BVDV of calves vaccinated with MLV BVDV vaccines has been commonly associated with activation of T cell mediated immune responses independent of the induction of an adequate antibody response [11,13,14]. A previous study reported the depletion of CD4+ lymphocytes in calves acutely infected with BVDV could prolong the duration of viral shedding [24]. Additionally, in another study, 80% of calves vaccinated at 3 days of age with a MLV BVDV vaccine and challenged 7-9 months later with virulent BVDV 2 became viremic after challenge; however, calves were protected against severe clinical disease in the absence of antibody responses at initial vaccination [17]. This indicates that induction of specific T cell memory responses after early vaccination may not always prevent viremia and virus shedding in young calves after challenge with BVDV. In the current study we did not evaluate BVDV-specific T cell responses to vaccination and challenge; however, it is possible that a stronger activation of T cell memory responses in calves vaccinated with D that became viremic could have reduced the duration of viremia to only 2 days; additionally, T cell memory responses in groups B and C could have been associated with the reduced proportion of calves with viremia and nasal shedding.

Previous reports have demonstrated that acute BVDV infection in young calves can result in decreased weight gains and decreased performance [9,11]. In the current study, control calves had lower mean body weights at day 0 and at the end of the study compared with calves from groups B and C. Mean body weights of control and group D calves were similar during the study. It is possible that vaccines B and C had a positive effect on weight gain after vaccination as previously reported [25]. Additionally, the higher frequency of viremia in control and group D calves could have had a negative effect on performance and weight gain. Another study demonstrated that young calves vaccinated with a MLV BVDV vaccine and subsequently challenged with virulent BVDV have higher mean body weights and average daily gains

compared with non-vaccinated calves [9]. The higher mean body weights observed in calves from groups B and C at the end of the study suggest that higher levels of BVDV antibodies before challenge and prevention of viremia could have a positive effect on performance, although this observation would need further research using larger numbers of experimental subjects. Prevention of weight loss could be a highly desirable outcome of vaccination programs for early weaned beef calves.

Conclusions

Vaccination of young calves possessing maternally-derived immunity with multivalent MLV vaccines was demonstrated to be beneficial in reducing viremia and virus shedding following BVDV challenge at 45 days after vaccination. Moderate to low levels of maternally-derived BVDV antibodies protected early weaned beef calves against severe clinical disease induced by challenge with virulent BVDV 2. Decay of maternally-derived BVDV antibodies was observed in all groups and just a small proportion of calves seroconverted to BVDV 2 after vaccination; however, the ability of MLV BVDV vaccines to prime B cell responses, induce antibody production, or delay the decay of maternal immunity could result in reduced numbers of viremic calves and prevent virus shedding as was observed in calves from groups B and C in the present study. Reduction of viremia and BVDV shedding could result in decreased BVDV transmission and disease by increasing calf-herd immunity and reducing environmental load of free virus as has been suggested by a previous study [26]. Additionally, MLV BVDV vaccines that reduce viremia after BVDV challenge could have a positive effect on calf performance and would be of most benefit when establishing health programs for early weaned beef calves.

Methods
Animals
Forty-eight crossbred steer calves born and raised at the Upper Coastal Plain Agricultural Research Center, Winfield, AL were utilized in this study. Calves were born in September-October 2012 to cows that had received at least one dose of a modified-live BVDV vaccine D[a] prior to breeding during the 2 years previous to the start of the study. At birth, calves were identified by an ear tattoo and ear tag. All calves remained with their dams and consumption of colostrum occurred under natural conditions in the pasture. A blood sample for detection of neutralizing antibodies against BVDV 1 and BVDV 2 was collected from all calves at day −75 of the study at a median calf age of 44 days to determine the initial maternally-derived BVDV antibody levels.

Experimental design

All calves were early weaned on study day −45, which corresponded to calf ages between 62–92 days (2–3 months) with a median age of 72.2 days. To prepare for early weaning, creep feeding was offered for 3 weeks prior to weaning in order to train calves to the weaning diet. The weaning diet was an energy dense (65-75% of total digestible nutrients), relatively high protein (14-17%), and highly palatable ration to meet all nutritional requirements of young growing calves. Calves were stratified by initial maternally-derived BVDV 2 serum antibody titers and assigned by the use of a random number generator [b] to 1 of 4 different vaccination groups. The stratification by initial levels of BVDV 2 antibodies ensured that each group received similar numbers of calves with different levels of maternally-derived BVDV 2 antibody levels. All calves underwent abrupt weaning on day −45 of the study and were vaccinated according to their assigned treatment group A (n = 12), B (n = 12), C (n = 12), or D (n = 12). Following vaccination, calves were separated in isolated pastures to prevent transmission of vaccine strains between groups. During this time, daily observation of the calves was performed to evaluate for adverse vaccine reactions. Forty-four days after weaning, calves were transported 192 miles to the North Auburn BVDV Unit located in Auburn, AL. Upon arrival to the North Auburn BVDV Unit, calves were rested and given access to fresh water, hay, and supplement. On the next day (day 0), all calves were challenged with virulent BVDV 2 1373 and placed in the same pasture for the remainder of the study. Clinical evaluation and sampling of calves was performed until day 28 after challenge. All calf protocols were reviewed and approved by the Institutional Animal Care and Use Committee of Auburn University (PRN # 2012–2157).

Vaccines

All vaccines used were commercially available, USDA-licensed stock material and were administered to calves at weaning (day −45). Group A was the control group and received 2 mL of 0.9% phosphate buffered saline subcutaneously once. Group B received 2 mL of vaccine B[c] subcutaneously once, group C received 2 mL of vaccine C[d] subcutaneously once, and group D received 2 mL of vaccine D[a] subcutaneously once. All vaccines were modified-live and multivalent containing modified-live types 1 and 2 of BVDV, parainfluenza virus 3, bovine herpesvirus 1, and bovine respiratory syncytial virus. All calves in this study were under 6 months of age and vaccination with vaccines B, C, and D was considered off-label.

BVDV challenge

Forty-five days after vaccination (day 0), all calves were experimentally inoculated with the noncytopathic (NCP) BVDV 2 strain 1373. The NCP BVDV 2 strain 1373 has been previously used in experimental BVDV inoculation of calves and shown to induce severe clinical disease, leukopenia, and thrombocytopenia [27]. The BVDV 2 strain 1373 was propagated in Madin-Darby bovine kidney (MDBK) cells in minimum essential medium [j] (MEM), supplemented with 10% equine serum, L-glutamine, penicillin G (100 units/ml), and streptomycin (100 μg/ml). Virus was harvested from cells by a single freeze-thaw method, aliquoted, and stored (−80°C) until needed. Aliquots were enumerated using the method of Reed and Muench [28], prior to inoculation of calves. All calves were inoculated by intranasal aerosol administration of 1×10^6 $TCID_{50}$ of the BVDV 2 strain 1373.

Sample and data collection

Daily clinical observations were performed by the same person, who was blinded to study group allocation, on days 0, 3, 6, 8, 10, 14, 21, and 28. Additionally, individual rectal temperatures, serum, whole blood, and deep nasal swab samples were collected on those same days. Whole blood samples were subjected to hematologic analysis on day 0 prior to challenge and on days 6, 8, 10, and 28 after challenge for individual white blood cell and platelet counts.

During sampling days, each calf was scored prior to handling for signs of abnormal respiration, diarrhea, and depression using a scale of 0 to 3, with the absence of a clinical sign scored as 0 and the most severe clinical sign scored as 3 [17]. Briefly, an abnormal respiratory score was given if an animal presented with a cough, labored breathing, nasal, or ocular discharge. Nasal and ocular discharges were judged as being serous, mucous, or mucopurulent. Diarrhea scores were judged as being normal feces, pasty feces, runny feces, or severe diarrhea with or without blood. Depression scores ranged from no depression, mild depression, moderate depression, or severe depression. In addition to visual examination, individual body weights were obtained on day −45 (vaccination/weaning day), day 0 (challenge day), and days 14, and 28 after challenge using a portable livestock electric scale [f] that was validated prior to and after each weighing.

Virus Isolation (VI)

Whole blood, serum, and deep nasal swab samples collected on days 0, 3, 6, 8, 10, 14, 21, and 28 after challenge were used for BVDV VI using the immunoperoxidase monolayer assay with techniques previously described [29]. Briefly, the isolated samples were suspended in 24-well plates and subsequently seeded in 50 μL culture medium. The cell suspension was subjected to co-cultivation on 25 cm^3 flasks containing monolayers of MDBK cells and was incubated for 24 hours at 38.5°C and 5% CO_2. Following cultivation, 50 μl of the cell culture supernatant was inoculated in triplicate into wells on 96-well microtiter plates containing monolayers of MDBK cells in culture medium. After 96 hours of incubation at 38.5°C and 5% CO_2, all samples were frozen at −80°C and subsequently thawed to detect BVDV using the immunoperoxidase monolayer assay as previously described [29].

Virus Neutralization (VN)

The standard virus neutralization microtiter assay was used to detect antibodies against BVDV in serum of calves collected on days −75, −45, 0 (prior to challenge), and 28 [28]. The BVDV 1 cytopathic strain NADL and BVDV 2 cytopathic strain 125c were used. For samples collected on days 0 and 28, the challenge BVDV 2 1373 non-cytopathic strain was also used. Briefly, following heat inactivation at 56°C for 30 minutes, serial 2-fold dilutions (1:2 to 1:4096) were made in 50 μL of culture medium. For each dilution, 3 wells of a 96-well plate were inoculated with an equal volume (50 μL) of culture medium containing 100–500 $TCID_{50}$ of the test strain. After inoculation, the plate was incubated at 38.5°C in a humidified atmosphere of 5% CO_2 and room air for 1 hour. Then, 2.5×10^3 MDBK cells in 50 μL of culture medium were added to each well. Plates were incubated for 72 hours and evaluated visually for cytopathic effect for the BVDV 1 and 2 cytopathic strains [29,30] or by staining the plates using the immunoperoxidase assay for the BVDV 2 1373 non-cytopathic strain. The geometric mean of antibody titers was calculated from the endpoint Log_2 titers of the animals in each group. Seronegativity to BVDV 1 and BVDV 2 was defined as a serum antibody titer less than 2 which equates to a Log_2 antibody titer of 0.

Statistical analysis

All statistical analyses were performed using the GLIMMIX procedure in the SAS 9.3 software package [g]. To detect changes in Log_2 transformed antibody levels, virus isolation, rectal temperatures, white blood cell counts, platelet counts, and body weights, a repeated measures generalized linear mixed model [Response = Group + Time (day) + Group * Day] was performed using an appropriate distribution function. The repeated nature of this experiment, viz. multiple observations on the same experimental unit = animal over time, implies non-independence of residuals. Hence, the residual variance was modelled to arrive at a reasonable residual covariance structure using Akaike's Information criterion corrected for small sample sizes (AICc) to determine the best structure. A first-order autoregressive structure with heterogeneous variances (ARH 1) was most commonly fitted. This structure allows for a separate residual variance at each time point and a correlation among time points that diminishes with the lag. Because clinical scores for respiratory distress and diarrhea were binary in nature (only scores 1 and 2 were given) the binary

distribution function was used in the abovementioned procedure; this analysis approach is commonly referred to as logistic regression. No analysis was performed for clinical depression score as all scores equalled zero. Dunnett's test for multiple comparisons was used to detect differences between vaccinated groups and the control group; a probability of $P \leq 0.05$ was considered statistically significant for all tests. The FREQ procedure in the abovementioned software package [h] was used to analyze the proportion of calves with viremia and virus shedding with a χ^2 test.

Endnotes

[a]Bovi-Shield Gold 5, Zoetis Animal Health, Florham Park, NJ
[b]Microsoft Excel 2010, Redmond, WA
[c]BRD-Shield, Novartis Animal Health, Larchwood, IA
[d]Express 5, Boehringer Ingelheim Vetmedica, Ridgefield, Conn.
[e]Powder River Cattle & Livestock Equipment, Provo, UT
[f]True-test Inc. Mineral Wells, TX
[g]SAS Institute Inc., Cary, NC
[h]PROC FREQ SAS 9.2, SAS Institute Inc., Cary, NC

Abbreviations

BVDV: Bovine viral diarrhea virus; MLV: Modified- live virus; CP: Cytopathic; NCP: Non-cytopathic; VI: Virus isolation; VN: Virus neutralization.

Competing interests

The authors declare that they have no competing interests.

Authors' contributions

MFC, PHW, and TP developed the experimental design of this study and co-wrote the manuscript. EvS performed the statistical analysis of the data and revised the manuscript. KPR, JG, and SPR collaborated with animal experiments, sampling, and data collection. PG and YZ performed laboratory testing. All authors read and approved the final manuscript.

Acknowledgements

The authors would like to thank Mr. George Fincher and Mr. Steven Ledbetter for animal care assistance.

Funding

Funds for this research project were obtained from the Alabama Agricultural Experiment Station, Auburn, AL.

Author details

[1]Department of Clinical Sciences, College of Veterinary Medicine, Auburn University, Auburn, AL, USA. [2]Department of Pathobiology, College of Veterinary Medicine, Auburn University, Auburn, AL, USA. [3]Department of Animal Sciences, College of Agriculture, Auburn University, Auburn, AL, USA. [4]Department of Crop, Soils, and Environmental Sciences, College of Agriculture and Alabama Agricultural Experiment Station, Auburn University, Auburn, AL, USA.

References

1. Houe H. Epidemiology of bovine viral diarrhea virus. Vet Clin North Am Food Anim Pract. 1995;11:521–47.
2. Ridpath JF. Immunology of BVDV vaccines. Biologicals. 2013;41:14–9.
3. Cortese VS, West KH, Hassard LE, Carman S, Ellis JA. Clinical and immunologic responses of vaccinated and unvaccinated calves to infection with a virulent type-II isolate of bovine viral diarrhea virus. J Am Vet Med Assoc. 1998;213:1312–9.

4. Ellis J, West K, Cortese V, Konoby C, Weigel D. Effect of maternal antibodies on induction and persistence of vaccine-induced immune responses against bovine viral diarrhea virus type II in young calves. J Am Vet Med Assoc. 2001;219:351–6.

5. Menanteau-Horta AM, Ames TR, Johnson DW, Meiske JC. Effect of maternal antibody upon vaccination with infectious bovine rhinotracheitis and bovine virus diarrhea vaccines. Can J Comp Med. 1985;49:10–4.

6. Munoz-Zanzi CA, Thurmond MC, Johnson WO, Hietala SK. Predicted ages of dairy calves when colostrum-derived bovine viral diarrhea virus antibodies would no longer offer protection against disease or interfere with vaccination. J Am Vet Med Assoc. 2002;221:678–85.

7. Fulton RW, Briggs RE, Payton ME, Confer AW, Saliki JT, Ridpath JF, et al. Maternally derived humoral immunity to bovine viral diarrhea virus (BVDV) 1a, BVDV1b, BVDV2, bovine herpesvirus-1, parainfluenza-3 virus bovine respiratory syncytial virus, Mannheimia haemolytica and Pasteurella multocida in beef calves, antibody decline by half-life studies and effect on response to vaccination. Vaccine. 2004;22:643–9.

8. Howard CJ, Clarke MC, Brownlie J. Protection against respiratory infection with bovine virus diarrhoea virus by passively acquired antibody. Vet Microbiol. 1989;19:195–203.

9. Platt R, Widel PW, Kesl LD, Roth JA. Comparison of humoral and cellular immune responses to a pentavalent modified live virus vaccine in three age groups of calves with maternal antibodies, before and after BVDV type 2 challenge. Vaccine. 2009;27:4508–19.

10. Woolums AR, Berghaus RD, Berghaus LJ, Ellis RW, Pence ME, Saliki JT, et al. Effect of calf age and administration route of initial multivalent modified-live virus vaccine on humoral and cell-mediated immune responses following subsequent administration of a booster vaccination at weaning in beef calves. Am J Vet Res. 2013;74:343–54.

11. Ridpath JF, Neill JD, Endsley J, Roth JA. Effect of passive immunity on the development of a protective immune response against bovine viral diarrhea virus in calves. Am J Vet Res. 2003;64:65–9.

12. Endsley JJ, Roth JA, Ridpath J, Neill J. Maternal antibody blocks humoral but not T cell responses to BVDV. Biologicals. 2003;31:123–5.

13. Zimmerman AD, Boots RE, Valli JL, Chase CC. Evaluation of protection against virulent bovine viral diarrhea virus type 2 in calves that had maternal antibodies and were vaccinated with a modified-live vaccine. J Am Vet Med Assoc. 2006;228:1757–61.

14. Endsley JJ, Quade MJ, Terhaar B, Roth JA. Bovine viral diarrhea virus type 1- and type 2-specific bovine T lymphocyte-subset responses following modified-live virus vaccination. Vet Ther. 2002;3:364–72.

15. Endsley JJ, Ridpath JF, Neill JD, Sandbulte MR, Roth JA. Induction of T lymphocytes specific for bovine viral diarrhea virus in calves with maternal antibody. Viral Immunol. 2004;17:13–23.

16. Step DL, Krehbiel CR, Burciaga-Robles LO, Holland BP, Fulton RW, Confer AW, et al. Comparison of single vaccination versus revaccination with a modified-live virus vaccine containing bovine herpesvirus-1, bovine viral diarrhea virus (types 1a and 2a), parainfluenza type 3 virus, and bovine respiratory syncytial virus in the prevention of bovine respiratory disease in cattle. J Am Vet Med Assoc. 2009;235:580–7.

17. Stevens ET, Brown MS, Burdett WW, Bolton MW, Nordstrom ST, Chase CC. Efficacy of a non-adjuvanted, modified-live virus vaccine in calves with maternal antibodies against a virulent bovine viral diarrhea virus type 2a challenge seven months following vaccination. Bovine Pract. 2011;45:23–31.

18. Palomares RA, Givens MD, Wright JC, Walz PH, Brock KV. Evaluation of the onset of protection induced by a modified-live virus vaccine in calves challenge inoculated with type 1b bovine viral diarrhea virus. Am J Vet Res. 2012;73:567–74.

19. Ridpath JF, Dominowski P, Mannan R, Yancey Jr R, Jackson JA, Taylor L. Evaluation of three experimental bovine viral diarrhea virus killed vaccines adjuvanted with combinations of Quil A cholesterol and dimethyldioctadecylammonium (DDA) bromide. Vet Res Commun. 2010;34:691–702.

20. Stoffregen BL, Bolin SR, Ridpath JF, Pohlenz J. Morphologic lesions in type 2 BVDV infections experimentally induced by strain BVDV2-1373 recovered from a field case. Vet Microbiol. 2000;77:157–62.

21. Moya A, Elena SF, Bracho A, Miralles R, Barrio E. The evolution of RNA viruses: A population genetics view. Proc Natl Acad Sci U S A. 2000;97:6967–73.

22. Deregt DL, Jacobs RM, Carman PS, Tessaro SV. Attenuation of a virulent type 2 bovine viral diarrhea virus. Vet Microbiol. 2004;100:151–61.

23. Dubey P, Mishra N, Rajukumar K, Behera SP, Kalaiyarasu S, Nema RK, et al. Development of a RT-PCR ELISA for simultaneous detection of BVDV-1, BVDV-2 and BDV in ruminants and its evaluation on clinical samples. J Virol Methods. 2014;213C:50–6.

24. Howard CJ, Clarke MC, Sopp P, Brownlie J. Immunity to bovine virus diarrhoea virus in calves: the role of different T-cell subpopulations analysed by specific depletion in vivo with monoclonal antibodies. Vet Immunol Immunopathol. 1992;32:303–14.

25. Tait Jr RG, Downey ED, Mayes MS, Park CA, Ridpath JF, Garrick DJ, et al. Evaluation of response to bovine viral diarrhea virus type 2 vaccination and timing of weaning on yearling ultrasound body composition, performance, and carcass quality traits in Angus calves. J Anim Sci. 2013;91:5466–76.

26. Thurmond MC, Munos-Zansi CA, Hietala SK. Effect of calfhood vaccination on tranmission of bovine viral diarrhea virus under typical drylot dairy conditions. J Am Vet Med Assoc. 2001;219:968–75.

27. Brock KV, Widel P, Walz P, Walz HL. Onset of protection from experimental infection with type 2 bovine viral diarrhea virus following vaccination with a modified-live vaccine. Vet Ther. 2007;8:88–96.

28. Reed LJ, Muench H. A simple method of estimating fifty per cent endpoints. Am J Hyg. 1938;27:493–7. 71:5–6822.

29. Walz PH, Givens MD, Cochran A, Navarre CB. Effect of dexamethasone administration on bulls with a localized testicular infection with bovine viral diarrhea virus. Can J Vet Res. 2008;72:56–62.

30. Larska M, Polak MP, Liu L, Alenius S, Uttenthal A. Comparison of the performance of five different immunoassays to detect specific antibodies against emerging atypical bovine pestivirus. J Virol Methods. 2013;187:103–9.

3

Cloning, expression and antiviral activity of mink alpha-interferons

Hai-ling Zhang[1], Jian-jun Zhao[1], Xiu-li Chai[1], Lei Zhang[1], Xue Bai[1], Bo Hu[1], Hao Liu[1], Dong-liang Zhang[2], Ming Ye[2], Wei Wu[2] and Xi-jun Yan[1*]

Abstract

Background: As a key link between innate and adaptive immune responses, the interferon (IFN) system is the first line of defense against viral infection. IFN, and in particular, IFN-α, has been used clinically as an effective therapeutic agent for viral infections. However, different subtypes of IFN-α demonstrate distinct antiviral activity. Therefore, it is important to identify IFN-α subtypes with high antiviral activity for the development of genetically engineered antiviral drugs.

Results: In this study, we cloned the genes for 13 IFN-α subtypes from peripheral blood lymphocytes of the mink. The homologies of the 13 mink IFN-α genes were 93.6–99.3% and 88.8–98.4% at the nucleotide and amino acid sequence levels, respectively. In contrast to human and canine IFN-α subtypes, most mink IFN-α subtypes contained two N-glycosylation sites. We expressed and purified 13 mink IFN-α subtypes in *Escherichia coli*. The cytopathic effect inhibition assay showed that all the 13 recombinant mink IFN-α subtypes inhibited the propagation of vesicular stomatitis virus in WISH cells, with IFN-α2 and IFN-α12 demonstrating the highest activities. Furthermore, recombinant mink IFN-α2 and IFN-α12 significantly suppressed the propagation of canine distemper virus in Vero cells, with IFN-α2 demonstrating the highest activity.

Conclusions: We identified the mink IFN-α2 subtype as a promising candidate for the development of effective antiviral drugs.

Keywords: Mink, Interferon subtype, Antiviral activity

Background

Interferon (IFN) was first identified by Isaacs in 1957 [1]. IFN belongs to the cytokine family of proteins and has a wide range of physiological functions, such as inhibiting viral infection, regulating cell proliferation and differentiation, and modulating immune responses [2]. The IFN system is one of the first defensive barriers against viral infection and is an important component of natural antiviral immunity [3,4].

IFNs are key cytokines with antiviral, antitumor, and immunomodulatory activities. Based on gene sequences, chromosome location, and receptor specificity, the members of the IFN family are classified into I, II, and III subtypes. Subtype I includes IFN-α, β, ω, ε, κ, δ and ζ

[5-8], and type I IFNs have been shown to possess effective antiviral activity. Type II IFN is also known as immune IFN (IFN-γ) [9]. Interferon-γ, a cytokine produced by T lymphocytes and natural killer cells, plays a central role in the modulation of the immune response [10]. The type III interferons are also known as the IFN-λs and are more related to type I IFNs based on their amino acid sequence and protein function. However, the more limited tissue expression of IFN-λ receptors suggests that type III IFNs do not simply recapitulate the type I IFN antiviral system. They have antiviral effects in the respiratory tract, gastrointestinal tract, skin mucosa, epithelial cells, and some tumor cells. Among the IFN family, IFN-α is one of the major modulators of the defensive system against viral infection in mammals and has been widely used in the clinic as a therapeutic for viral infection [11,12]. All IFNs identified in vertebrates are secreted proteins, with IFN-α being secreted from virus-infected white blood cells. The human IFN family

* Correspondence: yanxijun@163.com
[1]Division of Infectious Diseases of Special Economic Animal, Institute of Special Animal and Plant Sciences, Chinese Academy of Agricultural Sciences, 4899 Juye Street, Changchun 130112, China
Full list of author information is available at the end of the article

consists of 13 subtypes. Despite differences in their amino acid sequences, the subtypes of human IFN-α have similar 3D structures and similar physiological and biochemical characteristics, such as stability and recognition by surface receptors. Human IFN-α is composed of 166–172 amino acids and has no glycosylation sites. The average molecular weight of IFN-α is about 19 kDa. The homology of amino acids among IFN-αs from different subtypes ranges from about 75–95% [13]. The IFN-αs can be further classified into subtypes, which have different biological functions.

IFN is a conserved molecule that has been found in humans, mouse, sheep, rabbits, dogs, weasels and other mammals, as well as in fish, turtles and insects. IFNs have been used in both human and veterinary medicine, not only for the treatment of viral infections but also for cancer. Mink (*Neovison vison*) is one of the major fur animals and its health problems have become an important issue for the fur industry. Infection by the canine distemper virus, Parvovirus, and Aleutian mink disease virus among minks has caused serious economic losses to the fur animal industry [14]. Therefore, there is an urgent need to develop effective, non-toxic, and environmentally friendly antiviral drugs to control viral infections in mink. In this study, we cloned and expressed the genes for 13 IFN-α subtypes in the mink and characterized their antiviral activity.

Results

Analysis of mink IFN-α genes

By reverse transcription polymerase chain reaction (RT-PCR), we successfully amplified the predicted 564 bp mink IFN-α (MiIFN-α) cDNA. Restriction enzyme analysis confirmed that we had correctly subcloned MiIFN-α cDNAs into recombinant plasmids. DNAStar software analysis demonstrated that the cDNAs of 13 subtypes of MiIFN-α were 564 bp long and encoded 187 amino acids. Due to the different amino acids components, there were slight variations in molecular weight among the 13 MiIFN-α subtypes. The GenBank registration number and molecular weight of the cloned 13 MiIFN-α subtypes are listed in Table 1.

SignalP 4.1 server software (http://www.CBS.DTU.DK/Services/SignalP) analysis predicted that the N terminal 23 amino acids represented the signal peptide. The homologies of 13 MiIFN-α subtypes were 93.6–99.3% and 88.8–98.3% at the nucleotide and amino acid sequence levels, respectively (Table 2).

Most secreted proteins in eukaryotes are modified on the amino acid Asn located in the consensus sequence Asn.Xaa.Ser/Thr (NXS/T) by an N-glycan, a process known as N-glycosylation [15]. Analysis using NetNGlyc Server 1.0 (http://www.CBS.DTU.DK/Services/NetNGlyc)

Table 1 The 13 MiIFN-α subtypes cloned in this study

IFN-α subtype	MW (Da)	Accession number
MiIFN-α1	20956	EU863613
MiIFN-α2	20999	EU863614
MiIFN-α3	20958	EU863615
MiIFN-α4	21031	EU863616
MiIFN-α5	21089	EU863617
MiIFN-α6	21204	EU863618
MiIFN-α7	21002	EU863619
MiIFN-α8	21032	EU863620
MiIFN-α9	21021	EU863621
MiIFN-α10	21146	EU863622
MiIFN-α11	21248	EU863623
MiIFN-α12	21060	EU863624
IFN-α13	20983	EU091340

predicted that IFN-α1–3 contained one glycosylation site at ^{54}NYTN^{57}, whereas IFN-α4–13 contained two glycosylation sites. In addition to the glycosylation site at ^{54}NYTN^{57}, IFN-α4–9 and IFN-α13 contained a glycosylation site at ^{101}NTTL^{104}, whereas IFN-α10–12 contained a glycosylation site at ^{101}NMTL^{104}. Further analysis demonstrated that the number and position of cysteines were not the same among the 13 subtypes. IFN-α1–3, IFN-α5, IFN-α7, IFN-α10, IFN-α11 and IFN-α13 contained 8 cysteine residues at the same positions of 5, 16, 24, 52, 92, 109, 122 and 160. IFN-α4, IFN-α6, IFN-α8, IFN-α9 and IFN-α12 contained only 7 cysteine residues with a cysteine residue at position 16 replaced by serine (Figure 1). These data demonstrate the existence of a single nucleotide polymorphism (SNP) among MiIFN-α subtypes, in agreement with previous reports on SNPs of IFN-α in other species [15,16].

Both mink and ferret belong to *Mustelidae*. The homology between IFN-α1–13 and the published sequences for ferret (GenBank registration number: EF368207) were 95.0–97.3% and 91.5–94.2% at the nucleotide and amino acid sequence levels, respectively. The amino acid sequence analysis showed that fox (EF990625), raccoon (EF543192), and canine (EF28625) IFN-α each contained only one potential N-glycosylation site at ^{101}NMTL^{104}, which is the same site in MiIFN-α10–12. The homologies between mink, fox, raccoon and canine IFN-α were 79.1–80.9% and 68.8–71.4% at the nucleotide and amino acid sequence levels, respectively. Nucleotide evolution tree analysis showed significant differences in the nucleotide sequences among the 13 subtypes of MiIFN-α and those of other species of animals and human IFN-αs (Figure 2).

Table 2 Homology (%) of amino acids and nucleotides among MiIFN-α subtypes

	IFN-α1	IFN-α2	IFN-α3	IFN-α4	IFN-α5	IFN-α6	IFN-α7	IFN-α8	IFN-α9	IFN-α10	IFN-α11	IFN-α12	IFN-α13
IFN-α1	–	99.3	97.0	95.0	96.3	94.5	94.7	94.7	93.8	94.7	94.3	96.1	95.4
IFN-α2	98.4	–	96.6	95.7	97.0	95.2	94.7	94.9	94.0	94.3	94.0	95.7	95.0
IFN-α3	94.7	94.1	–	96.3	96.8	94.7	96.3	96.6	95.7	96.3	95.2	98.0	95.6
IFN-α4	90.4	92.0	93.0	–	98.8	98.4	96.5	96.3	95.4	96.6	95.0	95.7	96.1
IFN-α5	93.0	94.7	93.6	97.3	–	97.2	97.0	96.1	95.2	97.0	95.6	95.6	96.1
IFN-α6	89.3	90.9	91.4	98.4	95.7	–	95.2	95.0	94.3	95.0	96.3	94.7	95.6
IFN-α7	91.4	90.9	93.0	93.6	94.1	92.5	–	96.8	96.3	97.9	97.2	95.2	96.3
IFN-α8	90.9	90.9	94.1	92.5	92.0	91.4	94.1	–	99.1	95.9	94.3	97.3	95.6
IFN-α9	89.3	89.3	92.5	90.9	90.4	89.8	93.6	98.4	–	95.0	93.6	96.5	94.7
IFN-α10	91.4	90.9	94.1	94.7	95.2	93.0	96.8	92.0	90.4	–	97.2	96.3	96.3
IFN-α11	89.8	89.3	92.0	92.5	93.0	94.1	95.2	90.4	88.8	96.8	–	94.9	95.7
IFN-α12	93.0	92.5	97.3	92.5	92.0	91.4	92.0	95.2	93.6	93.6	92.0	–	95.6
IFN-α13	91.4	90.9	91.4	92.0	92.5	91.4	93.6	90.4	88.8	93.6	93.0	90.4	–

"–" same sequence. The upper line shows identities at the nucleotide level; The lower line shows identities at the amino acid level. The sequences for alignment were from the following GenBank accession numbers: IFN-α1(MiIFN-α1, EU863613), IFN-α2 (MiIFN-α2, EU863614), IFN-α3 (MiIFN-α3, EU863615), IFN-α4 (MiIFN-α4, EU863616), IFN-α5 (MiIFN-α5, EU863617), IFN-α6 (MiIFN-α6, EU863618), IFN-α7(MiIFN-α7, EU863619), IFN-α8 (MiIFN-α8, EU863620), IFN-α9 (MiIFN-α9, EU863621), IFN-α10 (MiIFN-α10, EU863622), IFN-α11 (MiIFN-α11, EU863623), IFN-α12 (MiIFN-α12, EU863624), IFN-α13 (MiIFN-α13, EU091340).

Expression and purification of MiIFN-α in *E. coli*

To evaluate the biological activity of MiIFN-α, we subcloned 13 MiIFN-α cDNAs into a prokaryotic expression vector pProEX HTb and induced their expression by isopropyl-beta-D-thiogalactopyranoside (IPTG) in *E. coli* BL21. Sodium dodecyl sulfate (SDS)-polyacrylamide gel electrophoresis (PAGE) analysis showed the presence of protein bands at 19 kDa (Figure 3A), consistent with the predicted molecular weights of MiIFN-α. Protein solubility analysis showed that MiIFN-α recombinant proteins were in the form of inclusion bodies. SDS-PAGE analysis of the isolated inclusion bodies showed that 80% of recombinant proteins were in inclusion bodies. Western blot analysis of partially purified MiIFN-α with an anti-6xHis antibody showed a specific band of about 19 kDa (Figure 3B).

Antiviral activity of recombinant MiIFN-α

To examine the antiviral activity of recombinant MiIFN-αs, we first used the WISH/ vesicular stomatitis virus (VSV) system. Compared to the cells without virus infection, challenge of WISH cells with 100 $TCID_{50}$ VSV for 24 h resulted in significant cell lesions. However, pretreatment with 13 subtypes of MiIFN-α attenuated VSV-induced cell lesions, with MiIFN-α2 and MiIFN-α12 demonstrating the strongest effects. Further analysis showed that the effective antiviral concentrations of MiIFN-α2 and MiIFN-α12 in WISH cells were 0.18×10^4 IU/mg and 0.3×10^3 IU/mg, respectively.

To confirm that the antiviral activity of recombinant MiIFN-α is not limited to VSV, we employed the canine distemper virus (CDV)/Vero system. We selected MiIFN-α2 and MiIFN-α12, because these two subtypes exhibited the strongest antiviral activity against VSV. The results showed that recombinant MiIFN-α2 and MiIFN-α12 significantly inhibited CDV-induced cell lesions. Further analysis showed that 0.145 μg purified MiIFN-α2 protein and 0.28 μg purified MiIFN-α12 could suppress 100 $TCID_{50}$ CDV-mediated cell lesions. These data indicate that MiIFN-α2 exhibits the strongest antiviral activity against VSV and CDV.

Discussion

The fur animal industry is expanding in the Northeast and Western parts of China. However, the health of fur animals has been compromised by viral infections, such as those with CDV, Parvovirus, and Aleutian mink virus. IFN was first recognized on the basis of its anti-viral activity and only later shown to act primarily as an immunomodulator. IFN-α has been identified from different species, but the biological activity of MiIFN-α has not been tested until now. To determine whether MiIFNα also exhibits antiviral activity similar to IFNs from other species, we examined the ability of recombinant MiIFN-αs to inhibit the replication of VSV.

Using RT-PCR, we successfully amplified the predicted 564 bp mink IFN-α cDNA. The homologies of 13 MiIFN-α subtypes were 93.6–99.3% and 88.8–98.3% at the nucleotide and amino acid sequence levels, respectively. It is surprising that all the subtypes have the same size, whereas size differences have been reported in other species. In 14 pig IFN-αs, multiple sequence alignment revealed a C-terminal deletion of 8 residues in six IFN-α subtypes (IFN-α1, α2, α3, α7, α10 and α11) [17].

Figure 1 Analysis of amino acid sequences of 13 MiIFN-α subtypes. Red underlining indicates the predicted signal sequence of MiIFN-αs. Shaded areas represent the predicted cysteine residues, and boxed areas indicate potential N-glycosylation sites.

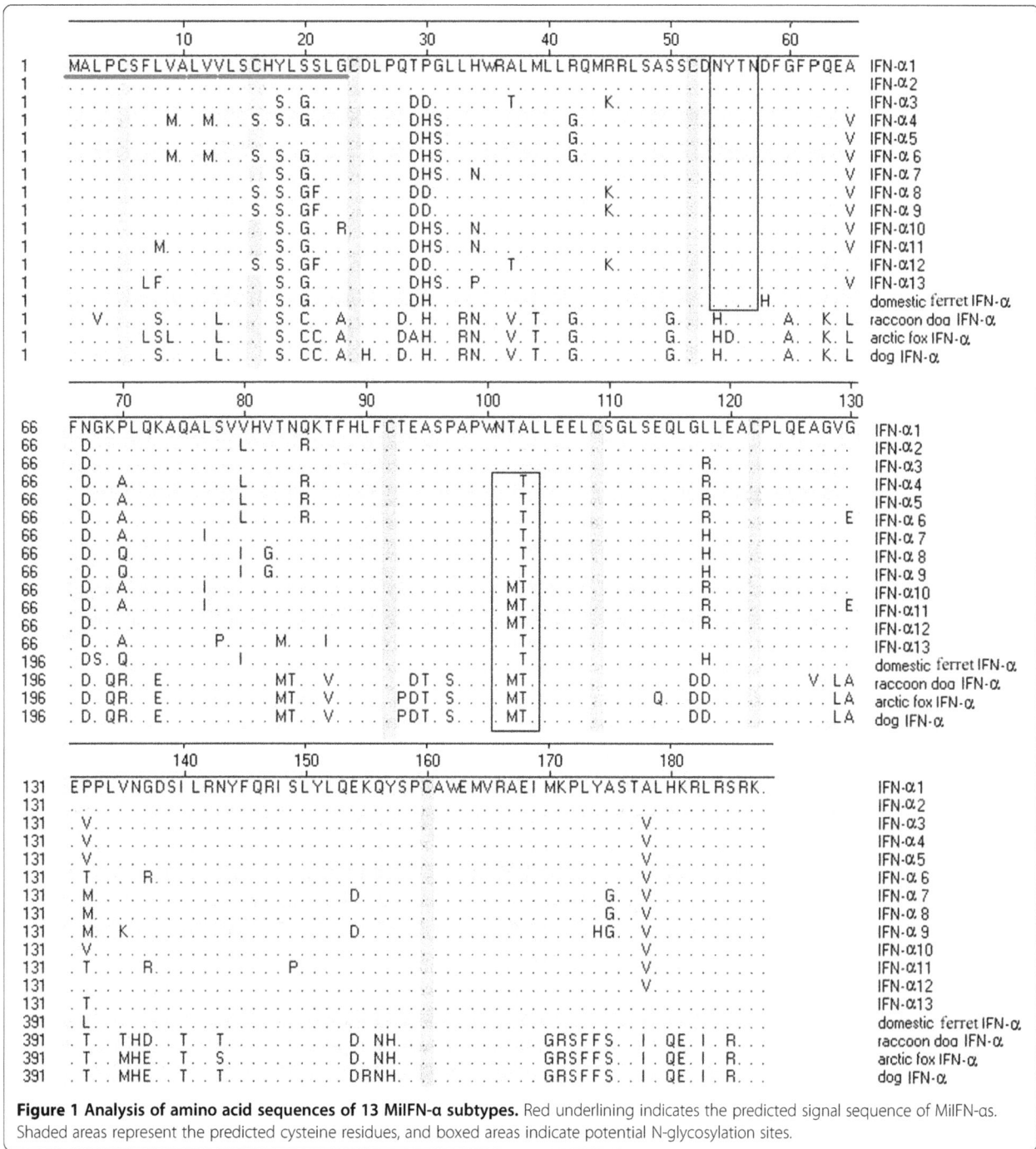

The antiviral activities of intact porcine IFN-α genes are approximately 2–50 times higher than those of the subtypes with C-terminal deletions in WISH cells and 15–55 times higher in PK15 cells. In addition, the size of feline IFN-α subtypes are different; feline IFN-α5 has five additional amino acids inserted at position 139, which are not present in the other four subtypes [18]. More than 10 different subtypes of IFN-α have been reported in mice and 16 or more subtypes have been reported to exist in humans. In mouse, the size of IFN-α subtypes is variable. However, the size of the human IFN subtypes is consistent. In mice injected with plasmids encoding murine (Mu)IFN-α1, muIFN-α4 or muIFN-α9, and subsequently challenged with murine cytomegalovirus (MCMV), muIFN-α1 exerted the greatest antiviral effect. In another study, eight different human cell-derived IFN-α subtypes were tested for their antiviral activities. Human (Hu)IFN-α8 was found to be the most

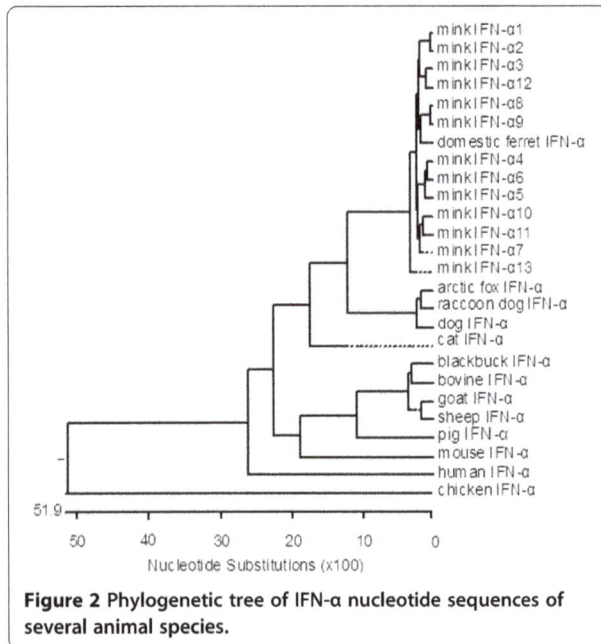

Figure 2 Phylogenetic tree of IFN-α nucleotide sequences of several animal species.

potent, whereas HuIFN-α1 exhibited the least antiviral activity. In the current study, we compared the antiviral effects of the MiIFN-α subtypes. There is no evidence to prove that the strength of antiviral activity is related to the size of the IFN-α subtype. Phylogenetic analysis (Figure 2) further indicated that IFN-α was subdivided into two monophyletic lineages: chicken (avian) and mammalian. The mammalian branch can be divided into carnivores and herbivores. The similarity of mink, domestic ferret, Eurasian badger, giant panda, dog, fox, and cat IFN-αs is consistent with their grouping within the carnivore monophyletic group (which is distinct from other herbivores IFN-αs). Indeed, both gene conversion and gene duplication have shaped the evolution of the IFN-α gene family in eutherian species [19]. The features of MiIFN-α subtype sequences provide more support for this view.

IFN has a broad-spectrum of antiviral effects and represents an ideal choice for the development of antiviral drugs. IFN was the first cytokine approved by the US Food and Drug Administration for clinical application. Among the members of the IFN family, IFN-α has relatively higher antiviral activity. IFN-α has been identified from different species, including birds, rodents, and primates [20]. IFN-α is a multi-gene family, with each member located on the same chromosome within a certain region [19]. One unique characteristic of the IFN-α gene is that it has only one open reading frame (ORF) without any introns. For example, dog has 8 IFN-α genes, cat has 5 IFN-α genes, giant panda has 12 IFN-α genes, and the marmot has 10 IFN-α genes. For each subtype of IFN-α gene of the same species, the sequence of the PCR product is the same whether using genomic DNA or cDNA as the template. In this study, we cloned 13 MiIFN-α genes, including six functional genes and two pseudogenes. In vitro assays showed that only the product of the functional IFN gene had antiviral activity. The reason for the genetic diversity of IFN-α during evolution is still unclear, but different subtypes have distinct biological activities [18]. Tan *et al.* cloned 12 IFN-α genes from the giant panda and found that IFN-α8, IFN-α4, and IFN-α10 had higher activity whereas IFN-α11 had low biological activity in 293 cells (human renal epithelial cells transfected with adenovirus E1A gene) [17]. Furthermore, IFN-α3, IFN-α4, and IFN-α8 demonstrated higher activity in B6 cells, whereas IFN-α3, IFN-α7, and IFN-α10 showed higher activity in K562 cells [18]. Taira *et al.* cloned 5 dog IFN-α genes and found that rCaIFN-α8 demonstrated high anti-VSV activity. In addition, the anti- canine adenovirus (CAV)-1 activity of rCaIFN-α8 in Madin-Darby canine kidney (MDCK) cells was 33–666 times higher than the anti-VSV activity, but rCaIFN-α8 had no effects on CHV-1 [21]. Taken together, these data suggest that IFN-α has many subtypes, most of which have antiviral activity in different types of cells. Although the IFN-α family has many pseudogenes that can be transcribed into mRNA, these pseudogenes have no anti-viral function. The potential roles of the pseudogenes of IFN-α remain to be determined.

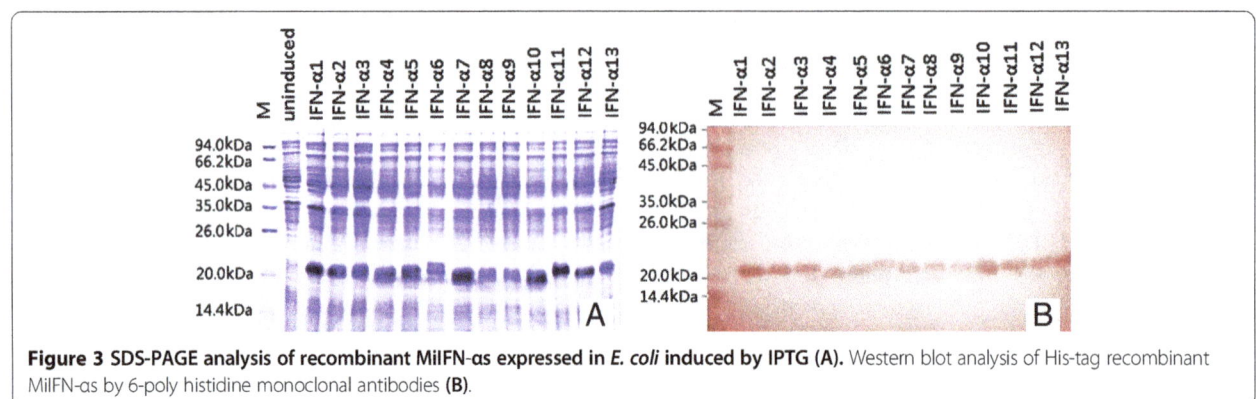

Figure 3 SDS-PAGE analysis of recombinant MiIFN-αs expressed in *E. coli* induced by IPTG (A). Western blot analysis of His-tag recombinant MiIFN-αs by 6-poly histidine monoclonal antibodies **(B)**.

Effective induction of IFN expression plays an important role during the immune response to viral infection. IFN-α is a multi-gene family consisting of different subtypes with high homology and similar function. However, recent studies have demonstrated that there are functional differences among the subtypes, probably due to the different amino acid sequences. Indeed, our 13 cloned MiIFN-αs demonstrated a variety of constituent amino acids in each subtype. MiIFN-α4–13 had two N-glycosylation sites, whereas MiIFN-α1–3 had only one N-glycosylation site. IFN-α1–3, IFN-α5, IFN-α7, IFN-α10, IFN-α11, and IFN-α13 had 9 cysteine residues, whereas IFN-α4, IFN-α6, IFN-α8, IFN-α9, and IFN-α12 contained only 8 cysteine residues. Antiviral activity analysis showed that only IFN-α1, IFN-α2, IFN-α3, IFN-α8, IFN-α9, and IFN-α12 had antiviral function. It will be interesting to investigate whether N-glycoslylation sites are essential for the antiviral activity of IFN-α.

Conclusions

In summary, in this study for the first time, we have cloned 13 subtypes of the MiIFN-α gene and successfully expressed them in *E. coli*. Most of the purified recombinant MiIFN-α subtypes demonstrated antiviral activity against VSV and CDV, and MiIFN-α2 exhibited the highest antiviral activity. Therefore, the MiIFN-α2 subtype is a promising candidate for the development of effective antiviral drugs for the fur animal industry.

Methods
Reagents
VSV was provided by Dr. Haidong Zhi from the Institute of Harbin Veterinary Research, Chinese Academy of Agricultural Sciences (CAAS). Canine distemper virus (CDV) strains were from commercial CDV-3 vaccine strains. WISH and Vero cells were purchased from the Chinese Academy of Sciences Shanghai Cell Bank. Plasmid pProEX HTb, *E. coli* JM109/BL21, and TRIzol were purchased Invitrogen (USA). RPMI 1640 medium was purchased from GIBCO. Lymphocyte isolation reagent was from the Chinese Academy of Medical Sciences. ExTaq polymerase, AMV reverse transcriptase, and Concanavalin A (Con A) were purchased from Sigma (USA). The Ni-NTA protein purification system and anti-6xHis monoclonal antibodies were purchased from Invitrogen.

PCR primers were synthesized by Shanghai Ying-Jun Biotech.

Six-month-old minks were purchased from a fur animal farm in the Jilin Province of China and housed in boxes at the animal house of the Central Laboratory for Animal Diseases of the Institute of Special Animal and Plant Sciences. All animal work and experimental procedures were performed according to the regulations for the administration of affairs concerning experiental animals, which was approved by the state council on October 21, 1988 and promulgated by decree No. 2 of the State Science and Technology Commission on November 14, 1988.

RT-PCR and analysis of IFN-α sequences
Peripheral blood lymphocytes (PBMCs) were separated under sterile conditions from healthy minks, stimulated with 25 µg/mL ConA for 24 h, centrifuged, and resuspended in 1 mL TRIzol reagent. Total RNA was isolated by the phenol/chloroform method as described previously [22,23]. cDNA was synthesized from total RNA using Oligod (T)$_{15}$ primer, and PCR was performed with cDNA and primers to amplify IFN-α cDNA [16]. The primer sequences are shown in Table 3. The PCR products were subcloned into the pGEM-T vector for sequencing at Shanghai Ying-Jun BioTech (Invitrogen). The amino acid sequences of the MiIFN-αs ORF were aligned with that of IFN-αs of arctic fox, raccoon, and dog IFN-α from GenBank using DNAStar 5.0 software. A multi-species phylogenetic tree based on the nucleotide sequences of the various IFNs was constructed with DNAStar 5.0 MegAlign software. Signal peptides were predicted using online SignalP 4.1 server (http://www.cbs.dtu.dk/Services/SignalP/). The glycosylation sites were predicted using the online 1.0 NetNGlyc Server.

Construction of mMiIFN-α1–13 expression vector
The PCR products were separated by 1.5% agarose gel electrophoresis. The gel purified DNA was cut with *Bam*H I and *Hin*d III, ligated into the pProEX HTb vector, and transformed into competent *E. coli* /BL 21 cells. Positive clones were validated by PCR and restriction enzymes digestion and sequenced by Shanghai Ying-Jun BioTech. The recombinant plasmid was named pHTb/MiIFN-α.

Table 3 Primers used in MiIFN-α and mature peptide (mMiIFN-α) gene PCR assays

Gene fragment	Predicted size (bp)	Primers	Tm(°C)
MiIFN-α1–13	564	P1 5'-ATGGCCCTGCCCTGCTCCT- 3'	50.1
		P2 5'-TCACTTCCTGCTCCGCAATC-3'	
mMiIFN-α1–13	495	P3 5'- CGGGATCCTGTGACCTGCCTCAG-3'	55
		P4 5'- CCAAGCTTTCACTTCCTGCTCCGCAAT-3'	

Expression and purification of recombinant mMiIFN-α1–13

pHTb/MiIFN-αs were transformed into *E. coli* BL21 competent cells and selected with ampicillin. Positive clones were inoculated in 5 ml liquid Luria broth (LB) media and cultured at 37°C. When the optical density at 600 nm (OD_{600}) reached 0.5, 1 mmol/L IPTG was added to induce protein expression. For purification, the bacteria were centrifuged at 10,000 rpm for 10 min. Following several cycles of freezing and thawing, the bacterial pellet was mixed with 1 mg/mL lysozme and lysed by sonication on ice. After collection by centrifuging at 4°C at 10,000 rpm for 10 min, the pellet was washed with buffer (1% Triton X-100, 50 mmol/ml Tris · HCl pH 8.0, 100 mmol/mL NaCl) and dissolved in 8 mol/L urea buffer. Then 50% NI −NTA (4:1) was added and incubated on ice with slow mixing using a magnetic stirrer blender. Finally, the mixture was loaded onto a chromatography column (Novagen) and eluted by serial washing (using pH 8.0, pH 6.3, and pH 4.5 50 Mm Tris · HCl buffer containing 8 M urea). The eluents were separated by 12% SDS-PAGE and transferred onto a PVDF membrane. The membrane was blocked with 5% milk in TBST (0.1 phosphate buffer contain 0.5% Tween20) and incubated with mouse anti-6xHis monoclonal antibody (1:300) at 4°C overnight, followed by incubation with goat anti-mouse IgG-HRP (1:2000) at room temperature for 1 h. Finally, the membrane was developed using the TMB Chromogenic Reagent (Sigma, USA).

Antiviral activity assay

The antiviral activity of 0.5 mg/mL recombinant IFN-α was determined by cytopathic inhibition assay. WISH cells were plated in 96-well plates and incubated at 37°C with 5% CO_2 for 12–18 h. Diluted recombinant IFN-α was added to the cell monolayer and incubated at 37°C with 5% CO_2 overnight. Next, the cells were challenged with 100 $TCID_{50}$ VSV, and the plates were incubated at 37°C for 1–2 days. VSV-induced cytopathic effects were assessed by microscopic examination, and IFN-α concentrations were expressed as the inverse dilution that provided protection of 50% of the cells from VSV-induced cytopathic effects (CPE_{50}).

In addition, the antiviral activity of recombinant IFN-α was determined by the inhibition of CDV propagation in Vero cells. The titer of CDV TCID 50 was determined by reference for Reed-Muench method. Vero cells were plated in 24-well plates until the formation of a monolayer. Diluted recombinant IFN-α was added to the cell monolayer and incubated at 37°C with 5% CO_2 overnight. Next, the cells were challenged with 100 $TCID_{50}$ CDV, and the plates were incubated at 37°C for 1–2 days. The CDV-induced cytopathic effects were assessed by microscopic examination, and IFN-α concentrations were expressed as the inverse dilution that provided protection of 50% of the cells from CDV-induced cytopathic effects (CPE_{50}).

Competing interest

The authors declare that they have no competing interest.

Authors' contributions

HZ designed the study, performed the experiments, and wrote the manuscript; JZ constructed the plasmids; XC purified the protein; LZ performed sequence analysis; XB, HB, and HL evaluated the antiviral activity of recombinant proteins; DZ and MY cultured cells and virus; XY and WW wrote the manuscript and put forward reasonable proposals. All authors read and approved the final manuscript.

Acknowledgments

This study was supported by Jilin Science and Technology Development Project (No. 20140520172JH), and Jilin City Outstanding Youth Project (No. 2013625018).

Author details

[1]Division of Infectious Diseases of Special Economic Animal, Institute of Special Animal and Plant Sciences, Chinese Academy of Agricultural Sciences, 4899 Juye Street, Changchun 130112, China. [2]Jilin Teyan Biotechnological Co. Ltd, 388 Liuying West Road, Changchun 130122, China.

References

1. Chelbi-Alix MK, Wietzerbin J. Interferon, a growing cytokine family: 50 years of interferon research. Biochimie. 2007;89:713–8.
2. Huang L, Cao RB, Wang N, Liu K, Wei JC, Isahg H, et al. The design and recombinant protein expression of a consensus porcine interferon: CoPoIFN-α. Cytokine. 2012;57:37–45.
3. Janardhana V, Tachedjian M, Crameri G, Cowled C, Wang LF, Baker ML. Cloning, expression and antiviral activity of IFNγ from the Australian fruit bat, Pteropus alecto. Dev Comp Immunol. 2012;36:610–8.
4. Borden EC, Sen GC, Uze G, Silverman RH, Ransohoff RM, Foster GR, et al. Interferons at age 50: past, current and future impact on biomedicine. Nat Rev Drug Discov. 2007;6:975–90.
5. Takaoka A, Yanai H. Interferon signalling network in innate defence. Cell Microbiol. 2006;8:907–22.
6. Kotenko SV, Gallagher G, Baurin VV, Lewis-Antes A, Shen M, Shah NK, et al. IFN-lambdas mediate antiviral protection through a distinct class II cytokine receptor complex. Nat Immunol. 2003;4:69–77.
7. Sheppard P, Kindsvogel W, Xu W, Henderson K, Schlutsmeyer S, Whitmore TE, et al. IL-28, IL-29 and their class II cytokine receptor IL-28R. Nat Immunol. 2003;4:63–8.
8. Lopušná K, Režuchová I, Betáková T, Skovranová L, Tomašková J, Lukáčiková L, et al. Interferons lambda, new cytokines with antiviral activity. Acta Virol. 2013;57:171–9.
9. Li HT, Ma B, Mi JW, Jin HY, Xu LN, Wang JW. Molecular cloning and functional analysis of goose interferon gamma. Vet Immunol Immunop. 2007;117(1–2):67–74.
10. Hoegen B, Saalmüller A, Röttgen M, Rziha HJ, Geldermann H, Reiner G, et al. Interferon-gamma response of PBMC indicates productive pseudorabies virus (PRV) infection in swine. Vet Immunol Immunop. 2004;102(4):389–97.
11. Li L, Sherry B. IFN-alpha expression and antiviral effects are subtype and cell type specific in the cardiac response to viral infection. Viro. 2010;396:59–68.
12. Ma D, Jian D, Qing M, Weidner JM, Qu X, Guo H, et al. Antiviral effect of interferon lambda against West Nile virus. Antivir Res. 2009;83:53–60.
13. Kuruganti S, Accavitti-Loper MA, Walter MR. Production and characterization of thirteen human type-I interferon-α subtypes. Protein expres purif. 2014;103:75–83.
14. Wang J, Cheng S, Yi L, Cheng Y, Yang S, Xu H, et al. Evidence for natural recombination between mink enteritis virus and canine parvovirus. Virol J. 2012;9:252.
15. Song W, Mentink RA, Henquet MG, Cordewener JH, van Dijk AD, Bosch D, et al. N-glycan occupancy of Arabidopsis N-glycoproteins. J Proteomics. 2013;93:343–55.
16. Zhang H, Chai X, Luo G, Wang F, Yi L, Shao X, et al. Cloning, expression and antiviral activity of arctic fox (Alopex lagopus) interferon-gamma gene. J Biot China. 2008;24(9):1625–30.

17. Tan XM, Tang Y, Yang YF, Song HM, Zhang YZ. Gene cloning, sequencing, expression and biological activity of giant panda (Ailuropoda melanoleuca) interferon-alpha. Mol Immunol. 2007;44:3061–9.
18. Wonderling R, Powell T, Baldwin S, Morales T, Snyder S, Keiser K, et al. Cloning, expression, purification, and biological activity of five feline type I interferons. Vet Immunol Immunop. 2002;89:13–27.
19. Hughes AL. The evolution of the type I interferon gene family in mammals. J Mol Evol. 1995;41:539–48.
20. Hardy MP, Owczarek CM, Jermiin LS, Ejdebäck M, Hertzog PJ. Characterization of the type I interferon locus and identification of novel genes. Genomics. 2004;84:331–45.
21. Taira O, Watanugi I, Hagiwara Y, Takahashi M, Arai S, Sato H, et al. Cloning and expression of canine interferon-alpha genes in Escherichia coli. T J Vet Med Sci. 2005;67:1059–62.
22. Waldvogel AS, Lepage MF, Zakher A, Reichel MP, Eicher R, Heussler VT. Expression of interleukin 4, interleukin 4 splice variants and interferon gamma mRNA in calves experimentally infected with Fasciola hepatica. Vet Immunol Immunop. 2004;97(1–2):53–63.
23. Fung MC, Sia SF, Leung KN, Mak NK. Detection of differential expression of mouse interferon-alpha subtypes by polymerase chain reaction using specific primers. J Immunol Methods. 2004;284(1–2):177–86.

4

Novel adenovirus detected in captive bottlenose dolphins (*Tursiops truncatus*) suffering from self-limiting gastroenteritis

Consuelo Rubio-Guerri[1*], Daniel García-Párraga[2], Elvira Nieto-Pelegrín[1], Mar Melero[1], Teresa Álvaro[2], Mónica Valls[2], Jose Luis Crespo[2] and Jose Manuel Sánchez-Vizcaíno[1]

Abstract

Background: Adenoviruses are common pathogens in vertebrates, including humans. In marine mammals, adenovirus has been associated with fatal hepatitis in sea lions. However, only in rare cases have adenoviruses been detected in cetaceans, where no clear correlation was found between presence of the virus and disease status.

Case presentation: A novel adenovirus was identified in four captive bottlenose dolphins with self-limiting gastroenteritis. Viral detection and identification were achieved by: PCR-amplification from fecal samples; sequencing of partial adenovirus *polymerase (pol)* and *hexon* genes; producing the virus in HeLa cells, with PCR and immunofluorescence detection, and with sequencing of the amplified *pol* and *hexon* gene fragments. A causative role of this adenovirus for gastroenteritis was suggested by: 1) we failed to identify other potential etiological agents; 2) the exclusive detection of this novel adenovirus and of seropositivity for canine adenoviruses 1 and 2 in the four sick dolphins, but not in 10 healthy individuals of the same captive population; and 3) the virus disappeared from feces after clinical signs receded. The partial sequences of the amplified fragments of the *pol* and *hexon* genes were closest to those of adenoviruses identified in sea lions with fatal adenoviral hepatitis, and to a Genbank-deposited sequence obtained from a harbour porpoise.

Conclusion: These data suggest that adenovirus can cause self-limiting gastroenteritis in dolphins. This adenoviral infection can be detected by serology and by PCR detection in fecal material. Lack of signs of hepatitis in sick dolphins may reflect restricted tissue tropism or virulence of this adenovirus compared to those of the adenovirus identified in sea lions. Gene sequence-based phylogenetic analysis supports a common origin of adenoviruses that affect sea mammals. Our findings suggest the need for vigilance against adenoviruses in captive and wild dolphin populations.

Keywords: Adenovirus, Cetacean, Bottlenose dolphin, *Tursiops truncatus*

Background

Adenoviruses are common pathogens of vertebrates [1] that were first discovered in human adenoids [2], and were soon identified as a cause of canine hepatitis [3]. These icosahedral non-enveloped, double-stranded DNA viruses have genomes that range from 26 to 45 kbp [4], and have been demonstrated in all vertebrate classes [1,5]. Most adenoviral species show quite restricted host specificity and tend to be associated with a typical pathology [5]; for example, human adenovirus (HAdV) C causes respiratory disease and HAdV-D provokes conjunctivitis, whereas these two pathologies can also be the result of HAdV-B infection. In contrast, HAdV-F and HAdV-G produce gastroenteritis in most cases [1]. Similarly to human adenoviruses, other adenoviruses that affect mammals (forming the *Mastadenovirus* genus) have been reported to cause respiratory, ocular and gastrointestinal pathologies, although some present as hepatitis [3] or encephalitis as the chief manifestations [5].

In addition to their role in pathology, adenoviruses are very important vectors in the gene therapy of genetic disorders and cancer [6], as they can accommodate a large DNA cargo, exhibit tropisms for multiple organs and can be engineered to decrease virulence. Nonetheless, they still

* Correspondence: consuelo@sanidadanimal.info
[1]VISAVET Center and Animal Health Department, Veterinary School, Complutense University of Madrid, Av Puerta del Hierro s/n, 28040 Madrid, Spain
Full list of author information is available at the end of the article

present toxicity problems [7], which has led to investigation of the potential of using animal adenoviruses as vectors for gene delivery to humans [8-10]. In line with this, the identification of new animal adenoviruses, in addition to being interesting from an animal health perspective may be promising for gene therapy.

Sea lions are the only marine mammals in which adenoviruses have been recognized as pathogens. Adenovirus-like viral particles have been long since associated with hepatitis in stranded California sea lions (Zalophus californianus) [11,12]. More recently, a novel adenovirus (otarine adenovirus 1) was isolated from two stranded California sea lions with fatal hepatitis [13]. This adenovirus caused an outbreak of fatal hepatitis and enteritis in three captive sea lions of different species: California sea lion (Zalophus californianus), South African fur seal (Arctocephalus pusillus) and South American sea lion (Otaria flavescens) [14]. In rare cases, adenoviruses have been isolated from gastrointestinal samples of other marine mammals, including a sei whale (Balaenoptera borealis) [15], two bowhead whales (Balaena mysticetus) [16] and a beluga whale (Delphinapterus leucas) [17]. Serological studies in Canadian fauna have also revealed antibodies against canine adenovirus 2 in 17% of the walruses (Odobenus rosmarus) examined [18]. However, only in the case of sea lion hepatitis, has a clear association been established between the presence of virus and disease status. The partial sequence of the adenoviral DNA polymerase (pol) gene deposited in the Genbank (JN377908) was annotated as having been obtained from a harbour porpoise (Phocoena phocoena). However, there is no further information or referred publication available.

Here we identify a novel adenovirus in fecal samples of four captive bottlenose dolphins (Tursiops truncatus) which presented with self-limiting gastroenteritis. Gastric lesions, ulceration and parasitism are common in captive and free-ranging dolphins [19-21]. However, reports of dolphin gastroenteritis are rare and the disease has never been associated with adenovirus. Pathological evidence for gastroenteritis has been reported [22] in two necropsies of common dolphins from the Black Sea (Delphinus delphis ponticus) that showed evidence of systemic infection with Cetacean morbillivirus infection. Nevertheless, infections with this virus do not typically manifest as gastroenteritis and instead affect primarily the lungs and brain [23]. Fatal gastroenteritis and toxic shock-like syndrome in dolphins has been attributed to enterotoxigenic Staphylococcus aureus [24]. This animal concomitantly suffered brucellar osteomyelitis and was treated with antibiotics for nearly 1 year.

The present report describes several lines of evidence suggesting that adenovirus can be responsible for gastroenteritis in dolphins. Sequencing of PCR-amplified regions of adenoviral DNA (pol) and hexon genes revealed genetic closeness, but was not identical with the previously deposited sequences of sea lions and harbour porpoise adenoviruses. This suggests a close common ancestral origin of these viruses in marine mammals.

Case presentation

At the end of September 2013, four captive bottlenose dolphins (Tursiops truncatus) in a total population of 14 individuals, all born at the Oceanográfic water park (www.cac.es/oceanografic) in the City of the Arts and the Sciences, Valencia (Spain), presented with anorexia, diarrhoea and vomiting. The four animals, aged 4-10 years, displayed no cough, respiratory disturbances or conjunctival infection. The other 10 dolphins in the same cohort remained healthy throughout this study. As soon as clinical signs became evident in the sick animals, they were isolated in a separate pool. The clinical signs of one dolphin (animal 1) appeared to be the mildest and it recovered in 1 week without treatment; in Figure 1A, the dark horizontal bar marks the period during which clinical manifestations were present. The other three dolphins (animals 2-4) were more severely affected and were administered oral rehydration therapy to compensate for fluid lost through vomiting and diarrhoea. They underwent longer disease-manifesting periods (Figure 1A). Day 1 was the day on which the first animal became overtly sick with vomiting and diarrhea.

Blood and fecal samples, obtained by rectal cannulation, were subjected to diagnostic tests. Animal sampling were conducted according to Spanish and European regulations (RD 53/2013, Directive 2010/63/UE) on animal welfare. No abnormalities were observed in the complete blood count, serum biochemistry or activity of serum enzymes such us aspartate and alanine aminotransferases. Blood samples gave negative serological results for several viruses (parvovirus, parainfluenza, coronavirus, influenza A) and for Leptospira interrogans (tests carried out by Penta Laboratories, Alicante, Spain). The microbiological analysis of feces performed at the Central Laboratory for Animal Health (Algete, Madrid, Spain) failed to reveal any bacterial pathogens using standard microbial growth assays in either sick or healthy animals. Fecal material also yielded negative results in a test for rotavirus antigen (Penta Laboratories) and in the fast immunoassays to detect canine parvovirus (VetScan Canine Parvovirus Rapid Test kit, Abaxis, Union City, CA, USA), bovine rotavirus, coronavirus and cryptosporidium (FASTest® D4T bovine; MEGACOR Diagnostik, Hörbranz, Austria), and in a real-time PCR (qPCR) assay for calicivirus [25]. The only differential finding between diseased and healthy animals was seropositivity for antibodies against canine adenoviruses 1 and 2 (ELISA kit D1003-AB01, European Veterinary Laboratory, The Netherlands) [26]. These antibodies were found exclusively in all four sick animals during the disease manifestation period (tested on days 2-4 of this period in animals 1-3, and on day 10 in animal 4). The other 10

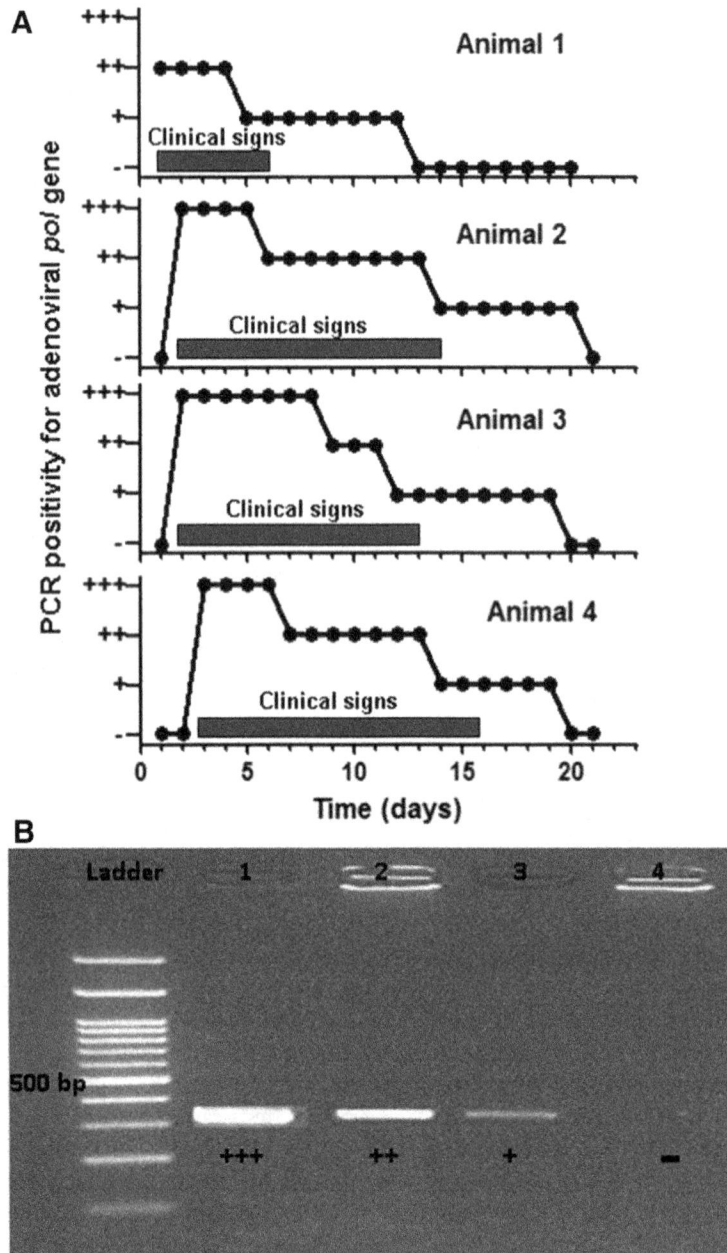

Figure 1 Presence of adenoviral DNA in fecal samples of four diseased bottlenose dolphins. A) Variation in the intensity of the adenoviral *polymerase (pol)* amplicon across different diseased animals and samples taken at the indicated times from the same animal. Black bars indicate the period during which each animal exhibited clinical manifestations. Day 1 was the day on which the first animal became overtly sick with vomiting and diarrhea. **B)** Representative results showing four levels of band intensity (- / + / ++ / +++) for the PCR amplicons of a region of the adenoviral *pol* gene. Line 1 corresponds to an amplification prepared from a fecal sample taken on day 2 from animal 2; Line 2, from a fecal sample taken on day 1 from animal 1; Line 3, on day 15 from animal 3; and Line 4, on day 20 from animal 4, used as negative controls. On the DNA ladder, the band of 500 bp is indicated.

healthy animals did not give a positive test (assayed on days 3-20 from the beginning of the outbreak; one animal was tested on both days 3 and 20). Before the outbreak, all 14 animals were seronegative for canine adenoviruses 1 and 2 (tested retrospectively on serum collected and kept frozen <4 months, usually around 2 months). Based on

retrospective sampling, one sick animal was negative 15 days before disease, and a healthy animal was negative 5 days before the beginning of the outbreak). These findings led us to search for adenoviruses in the fecal samples collected from all 14 animals in the cohort from the beginning of the outbreak. The feces of healthy animals were collected daily the first 5 days of the outbreak and then every 5-10 days during the outbreak. Fecal sampling in the diseased animals was carried out daily for 21 days from the beginning of the outbreak and then every 5 days for another 10 days. Afterward fecal samples were collected from all animals every 15 days for 3 months.

To detect adenoviral DNA in feces, parts of the adenoviral *DNA polymerase* (*pol*) and *hexon* genes were PCR-amplified using degenerate consensus primers. For *pol* amplification, a previously described [27] nested PCR assay was performed exactly as reported, on 25 µl the of amplification reaction. For the first PCR reaction 1 µg of DNA extracted from fecal samples with High Pure PCR Template Preparation Kit (Roche Diagnostics GmbH, Mannheim, Germany) was used as a template. The same volumes of PCR reaction and amount of DNA were used for the amplification of the *hexon* sequence, and previously reported PCR assay was followed exactly [28].

The results of these PCR assays were analyzed by agarose gel electrophoresis and staining with SYBR Safe stain (Invitrogen, Carlsbad, CA, USA). All sick animals were positive for the expected *pol* amplicon (320 bp) (Figure 1B) and the *hexon* amplicon (435 bp, not shown), while all healthy animals were negative for both. The identity of the amplified products was confirmed by purification (QIAquick PCR Purification kit, Qiagen, Hilden, Germany) and identified by Sanger sequencing (ABI Prism 3730, from Applied Biosystems, Foster City, CA, USA) using one of the consensus primers utilized in the amplification step as the sequencing primer.

Comparison of the amplification reactions on the same amounts of DNA from the fecal samples collected from different animals and from the same animal on distinct days revealed variable band intensities. These intensities could be visually graded semi-quantitatively as negative (-), low (+), intermediate (++) or high (+++) (shown for *pol* in Figure 1B). Figure 1A plots these intensities for the *pol* band in relation to the presence of disease manifestations in each animal. Band intensity was strongest as soon as clinical signs were patent, and they remained at this initial high level for 4-7 days, finally decreasing before clinical signs subsided. The signal decreased to the lowest level around the same time as the clinical signs disappeared. Nevertheless, the virus remained detectable at low levels in feces for approximately 1 week after animals no longer manifested clinical signs. This suggests that, in order to prevent contagion, isolation of diseased animals should continue at least for 1 week after clinical cure. It is noteworthy that the animal with the mildest disease manifestations (animal 1) exhibited lower band intensity at peak infection than the more severely affected animals.

The sequences of the PCR-amplified *pol* and *hexon* gene fragments (Genbank entries KJ126836 and KJ126837,

respectively) were identical for all four animals, which indicates that they were all infected with the same adenovirus. Similarity searches of all adenoviral sequences in Genbank (www.ncbi.nlm.nih.gov/nuccore) using BLASTN (http://blast.ncbi.nlm.nih.gov) showed that the *pol* amplicon in the present work exhibited the highest nucleotide identity (78%) with entry JN377908, this being a deposited, but unpublished, sequence from an adenovirus detected in a harbour porpoise (*Phocoena phocoena*) on the coast of Florida (USA). The *hexon* amplicon showed the highest identity (72%) with otarine adenovirus strain MJ12 (entry AB714142) [14]. We conclude that the adenovirus in the four bottlenose dolphins closely resembles, but differed from previously detected adenoviruses in marine mammals. We designate this apparently novel adenovirus as tursiops adenovirus 1. The phylogenetic analysis [29] of the amino acid sequences deduced from the *pol* and *hexon* amplicons further supports the closeness of tursiops adenovirus 1 to the adenoviruses isolated from other marine mammals, including harbour porpoises, seals and sea lions (Figure 2).

In an effort to confirm this tursiops adenovirus 1 and characterize it in greater detail, we attempted to grow it in HeLa cells. This human-derived cell line was used as specific-host cell lines were not available, and also because canine adenovirus 2 has been proven to infect HeLa cells [30]. Centrifuged (10 min, 2,000 × g, 4°C) fecal homogenates prepared by vortexing in 3 volumes of phosphate-buffered saline (PBS), were filtered through sterile 0.2 µm-pore filters (Sartorius, Goettingen, Germany) and were left to stand for 1 h at 4°C in the presence of 0.5 mg/ml gentamycin. 0.2 ml of this solution were added to subconfluent HeLa cell monolayers, which had been grown (37°C, 5% CO_2) in 6-well plastic plates in Dulbecco's Modified Eagle Medium (DMEM; Lonza, Basel, Switzerland) supplemented with 10% heat-inactivated fetal bovine serum (FBS) (Invitrogen, Carlsbad, CA, USA), 100 U/ml penicillin and 0.1 mg/ml streptomycin (Sigma-Aldrich, St. Louis, USA). Immediately before this inoculation, the medium was replaced with 0.3 ml of FBS-free medium. After 1 h, 1.5 ml of the 10% FBS-containing medium was added and the culture continued. Each day, a 0.2-ml sample of culture medium was taken for the PCR *pol* gene analysis. With the cultures inoculated with samples of diseased animals, the PCR assay on the culture medium was initially negative or very weakly positive, but became strongly positive on days 4-5. The cultures inoculated with samples of healthy dolphins, which had been processed in parallel, did not give a positive PCR reaction. The sequence of the *pol* fragment amplified by PCR from the positive cultures on day five after inoculation with the fecal material was identical to that obtained directly from fecal samples, which confirmed that the virus corresponded to the original adenovirus detected in feces. These results suggest that the virus can replicate to

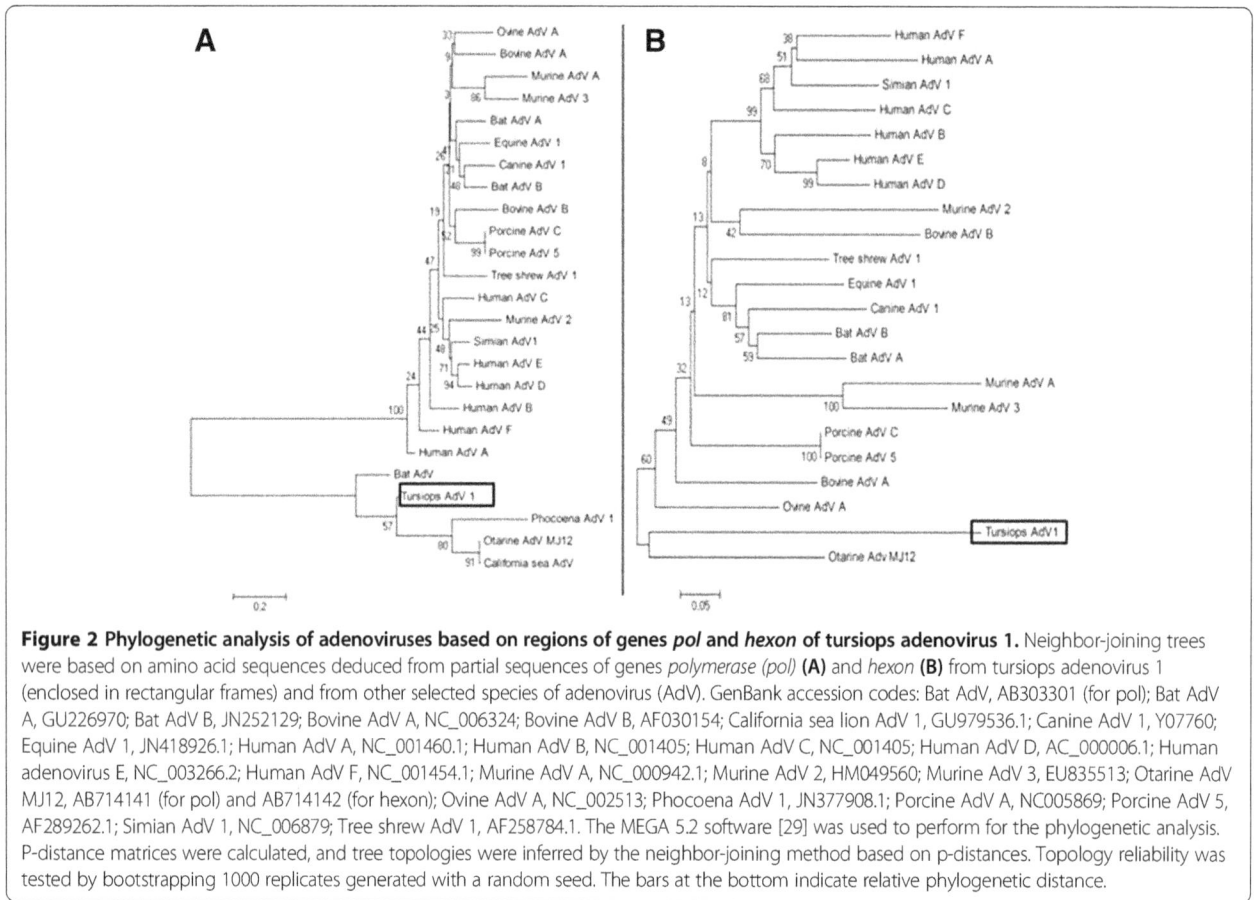

Figure 2 Phylogenetic analysis of adenoviruses based on regions of genes *pol* and *hexon* of tursiops adenovirus 1. Neighbor-joining trees were based on amino acid sequences deduced from partial sequences of genes *polymerase (pol)* **(A)** and *hexon* **(B)** from tursiops adenovirus 1 (enclosed in rectangular frames) and from other selected species of adenovirus (AdV). GenBank accession codes: Bat AdV, AB303301 (for pol); Bat AdV A, GU226970; Bat AdV B, JN252129; Bovine AdV A, NC_006324; Bovine AdV B, AF030154; California sea lion AdV 1, GU979536.1; Canine AdV 1, Y07760; Equine AdV 1, JN418926.1; Human AdV A, NC_001460.1; Human AdV B, NC_001405; Human AdV C, NC_001405; Human AdV D, AC_000006.1; Human adenovirus E, NC_003266.2; Human AdV F, NC_001454.1; Murine AdV A, NC_000942.1; Murine AdV 2, HM049560; Murine AdV 3, EU835513; Otarine AdV MJ12, AB714141 (for pol) and AB714142 (for hexon); Ovine AdV A, NC_002513; Phocoena AdV 1, JN377908.1; Porcine AdV A, NC005869; Porcine AdV 5, AF289262.1; Simian AdV 1, NC_006879; Tree shrew AdV 1, AF258784.1. The MEGA 5.2 software [29] was used to perform for the phylogenetic analysis. P-distance matrices were calculated, and tree topologies were inferred by the neighbor-joining method based on p-distances. Topology reliability was tested by bootstrapping 1000 replicates generated with a random seed. The bars at the bottom indicate relative phylogenetic distance.

some extent in HeLa cells. However, transmission electron microscopy (tFEI Tecnai G2 Spirit microscope, EM Service, Principe Felipe Research Centre, Valencia, Spain) of ultrathin sections of the glutaraldehyde-fixed, osmium tetroxide-stained, durcupan-embedded and lead citrate counterstained cell monolayers on day 5 of culture did not provide conclusive evidence of adenovirus (although a few suggestive images of rounded particles of around 125-160 nm were observed [31] in the infected cells nuclei, data not shown). Therefore, the inference from these results that the virus can replicate in HeLa cells was confirmed by immunofluorescence using a monoclonal antibody against canine adenovirus 1 (clone 2E10-H2, VMRD, Pullman, WA, USA) and, as secondary antibody, Alexa 488-conjugated goat anti-mouse IgG (Invitrogen). Cells were fixed with ice-cold methanol (methanol 100%, Sigma) at -20°C and permeabilized with 0.1% Triton X-100 for 5 min. After three washes with PBS, cells were blocked with 5% goat serum in PBS for 1 hour and stained at room temperature with anti-CAV1 MoAb for 1 h at a final concentration of 0.1 mg/ml. Then, cells were washed three times with PBS and incubated for 1 h with a secondary Alexa 488-conjugated goat anti-mouse Ab (diluted 1:800) for detection in the green channel. After three washes with PBS, cover glasses were dried at room temperature for

20 minutes followed by assembly of the cover glasses in the slides. Confocal Microscopy was performed at the Madrid Science Park microscopy facility using a Olympus FV1200 equipped and images were processed with Photoshop CS5.

The cells of a culture inoculated with material derived from a sick animal (animal 3, on third day of clinical manifestations), when examined on day four after inoculation, gave clear nuclear fluorescence and moderate diffuse cytoplasmic fluorescence (Figure 3, downright panel), as previously described for adenovirus [32]. In contrast, a parallel culture inoculated with an equivalent amount of FBS-medium free material (Mock) did not exhibit substantial fluorescence (Figure 3 topright panel).

Conclusions

In summary, we report herein self-limiting gastrointestinal disease in bottlenose dolphins, which appears to be due to a hitherto unknown adenovirus that is genetically close to the adenoviruses found previously in marine mammals, such as sea lions. Adenoviral causality is supported by the exclusive detection in the four diseased animals, concomitantly with the disease, of adenovirus in feces and of antibodies for canine adenoviruses 1 and 2 in the serum. While adenoviral infection of sea lions causes hepatitis

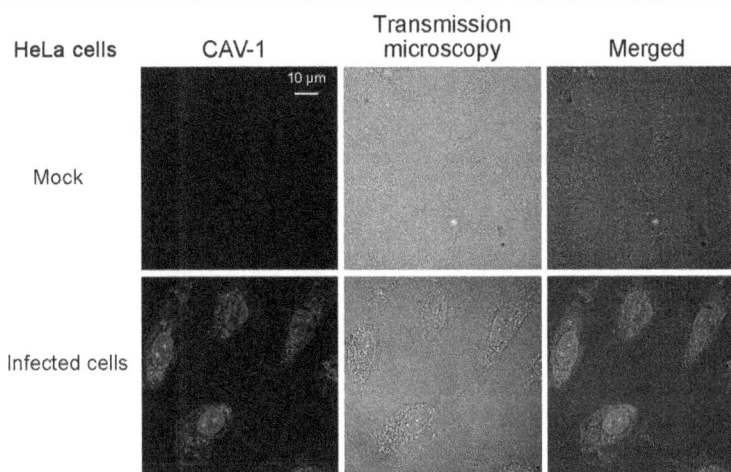

Figure 3 Immunofluorescence of HeLa cell cultures inoculated with FBS medium-free (top) and fecal extracts from diseased animals (below). The HeLa cells were fixed the day 4 after infection. Immunofluorescence staining was done using anti-Cav-1 MoAb (first column). Transmission microscopy images were used to see the location and structure of the HeLa cells (second column). The merged images shown in the last column were generated with Photoshop S5 software. Pictures were taken at 600x magnification and scale bar represents 10 um.

and death [13,14], the dolphins infected with putative tursiops adenovirus 1 suffered self-limiting disease, with no signs of hepatitis. In addition, the dolphins showed no apparent respiratory or ocular pathologies, which are frequent in adenoviral infections of many other species [1,5]. Thus this adenovirus may not show liver, lung or eye tropism. Full adenoviral genome sequencing might help predict tropism, since certain genetic elements have been associated with certain tropisms [33]. The full viral sequence might also be necessary to more broadly confirm our present inference, based on the limited phylogenetic analysis of partial *pol* and *hexon* gene sequences (Figure 2), and that this adenovirus is more closely related with adenoviruses of other marine mammals than with those of other taxonomic groups. This close relation suggests that a branch of the adenoviral tree evolved when marine mammals became adenoviral hosts. It remains to be elucidated whether adenoviruses represent a serious threat to dolphins. In any case, the present findings highlight the need to consider this adenovirus a causal agent of dolphin gastroenteritis, which should be taken into account in the differential diagnosis of this condition, at least for captive dolphins.

Abbreviations
Pol: Polymerase; HAdV: Human adenovirus; EM: Electron microscopy; CBC: Complete blood counts; qPCR: Real-time polymerase chain reaction; USA: United States of America; DMEM: Dulbecco's Modified Eagle Medium; PBS: Phosphate-buffered saline; FBS: Fetal bovine serum; OsO4: Osmium tetroxide.

Competing interests
The authors declare that they have no competing interests.

Authors' contributions
Clinical monitoring and sample collection were performed by DGP, MV and TA; viral study, phylogenetic study and cell culture were analyzed by CRG, EN and MM; the manuscript was prepared and critically discussed by CRG, DGP, EN, JLC and JMSV and all the other authors made contributions of. All authors read and approved the final manuscript.

Acknowledgments
This work has been carried out under the auspices of a collaborative agreement on virology studies in sea mammals between The Oceanogràfic of the Ciudad de las Artes y las Ciencias of Valencia and the VISAVET Center of Complutense University of Madrid. We thank Vicente Rubio (IBV-CSIC, Valencia) for critically reading the manuscript; Carmen Martín Espada for the assays to detect rotavirus, coronavirus, cryptosporidium and parvovirus; Belén Rivera and Rocío Sánchez for technical assistance; Francisco Javier García Peña (Laboratorio Central de Sanidad Animal de Algete) for bacteriological assays; Narcisa Martinez Quiles for providing HeLa cells; and Mario Soriano (Electron Microscopy service of the Centro de Investigación Principe Felipe de Valencia) for assistance with EM sample preparation and analysis. CRG is the recipient of a predoctoral fellowship from the FPU programme of the Spanish Ministry of Education. MM is the recipient of a predoctoral fellowship from the PhD student grant programme of Complutense University of Madrid.

Author details
[1]VISAVET Center and Animal Health Department, Veterinary School, Complutense University of Madrid, Av Puerta del Hierro s/n, 28040 Madrid, Spain. [2]Veterinary Services, Oceanographic Aquarium of the Ciudad de las Artes y las Ciencias, C/ Junta de Murs i Valls s/n, 46023 Valencia, Spain.

References
1. Wold WSM, Horwitz MS. Adenoviruses. In: Martin MA, Knipe DM, Fields BN, Howley PM, Griffin D, Lamb R, editors. Fields' virology, vol. 2. Philadelphia: Wolters Kluwer Health/Lippincott Williams & Wilkins; 2007. p. 2395–436.
2. Rowe WP, Huebner RJ, Gilmore LK, Parrott RH, Ward TG. Isolation of a cytopathogenic agent from human adenoids undergoing spontaneous degeneration in tissue culture. Proc Soc Exp Biol Med. 1953;84:570–3.
3. Cabasso VJ, Stebbins MR, Norton TW, Cox HR. Propagation of infectious canine hepatitis virus in tissue culture. Proc Soc Exp Biol Med. 1954;85:239–45.
4. Berk AJ. Adenoviridae: the viruses and their replication. In: Martin MA, Knipe DM, Fields BN, Howley PM, Griffin D, Lamb R, editors. Fields' virology, vol. 2. Philadelphia: Wolters Kluwer Health/Lippincott Williams & Wilkins; 2007. p. 2355–94.

5.   Knowles DP. Adenoviridae. In: MacLachlan NJ, Dubovi EJ, editors. Fenner's Veterinary Virology, Fourth Edition. Oxford, UK: Elsevier/Academic Press; 2011. p. 203–12.

6.   Wold WS, Toth K. Adenovirus vectors for gene therapy, vaccination and cancer gene therapy. Curr Gene Ther. 2013;13:421–33.

7.   Raper SE, Chirmule N, Lee FS, Wivel NA, Bagg A, Gao GP, et al. Fatal systemic inflammatory response syndrome in a ornithine transcarbamylase deficient patient following adenoviral gene transfer. Mol Genet Metab. 2003;80:148–58.

8.   Fernandes P, Peixoto C, Santiago VM, Kremer EJ, Coroadinha AS, Alves PM. Bioprocess development for canine adenovirus type 2 vectors. Gene Ther. 2013;20:353–60.

9.   Szelechowski M, Bergeron C, Gonzalez-Dunia D, Klonjkowski B. Production and purification of non replicative canine adenovirus type 2 derived vectors. J Vis Exp. 2013;3:50833.

10. Puig M, Piedra J, Miravet S, Segura MM. Canine adenovirus downstream processing protocol. Methods Mol Biol. 2014;1089:197–210.

11. Britt Jr JO, Nagy AZ, Howard EB. Acute viral hepatitis in California sea lions. J Am Vet Med Assoc. 1979;175:921–3.

12. Dierauf LA, Lowenstine LJ, Jerome C. Viral hepatitis (adenovirus) in a California sea lion. J Am Vet Med Assoc. 1981;179:1194–7.

13. Goldstein T, Colegrove KM, Hanson M, Gulland FM. Isolation of a novel adenovirus from California sea lions Zalophus californianus. Dis Aquat Organ. 2011;94:243–8.

14. Inoshima Y, Murakami T, Ishiguro N, Hasegawa K, Kasamatsu M. An outbreak of lethal adenovirus infection among different otariid species. Vet Microbiol. 2013;165:455–9.

15. Smith AW, Skilling DE. Viruses and virus diseases of marine mammals. J Am Vet Med Assoc. 1979;175:918–20.

16. Smith AW, Skilling DE, Benirschke K, Albert TF, Barlough JE. Serology and virology of the bowhead whale (Balaena mysticetus L.). J Wildl Dis. 1987;23:92–8.

17. De Guise S, Lagace A, Beland P, Girard C, Higgins R. Non-neoplastic lesions in beluga whales (Delphinapterus leucas) and other marine mammals from the St Lawrence Estuary. J Comp Pathol. 1995;112:257–71.

18. Philippa JD, Leighton FA, Daoust PY, Nielsen O, Pagliarulo M, Schwantje H, et al. Antibodies to selected pathogens in free-ranging terrestrial carnivores and marine mammals in Canada. Vet Rec. 2004;155:135–40.

19. Greenwood AG, Taylor DC, Wild D. Fibreoptic gastroscopy in dolphins. Vet Rec. 1978;102:495–7.

20. Goldstein JD, Reese E, Reif JS, Varela RA, McCulloch SD, Defran RH, et al. Hematologic, biochemical, and cytologic findings from apparently healthy atlantic bottlenose dolphins (Tursiops truncatus) inhabiting the Indian River Lagoon, Florida, USA. J Wildl Dis. 2006;42:447–54.

21. Lane EP, de Wet M, Thompson P, Siebert U, Wohlsein P, Plon S. A systematic health assessment of indian ocean bottlenose (Tursiops aduncus) and indo-pacific humpback (Sousa plumbea) dolphins incidentally caught in shark nets off the KwaZulu-Natal Coast, South Africa. PLoS One. 2014;9:e107038.

22. Birkun Jr A, Kuiken T, Krivokhizhin S, Haines DM, Osterhaus AD, van de Bildt MW, et al. Epizootic of morbilliviral disease in common dolphins (Delphinus delphis ponticus) from the Black sea. Vet Rec. 1999;144:85–92.

23. Rubio-Guerri C, Melero M, Esperon F, Belliere EN, Arbelo M, Crespo JL, et al. Unusual striped dolphin mass mortality episode related to cetacean morbillivirus in the Spanish Mediterranean sea. BMC Vet Res. 2013;9:106.

24. Goertz CE, Frasca Jr S, Bohach GA, Cowan DF, Buck JD, French RA, et al. Brucella sp. vertebral osteomyelitis with intercurrent fatal Staphylococcus aureus toxigenic enteritis in a bottlenose dolphin (Tursiops truncatus). J Vet Diagn Invest. 2011;23:845–51.

25. Reid SM, King DP, Shaw AE, Knowles NJ, Hutchings GH, Cooper EJ, et al. Development of a real-time reverse transcription polymerase chain reaction assay for detection of marine caliciviruses (genus Vesivirus). J Virol Methods. 2007;140:166–73.

26. Bulut O, Yapici O, Avci O, Simsek A, Atli K, Dik I, et al. The serological and virological investigation of canine adenovirus infection on the dogs. ScientificWorldJournal. 2013;2013:587024.

27. Wellehan JF, Johnson AJ, Harrach B, Benko M, Pessier AP, Johnson CM, et al. Detection and analysis of six lizard adenoviruses by consensus primer PCR provides further evidence of a reptilian origin for the atadenoviruses. J Virol. 2004;78:13366–9.

28. Thomson D, Meers J, Harrach B. Molecular confirmation of an adenovirus in brushtail possums (Trichosurus vulpecula). Virus Res. 2002;83:189–95.

29. Tamura K, Dudley J, Nei M, Kumar S. MEGA4: Molecular Evolutionary Genetics Analysis (MEGA) software version 4.0. Mol Biol Evol. 2007;24:1596–9.

30. Klonjkowski B, Gilardi-Hebenstreit P, Hadchouel J, Randrianarison V, Boutin S, Yeh P, et al. A recombinant E1-deleted canine adenoviral vector capable of transduction and expression of a transgene in human-derived cells and in vivo. Hum Gene Ther. 1997;8:2103–15.

31. Weber J, Stich HF. Electron microscopy of cells infected with adenovirus type 2. J Virol. 1969;3:198–204.

32. Whetstone CA. Monoclonal antibodies to canine adenoviruses 1 and 2 that are type-specific by virus neutralization and immunofluorescence. Vet Microbiol. 1988;16:1–8.

33. Vigne E, Dedieu JF, Brie A, Gillardeaux A, Briot D, Benihoud K, et al. Genetic manipulations of adenovirus type 5 fiber resulting in liver tropism attenuation. Gene Ther. 2003;10:153–62.

5

Development of a nanoparticle-assisted PCR (nanoPCR) assay for detection of mink enteritis virus (MEV) and genetic characterization of the *NS1* gene in four Chinese MEV strains

Jianke Wang[1], Yuening Cheng[2], Miao Zhang[2], Hang Zhao[1], Peng Lin[1], Li Yi[1], Mingwei Tong[1] and Shipeng Cheng[1*]

Abstract

Background: Mink enteritis virus (MEV) causes mink viral enteritis, an acute and highly contagious disease whose symptoms include violent diarrhea, and which is characterized by high morbidity and mortality. Nanoparticle-assisted polymerase chain reaction (nanoPCR) is a recently developed technique for the rapid detection of bacterial and viral DNA. Here we describe a novel nanoPCR assay for the clinical detection and epidemiological characterization of MEV.

Results: This assay is based upon primers specific for the conserved region of the MEV *NS1* gene, which encodes nonstructural protein 1. Under optimized conditions, the MEV nanoPCR assay had a detection limit of 8.75×10^1 copies recombinant plasmids per reaction, compared with 8.75×10^3 copies for conventional PCR analysis. Moreover, of 246 clinical mink samples collected from five provinces in North-Eastern China, 50.8% were scored MEV positive by our nanoPCR assay, compared with 32.5% for conventional PCR. Furthermore no cross reactivity was observed for the nanoPCR assay with respect to related viruses, including canine distemper virus (CDV) and Aleutian mink disease parvovirus (AMDV). Phylogenetic analysis of four Chinese wild type MEV isolates using the nanoPCR assay indicated that they belonged to a small MEV clade, named "China type", in the MEV/FPLV cluster, and were closely clustered in the same location.

Conclusions: Our results indicate that the MEV China type clade is currently circulating in domestic minks in China. We anticipate that the nanoPCR assay we have described here will be useful for the detection and epidemiological and pathological characterization of MEV.

Keywords: Nanoparticle-assisted PCR, Mink enteritis virus, Nonstructural protein 1 gene, Genetic characterization, China type

Background

Mink enteritis virus (MEV), a member of the genus *Parvovirus* within the family *Parvoviridae*, and a subspecies of the feline parvovirus (FPV), is a single-stranded DNA virus with a genome length of approximately 5,094 nt [1-3]. The MEV genome contains two major open reading frames (ORFs), a 3' half ORF encoding the nonstructural proteins NS1 and NS2, and a 5' half ORF encoding the capsid proteins VP1 and VP2.

MEV causes mink viral enteritis, an acute and highly contagious disease whose symptoms include violent diarrhea, and which is characterized by high morbidity and mortality [4]. The initial description of the disease in Canadian minks in 1949 [5] was followed by the isolation and identification of the viral pathogen and development of a vaccine in 1952 [6]. The disease has since been reported in a number of other countries worldwide [2], including China [7], and poses a serious economic threat to the global mink fur farming industry [8].

Diagnosis of MEV constitutes an important measure for the control of the disease, and although a broad number of approaches have been adopted, they have

* Correspondence: tcscsp@126.com
[1]State Key Laboratory for Molecular Biology of Special Economic Animals, Institute of Special Animal and Plant Sciences, Chinese Academy of Agricultural Sciences, Changchun 130112, China
Full list of author information is available at the end of the article

their own disadvantages [4,9-16]. For example, although electron microscopy and virus isolation are highly specific and sensitive, they are often too time-consuming and expensive for routine clinical use. Moreover, the latex agglutination test is rapid but lacks specificity, and the haemagglutination inhibition test requires a continuous supply of fresh erythrocytes and is unsuitable for the detection of non-haemagglutinating MEV isolates [15].

Conventional polymerase chain reaction (PCR) has been widely used for the detection of MEV and other viruses [17] through amplification of the highly conserved *NS1* and *VP2* genes [13,14] and, together with restriction fragment length polymorphism (RFLP), has been used for differentiation of MEV vaccine and wild type strains [13]. In addition, real-time PCR have been developed for the detection and quantification of other parvoviruses, including canine [18-20], porcine [21-23], human B19 [24,25] and human 4 [26] parvoviruses.

Nanoparticle-assisted PCR (nanoPCR) [27] incorporates nanoparticles to improve the specificity and speed of the reaction, and has been successfully applied for the detection of pseudorabies virus [28], bacterial aerosols [29], porcine parvovirus [17] and porcine bocavirus [30]. Here we describe the development of a nanoPCR-based assay for rapid clinical detection and epidemiological characterization of MEV.

Results

Optimization of MEV nanoPCR assay conditions

Optimization of the nanoPCR assay encompassed adjustment of primer pairs, annealing temperature and the volumes of primer and plasmid DNA. Three primer pairs with fragment lengths of 194 bp, 163 bp and 389 bp, respectively, were compared, and based on gel quantification analysis by ImageJ 1.46r software, primer pair No. 1 (P1 and P2) was selected for use in conventional PCR and nanoPCR assays (data not shown). Band density was found to be optimal at an annealing temperature of 54.9°C, which was chosen for subsequent studies (Figure 1a). Using this annealing temperature, band density was found to be maximal at a primer volume of 0.6 μL (10 μmol/L) (Figure 1b) and a plasmid DNA volume of 1.0 μL (Figure 1c). Gel quantification analysis of all bands has been carried out using ImageJ 1.46r software (see Additional file 1).

Based on the results obtained with different annealing temperatures, primer volumes and plasmid DNA volumes for the MEV nanoPCR assay, an optimal 12 μL reaction volume was established, containing 6.0 μL of 2× nanobuffer, 0.6 μL each of the upstream and downstream primers (10 μmol/L), 1.0 μL of extracted DNA or standard plasmid, 0.2 μL of Taq DNA polymerase (5 U/μL) and ddH$_2$O up to 12 μL. The reaction conditions were as follows: 3 min at 94°C, followed by 31 cycles at 94°C for 30 s,

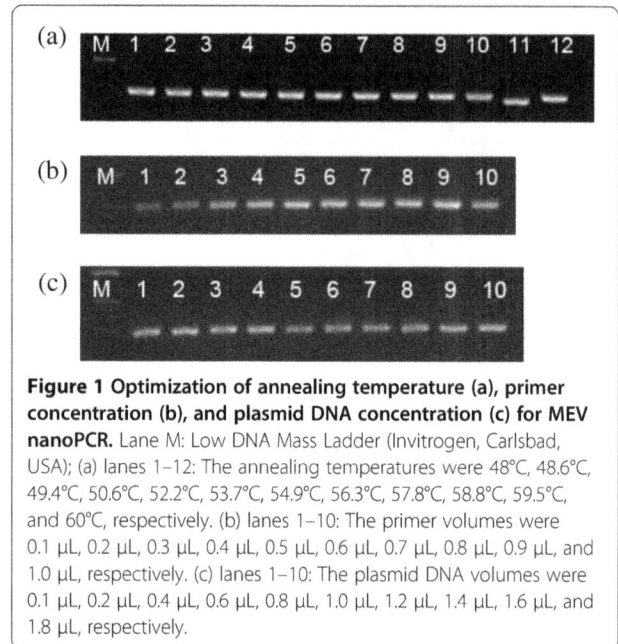

Figure 1 Optimization of annealing temperature (a), primer concentration (b), and plasmid DNA concentration (c) for MEV nanoPCR. Lane M: Low DNA Mass Ladder (Invitrogen, Carlsbad, USA); (a) lanes 1–12: The annealing temperatures were 48°C, 48.6°C, 49.4°C, 50.6°C, 52.2°C, 53.7°C, 54.9°C, 56.3°C, 57.8°C, 58.8°C, 59.5°C, and 60°C, respectively. (b) lanes 1–10: The primer volumes were 0.1 μL, 0.2 μL, 0.3 μL, 0.4 μL, 0.5 μL, 0.6 μL, 0.7 μL, 0.8 μL, 0.9 μL, and 1.0 μL, respectively. (c) lanes 1–10: The plasmid DNA volumes were 0.1 μL, 0.2 μL, 0.4 μL, 0.6 μL, 0.8 μL, 1.0 μL, 1.2 μL, 1.4 μL, 1.6 μL, and 1.8 μL, respectively.

54.9°C for 30 s and 72°C for 15 s, and a final elongation at 72°C for 10 min.

Sensitivity of the MEV nanoPCR assay

Evaluation of the sensitivity of MEV nanoPCR assay indicated that the detection limit of the MEV nanoPCR assay (8.75×10^1 copies/μL, Figure 2a) was 100-fold higher than that of conventional PCR analysis (8.75×10^3 copies/μL, Figure 2b).

Specificity of the MEV nanoPCR assay

Agarose gel electrophoresis analysis indicated no cross reaction of the nanoPCR assay with CDV or AMDV DNAs, nor DNA extracted from the tissues of healthy minks, but was positive for MEV-infected minks (Figure 3).

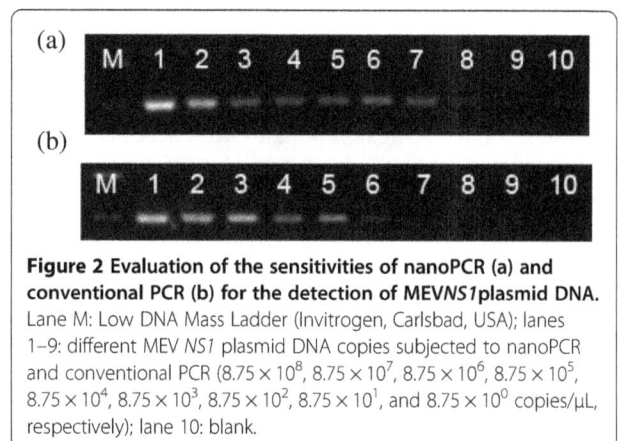

Figure 2 Evaluation of the sensitivities of nanoPCR (a) and conventional PCR (b) for the detection of MEV*NS1*plasmid DNA. Lane M: Low DNA Mass Ladder (Invitrogen, Carlsbad, USA); lanes 1–9: different MEV *NS1* plasmid DNA copies subjected to nanoPCR and conventional PCR (8.75×10^8, 8.75×10^7, 8.75×10^6, 8.75×10^5, 8.75×10^4, 8.75×10^3, 8.75×10^2, 8.75×10^1, and 8.75×10^0 copies/μL, respectively); lane 10: blank.

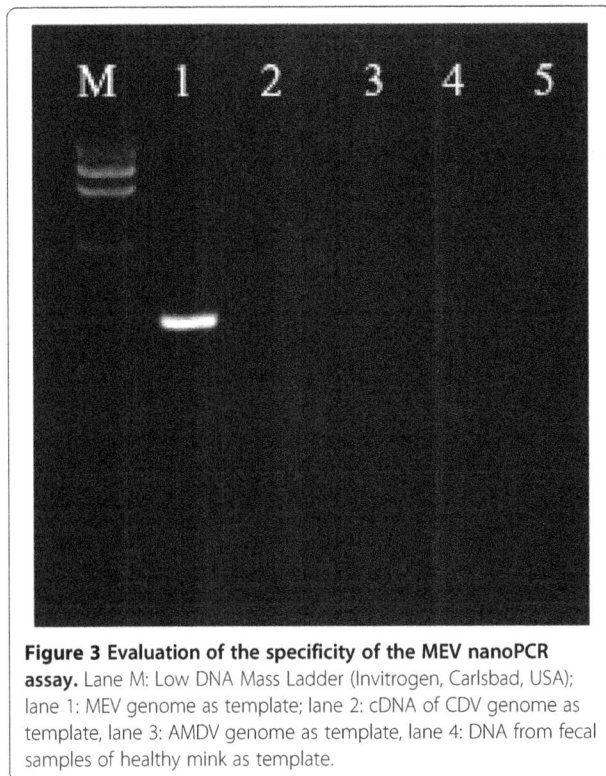

Figure 3 Evaluation of the specificity of the MEV nanoPCR assay. Lane M: Low DNA Mass Ladder (Invitrogen, Carlsbad, USA); lane 1: MEV genome as template; lane 2: cDNA of CDV genome as template, lane 3: AMDV genome as template, lane 4: DNA from fecal samples of healthy mink as template.

Diagnosis of MEV by nanoPCR assay

Clinical samples were subjected simultaneously to MEV nanoPCR and conventional PCR. Eighty samples (32.5%) were positive for MEV by both nanoPCR and conventional PCR, and 121 samples (49.2%) were negative by both nanoPCR and conventional PCR. Forty five (34.3%) samples that were positive by nanoPCR were negative by conventional PCR, while no sample that was negative by nanoPCR was found to be positive by conventional PCR (Table 1). Compared with the conventional PCR, the relative specificity and sensitivity of nanoPCR were 72.9% (121/166) and 100% (80/80), respectively. The ten fecal samples from experimentally infected minks were positive for MEV by both nanoPCR and conventional PCR. Parts of clinical samples detection by MEV nanoPCR were shown in Figure 4.

Table 1 Comparison of the sensitivity and specificity of nanoPCR and conventional PCR analysis for detection of MEV in fecal samples

nanoPCR	Conventional PCR		
	Positive	Negative	Total
Positive	80	45	125
Negative	0	121	121
Total	80	166	246

Percentage of agreement: (80 + 121)/246 = 81.7%; relative sensitivity: 80/80 = 100%; relative specificity: 121/166 = 72.9%.

DNA sequencing and phylogenetic analysis

Sequence analysis indicated high similarity between the products obtained with the nanoPCR amplification of the *NS1* gene of MEV (the object sequences) and the reference sequence of MEV, indicating that the MEV nanoPCR is specific. A phylogenetic tree was constructed by the Maximum Likelihood method, and the robustness of the phylogenetic analysis was determined by bootstrap analysis with 500 replications (Figure 5). Analysis of this tree demonstrated that carnivore parvoviruses were divided into FPLV/MEV and CPV clusters. The MEV Jlin/2010, MEV-SDNH, MEV SD07/09, and MEV SD12/01 strains were classified into a small MEV clade, named the China type, in the FPLV/MEV cluster. Moreover, MEV/LN-10, a natural recombination virus between mink enteritis virus and canine parvovirus [31], was found to be more distant from the small China clade. In general, strains from the same province shared a common clade.

Discussion

MEV is an important viral pathogen in the mink industry, causing high morbidity and mortality worldwide, and for which there are no effective treatments [32,33]. Accordingly, to improve epidemiological surveillance and prediction of the severity of MEV infection [4], we set out here to develop a simple and rapid diagnostic tool, targeting the conserved MEV *NS1* gene, for the detection and differentiation of MEV from other viruses.

A variety of methods currently exist for the detection of MEV, including the hemagglutination test and double antibody sandwich ELISA for the detection of MEV antigen [12], and the haemagglutination inhibition test, serum neutralisation test, and indirect ELISA for the detection of MEV antibodies [16]. These serological techniques, however, do not distinguish between vaccine or natural infection with wild-type virus as the cause of the antibody response. Moreover, although conventional PCR has been used to identify MEV infection [14,34], it is time-consuming and insensitive, and unsuitable for the detection of low viral loads in clinical samples. In addition, though LAMP assay is simple [4], it is readily subject to contamination.

The present study demonstrated that our nanoPCR assay is an effective and time-saving method for detecting MEV. This assay had 100-fold higher analytical sensitivity than conventional PCR, was specific for MEV, and exhibited no cross reactivity against other viruses. Of the 246 field samples in this study, 125 (50.8%) were positive for MEV when assayed by MEV nanoPCR, indicating the prevalence of MEV infection in China.

The results of our phylogenetic analysis, indicating that carnivore parvoviruses were divided into FPLV/MEV and CPV clusters, is similar to the results of a study based on VP2 gene sequences [31]. As shown in the phylogenetic

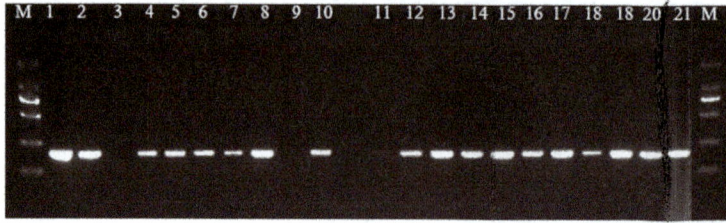

Figure 4 Detection of MEV in clinical samples by nanoPCR assay. Lane M: DL2000 DNA Maker (TaKaRa, Dalian, China); lane 1: MEV genome as template; lane 2: plasmid DNA as template; lanes 3: negtive control, lanes 4–21: DNA from clinical fecal samples as template.

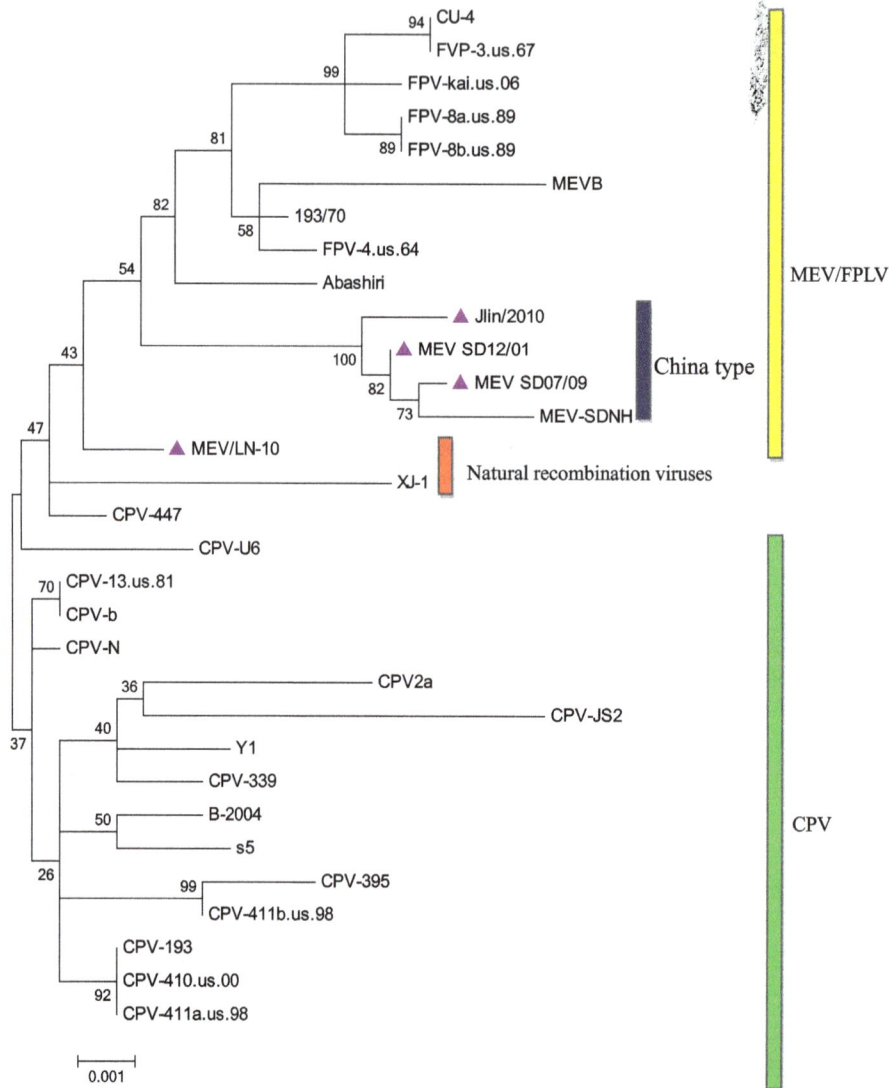

Figure 5 Phylogenetic analysis of MEV with other carnivore parvoviruses based on *NS1* gene nucleotide sequences. Nucleotide sequences were analyzed using the Maximum Likelihood method and Tamura-Nei model in MEGA6. Bootstrap values were calculated on 500 replicates. MEVs marked by solid triangles were isolated and preserved in our lab.

tree, The strains MEV Jlin/2010, MEV-SDNH, MEV SD07/09, and MEV SD12/01 were classified into a samll MEV clade, named China type, in the FPLV/MEV cluster. The nucleotide divergence of the *NS1* gene between strains in the China type clade was between 0.1% to 0.5%, and that between China type and other carnivore parvoviruses was between 0.7% to 1.8%, with the exception of the natural recombination virus strain MEV LN-10 strain [31](data not shown). Specifically, the 357G, 516A, 570 T, 897G, 999A, and 1149G nucleotide residues in the *NS1* gene of the China type strains differed from those of all previously described carnivore parvovirus strains. All new mutations which did not result in amino acid residue replacement were synonymous substitutions.

In summary, we have developed a convenient nanoPCR method for the detection of MEV that is rapid, sensitive, and specific, and which detects both MEV field strains and vaccine strains. Compared with conventional PCR, this nanoPCR assay requires minimal laboratory facilities and is relatively simple and inexpensive to perform. Although only limited numbers of clinical samples were used in the present study, further studies will evaluate its performance in different laboratories and with a larger cohort.

Conclusion

The nanoPCR assay developed in this study we have described here will be useful for the detection and epidemiological and pathological characterization of MEV. In addition, our results indicate that the MEV China type clade is currently circulating in domestic minks in China.

Methods

Viral strains and clinical samples

The viruses (MEV, CDV and AMDV) and 10 experimentally infected samples used in this study have been described in previous reports [4,35]. Animal experiments were approved by the Institute of Special Animal and Plant Sciences of CAAS, and animal experiments were performed in accordance with animal ethics guidelines and approved protocols. Fecal samples were obtained between 2007–2013 in Shandong, Hebei, Liaoning, Heilongjiang, and Jilin provinces, China, from 246 minks showing clinical and pathological signs of enteritis.

Viral DNA/RNA extraction

Fecal samples were collected and stored by our group as previously described [4]. The MEVB or ADMV strain was propagated in the feline kidney F81 cell line in MEM medium. Virus particles were isolated from infected F81 cells when a cytopathic effect was visible about 96 hours after inoculation. Total DNA was extracted from fecal samples and from MEV- or ADMV-infected (positive control) and mock-infected (negative control) cell cultures using a DNA extraction kit (TaKaRa, Dalian, China) according to the manufacturer's instructions. CDV RNA extraction and reverse transcription were performed as previously described [35].

Primers and construction of recombinant plasmid DNA

A consensus MEV *NS1* gene sequence was obtained by aligning the genomes of different MEV isolates collected from publicly available sequence data (GenBank Accession Nos. D00765, FJ592174). Primers were designed using Primer Premier5.0 software (Molecular Biology Insights, Inc., Cascade, CO, USA) to amplify the full-length MEV *NS1* gene, with a predicted fragment length of 2,013 bp). The complete coding sequence of the MEV *NS1* gene was cloned into the plasmid vector pEASY-T1 (TransGen Biotech Company, Beijing, China) as the standard plasmid. The resulting pEASY-T1-MEV-*NS1* construct was amplified in E.coli DH5α, and the recombinant plasmid pEASY-T1-MEV-*NS1* was purified with the EasyPure Plasmid MiniPrep Kit (TransGen Biotech Company, Beijing, China) and quantified using a BioSpectrometer (Eppendorf, Hamburg, Germany) (8.75×10^{10} DNA copies/μL). Constructs were then confirmed by PCR and sequencing and kept at −20°C until use. An additional set of primers was designed to amplify a conserved portion of the *NS1* gene specific to MEV (GenBank accession number: FJ592174) (Table 2), with a predicted amplicon length of 194 bp.

Conventional PCR

MEV conventional PCR analysis was carried out using a primer set (P1 and P2, see Table 2) yielding a PCR product with a predicted length of 194 bp. PCR was carried out in a 20 μL reaction volume containing 1 μL extracted DNA or standard plasmid, 10 μL of 2× *EasyTaq* PCR SuperMix containing *EasyTaq* DNA polymerase, deoxynucleoside triphosphate (dNTP) and buffer (TransGen Biotech Company, Beijing, China), 7 μL ddH$_2$O, and 1 μL of each of primers P1 and P2 (10 μM). The amplification regime was 5 min at 94°C followed by 31 cycles of 94°C for 30 s, 54°C for 30 s, and 72°C for 30 s, with a final elongation for 5 min at 72°C. PCR was carried out in a Life Express Thermal Cycler (HANGZHOU BIOER TECHNOLOGY CO., LTD, China). PCR products were subjected to electrophoresis on a 2% agarose gel.

Optimization of MEV nanoPCR assay conditions

Optimization of the annealing temperature, plasmid DNA volume and primer volume for the MEV nanoPCR assay was carried out using the same primer pair as in conventional PCR for the MEV nanoPCR assay. Annealing temperatures in the Life Express Thermal Cycler ranged

Table 2 NanoPCR and conventional PCR target gene and primers used for amplification of MEV

Primer name[a]	Length (nt)	Genome position[b]	Sequence (5'-3')	Melting temperature (°C)	Product (bp)
P1	20	1906-1925	ACAAGCGGCAAGCAATCCTC	54.9	194
P2	20	2080-2099	CTGCCTCTATTTCGGACCAT		
P3	23	151-173	CGCCATGTCTGGCAACCAGTATA	56	2013
P4	25	2139-2163	GGTTAATCCAAGTCGTCTCGAAAAT		

[a]P1 and P2 were used to amplify a portion of the *NS1* gene (194 bp). P3 and P4 were used to amplify the full-length MEV *NS1* gene (2,013 bp).
[b]The nucleotide positions of the nanoPCR and conventional PCR primers are according the genome sequence of mink enteritis virus strain MEVB (GenBank accession number FJ592174).

from 48°C to 60°C, the plasmid DNA volumes ranged from 0.1 to 1.8 µL, and the primer volumes ranged from 0.1 to 1.0 µL in increments of 0.1 µL. Products were visualized on 2% agarose gels at a voltage of 250 V for 15 min. The nanoPCR Kit (NPK02) was purchased from GREDBIO (Weihai, China). Gel quantification analysis of all bands was carried out using ImageJ 1.46r software (National Institutes of Health, Bethesda, MA, USA).

Sensitivity of MEV nanoPCR assay

The limits of detection of for the MEV nanoPCR assay detection were compared with conventional PCR using a

Table 3 Nucleotide sequence accession numbers of MEV, CPV and FPLV isolates analyzed in this study

No.	Strains	Accession no.	Genetic type	Host	Submitted year	Origin
1	Abashiri	D00765	MEV	mink	2007	Japan
2	MEVB	FJ592174	MEV	mink	2009	China
3	MEV/LN-10	HQ694567	MEV	mink	2011	China
4	MEV SD12/01	KC713592	MEV	mink	2012	China
5	MEV-SDNH	JX535284	MEV	mink	2013	China
6	MEV SD07/09	KM099273	MEV	mink	2014	China
7	CU-4	M38246	FPLV	feline	1996	USA
8	193/70	X55115	FPLV	feline	2005	USA
9	XJ-1	EF988660	FPLV	feline	2007	China
10	FPV-8a.us.89	EU659113	FPLV	feline	2008	USA
11	FPV-4.us.64	EU659112	FPLV	feline	2008	USA
12	FPV-3.us.67	EU659111	FPLV	feline	2008	USA
13	FPV-kai.us.06	EU659115	FPLV	feline	2008	USA
14	FPV-8b.us.89	EU659114	FPLV	feline	2008	USA
15	CPV-N	M19296	CPV-2	canine	1995	USA
16	CPV-b	M38245	CPV-2	canine	1996	USA
17	Y1	D26079	prototype CPV-2a	canine	2002	Japan
18	CPV2a	AJ564427	new CPV-2a	canine	2004	India
19	CPV-193	AY742932	new CPV-2b	canine	2005	USA
20	CPV-339	AY742933	new CPV-2a	canine	2005	New Zealand
21	CPV-447	AY742934	new CPV-2b	canine	2005	USA
22	CPV-U6	AY742935	new CPV-2a	canine	2005	Germany
23	CPV-395	AY742936	new CPV-2b	canine	2005	USA
24	B-2004	EF011664	new CPV-2a	canine	2006	China
25	CPV-13.us.81	EU659118	prototype CPV-2a	canine	2008	USA
26	CPV-410.us.00	EU659119	new CPV-2b	canine	2008	USA
27	CPV-411a.us.98	EU659120	new CPV-2b	canine	2008	USA
28	CPV-411b.us.98	EU659121	new CPV-2b	canine	2008	USA
29	CPV-JS2	KF676668	CPV-2a	canine	2013	China
30	s5	KF638400	CPV-2a	canine	2014	China

10-fold dilution series of the pEASY-T1-MEV-*NS1* plasmid (ranging from 8.75×10^8 to 8.75×10^0 copies/µL), and using ddH$_2$O was used as the negative control. PCR products were subjected to electrophoresis on a 2% agarose gel.

Specificity of MEV nanoPCR assay

Cross-reaction of the MEV nanoPCR assay with AMDV DNA and CDV cDNA was evaluated using pEASY-T1-MEV-*NS1* as the positive control, and DNA extracted from fecal samples of healthy minks as the negative control. PCR products were subjected to electrophoresis on a 2% agarose gel.

Detection of MEV in clinical samples

The sensitivity of the detection of MEV nanoPCR and conventional PCR assays was compared in clinical fecal samples from 246 minks in five provinces in North-Eastern China during the years 2007–2013. The location sources and the number of samples were as follows: Shandocng (122), Liaoning (31), Jilin (35), Heilongjiang (18), and Hebei (40) provinces. In addition, 10 fecal samples from experimentally infected animals were selected. Four of the positive products from the samples were sequenced.

NS1 gene sequencing and phylogenetic analysis

To determine the specificity of the MEV nanoPCR and the prevalence of MEV in China, the *NS1* genes from four MEVs (MEV Jlin/2010, MEV/LN-10, MEV SD07/09, and MEV SD12/01) detected by nanoPCR in the Jilin, Liaoning and Shandong province clinical samples were amplified, cloned, and sequenced as previously described [13,35]. The sequences of the full length 2,007 bp MEV *NS1* genes were assembled using the SeqMan and EditSeq functions of the DNAStar software package. Entire *NS1* gene sequences were aligned with the sequences of other carnivore parvovirus *NS1* genes collected from different locations worldwide (Table 3) and the consensus tree was edited in MEGA6. Phylogenetic analysis was performed using the Maximum Likelihood method, and setting the *p* distance algorithm of correction. Divergence was calculated by comparing sequence pairs in relation to the phylogeny reconstructed by MegAlign.

Additional file

> **Additional file 1: Gel quantification analysis of all bands by ImageJ.**

Competing interests

The authors declare that they have no competing interests.

Authors' contributions

JK Wang wrote the manuscript and carried out the experiments with the help of M Zhang who carried out primers design, L Yi contributed to the clinical samples collection, SP Cheng carried out sequence analysis, YN Cheng carried out PCR. P Lin, H Zhao and MW Tong revised the manuscript. All the authors have read and approved the final manuscript.

Acknowledgements

The study was supported by Jilin Provincial Special Economic Animal Biological Products Technology Innovation Center, Jilin Provincial Natural Science Foundation (No. 20140101029JC), and Jilin Provincial Key Science and Technology Project Fund (No. 20140204066NY and No. 20150204021NY).

Author details

[1]State Key Laboratory for Molecular Biology of Special Economic Animals, Institute of Special Animal and Plant Sciences, Chinese Academy of Agricultural Sciences, Changchun 130112, China. [2]Jilin Teyan Biological Technology Company, Changchun 130122, China.

References

1. Decaro N, Buonavoglia C. Canine parvovirus–a review of epidemiological and diagnostic aspects, with emphasis on type 2c. Vet Microbiol. 2012;155(1):1–12.
2. Steinel A, Parrish CR, Bloom ME, Truyen U. Parvovirus infections in wild carnivores. J Wildl Dis. 2001;37(3):594–607.
3. Kariatsumari T, Horiuchi M, Hama E, Yaguchi K, Ishigurio N, Goto H, et al. Construction and nucleotide sequence analysis of an infectious DNA clone of the autonomous parvovirus, mink enteritis virus. J Gen Virol. 1991;72(Pt 4):867–75.
4. Wang J, Cheng S, Yi L, Cheng Y, Yang S, Xu H, et al. Detection of mink enteritis virus by loop-mediated isothermal amplification (LAMP). J Virol Methods. 2013;187(2):401–5.
5. Schofield FW. Virus enteritis in mink. N Am Vet. 1949;30:651–4.
6. Wills CG. Notes on infectious enteritis of mink and its relationship to feline enteritis. Can J Comp Med Vet Sci. 1952;16(12):419–20.
7. Jiang TX, Pu HK, Wang L, Wang Y. Preliminary report about mink viral enteritis disease. Fur animals. 1981;2:4–6.
8. Hundt B, Best C, Schlawin N, Kassner H, Genzel Y, Reichl U. Establishment of a mink enteritis vaccine production process in stirred-tank reactor and Wave Bioreactor microcarrier culture in 1–10 L scale. Vaccine. 2007;25(20):3987–95.
9. Shen DT, Ward AC, Gorham JR. Detection of mink enteritis virus in mink feces, using enzyme-linked immunosorbent assay, hemagglutination, and electron microscopy. Am J Vet Res. 1986;47(9):2025–30.
10. Veijalainen PM, Neuvonen E, Niskanen A, Juokslahti T. Latex agglutination test for detecting feline panleukopenia virus, canine parvovirus, and parvoviruses of fur animals. J Clin Microbiol. 1986;23(3):556–9.
11. Uttenthal A, Larsen S, Lund E, Bloom ME, Storgard T, Alexandersen S. Analysis of experimental mink enteritis virus infection in mink: in situ hybridization, serology, and histopathology. J Virol. 1990;64(6):2768–79.
12. Wang JK, Cheng SP, Yi L, Yang S, Luo B, Xu HL, et al. Establishment of double antibody sandwich ELISA for detection of mink enteritis virus. Chin Vet Sci. 2011;41(2):183–7.
13. Wang JK, Cheng SP, Yang S, Yi L, Xu HL, Cheng YN, et al. Establishment of PCR-RFLP for differentiation of mink enteritis virus vaccine strain and wild strain. Chin Vet Sci. 2012;42(3):264–7.
14. Zhang HL, Yan XJ, Chai XL, Wu W, Yi L, Luo GL, et al. Establishment and application of PCR for detection of mink enteritis virus. Special Wild Econ Animal Plant Res. 2007;29(2):1–3.
15. Rivera E, Sundquist B. A non-haemagglutinating isolate of mink enteritis virus. Vet Microbiol. 1984;9(4):345–53.
16. Chen T, Zhao JJ, Zhang HL, Chai XL, Yan XJ, Wu W, et al. Prokaryotic expression of mink enteritis virus VP2 gene and establishment of indirect ELISA. Chin J Prev Vet Med. 2009;31(9):712–6.
17. Cui Y, Wang Z, Ma X, Liu J, Cui S. A sensitive and specific nanoparticle-assisted PCR assay for rapid detection of porcine parvovirus. Lett Appl Microbiol. 2014;58(2):163–7.
18. Elia G, Cavalli A, Desario C, Lorusso E, Lucente MS, Decaro N, et al. Detection of infectious canine parvovirus type 2 by mRNA real-time RT-PCR. J Virol Methods. 2007;146(1–2):202–8.

19. Kumar M, Nandi S. Development of a SYBR Green based real-time PCR assay for detection and quantitation of canine parvovirus in faecal samples. J Virol Methods. 2010;169(1):198–201.

20. Mech LD, Almberg ES, Smith D, Goyal S, Singer RS. Use of real-time PCR to detect canine parvovirus in feces of free-ranging wolves. J Wildl Dis. 2012;48(2):473–6.

21. Chen HY, Li XK, Cui BA, Wei ZY, Li XS, Wang YB, et al. A TaqMan-based real-time polymerase chain reaction for the detection of porcine parvovirus. J Virol Methods. 2009;156(1–2):84–8.

22. Perez LJ, Perera CL, Frias MT, Nunez JI, Ganges L, de Arce HD. A multiple SYBR Green I-based real-time PCR system for the simultaneous detection of porcine circovirus type 2, porcine parvovirus, pseudorabies virus and Torque teno sus virus 1 and 2 in pigs. J Virol Methods. 2012;179(1):233–41.

23. Song C, Zhu C, Zhang C, Cui S. Detection of porcine parvovirus using a taqman-based real-time pcr with primers and probe designed for the NS1 gene. Virol J. 2010;7:353.

24. Koppelman MH, van Swieten P, Cuijpers HT. Real-time polymerase chain reaction detection of parvovirus B19 DNA in blood donations using a commercial and an in-house assay. Transfusion. 2011;51(6):1346–54.

25. Zaki SA. Detection of human parvovirus B19 in cancer patients using ELISA and real-time PCR. Indian J Med Microbiol. 2012;30(4):407–10.

26. Vaisanen E, Lahtinen A, Eis-Hubinger AM, Lappalainen M, Hedman K, Soderlund-Venermo M. A two-step real-time PCR assay for quantitation and genotyping of human parvovirus 4. J Virol Methods. 2014;195:106–11.

27. Shen C, Zhang Z. An Overview of Nanoparticle-Assisted Polymerase Chain Reaction Technology. In: Bagchi D, Bagchi M, Moriyama H, Shahidi F, editors. Bio-Nanotechnology: A Revolution in Food, Biomedical and Health Sciences. Oxford: Blackwell Publishing Ltd; 2013. p. 97–106.

28. Ma XJ, Cui YC, Qiu Z, Zhang BK, Cui SJ. A nanoparticle-assisted PCR assay to improve the sensitivity for rapid detection and differentiation of wild-type pseudorabies virus and gene-deleted vaccine strains. J Virol Methods. 2013;193(2):374–8.

29. Xu SY, Yao MS. NanoPCR detection of bacterial aerosols. J Aerosol Sci. 2013;65:1–9.

30. Wang X, Bai A, Zhang J, Kong M, Cui Y, Ma X, et al. A new nanoPCR molecular assay for detection of porcine bocavirus. J Virol Methods. 2014;202:106–11.

31. Wang J, Cheng S, Yi L, Cheng Y, Yang S, Xu H, et al. Evidence for natural recombination between mink enteritis virus and canine parvovirus. Virol J. 2012;9(1):252.

32. Sun JZ, Wang J, Yuan D, Wang S, Li Z, Yi B, et al. Cellular microRNA miR-181b Inhibits Replication of Mink Enteritis Virus by Repression of Non-Structural Protein 1 Translation. PLoS One. 2013;8(12):e81515.

33. Zhang QM, Wang YP, Ji Q, Gu JM, Liu SS, Feng X, et al. Selection of antiviral peptides against mink enteritis virus using a phage display peptide library. Curr Microbiol. 2013;66(4):379–84.

34. Liu WQ, Fan QS, Jiang Y, Xia XZ, Huang G, Wang JG, et al. Establishment of a commonly used PCR technique for detection of carnivore parvoviruses. Chin J Vet Sci. 2001;21(3):249–51.

35. Yi L, Cheng S, Xu H, Wang J, Cheng Y, Yang S, et al. Development of a combined canine distemper virus specific RT-PCR protocol for the differentiation of infected and vaccinated animals (DIVA) and genetic characterization of the hemagglutinin gene of seven Chinese strains demonstrated in dogs. J Virol Methods. 2012;179(1):281–7.

6

Epidemiology of *Theileria bicornis* among black and white rhinoceros metapopulation in Kenya

Moses Y Otiende[1*], Mary W Kivata[4], Joseph N Makumi[4], Mathew N Mutinda[1], Daniel Okun[4], Linus Kariuki[1], Vincent Obanda[1], Francis Gakuya[1], Dominic Mijele[1], Ramón C Soriguer[2] and Samer Alasaad[2,3*]

Abstract

Background: A huge effort in rhinoceros conservation has focused on poaching and habitat loss as factors leading to the dramatic declines in the endangered eastern black rhinoceros (*Diceros bicornis michaeli*) and the southern white rhinoceros (*Ceratotherium simum simum*). Nevertheless, the role disease and parasite infections play in the mortality of protected populations has largely received limited attention. Infections with piroplasmosis caused by *Babesia bicornis* and *Theileria bicornis* has been shown to be fatal especially in small and isolated populations in Tanzania and South Africa. However, the occurrence and epidemiology of these parasites in Kenyan rhinoceros is not known.

Results: Utilizing 18S rRNA gene as genetic marker to detect rhinoceros infection with *Babesia* and *Theileria*, we examined blood samples collected from seven rhinoceros populations consisting of 114 individuals of black and white rhinoceros. The goal was to determine the prevalence in Kenyan populations, and to assess the association of *Babesia* and *Theileria* infection with host species, age, sex, location, season and population mix (only black rhinoceros comparing to black and white rhinoceros populations). We did not detect any infection with *Babesia* in the sequenced samples, while the prevalence of *T. bicornis* in the Kenyan rhinoceros population was 49.12% (56/114). White rhinoceros had significantly higher prevalence of infection (66%) compared to black rhinoceros (43%). The infection of rhinoceros with *Theileria* was not associated with animal age, sex or location. The risk of infection with *Theileria* was not higher in mixed species populations compared to populations of pure black rhinoceros.

Conclusion: In the rhinoceros studied, we did not detect the presence of *Babesia bicornis*, while *Theileria bicornis* was found to have a 49.12% prevalence with white rhinoceros showing a higher prevalence (66%) comparing with black rhinoceros (43%). Other factors such as age, sex, location, and population mix were not found to play a significant role.

Keywords: Ixodid, Ticks, Piroplasms, Diceros bicornis michaeli, Ceratotherium simum simum

Background

The populations and distribution ranges of the black rhinoceros (*Diceros bicornis*) and the white rhinoceros (*Ceratotherium simum*) have declined in the whole of Africa. The rate of their population decline is faster than any other large terrestrial mammal in recent times [1], a fact that supports their endangered status and calls for robust international efforts towards their recovery. These rhinoceros have been exterminated in the

majority of African countries, while their range among the remaining principal countries; Kenya, Tanzania, Namibia, Zimbabwe and South Africa [1] is greatly reduced and currently restricted in artificially created sanctuaries. Habitat loss and vicious poaching are the leading twin drivers of population decline of the rhinoceros [2]. However infectious diseases are also an incipient threat to endangered species [3] having been classified among the top five causes of species extinctions [4].

Piroplasms, which are blood-borne protozoan parasites in the genera *Babesia* and *Theileria* (Order Piroplasmidae), are globally distributed and transmitted by a diverse species of Ixodid ticks. These parasites infect a wide range of domesticated and wild mammals as well as humans. Infections may lead to severe disease and death or it may

* Correspondence: motiende@kws.go.ke; sameralasaad@hotmail.com
[1]Veterinary Services Department, Forensic and Genetics Laboratory Kenya Wildlife Service, P.O Box 40241–00100, Nairobi, Kenya
[2]Estación Biológica de Doñana, Consejo Superior de Investigaciones Científicas (CSIC), Avda. Américo Vespucio s/n 41092, Sevilla, Spain
Full list of author information is available at the end of the article

remain latent depending on virulence of the species and host immune status. Piroplasms have historically been known to infect rhinoceros with some infections associated with fatalities [5-7]. However the causal species were unknown until 10 years ago when *Babesia bicornis* and *Theileria bicornis* were independently associated with stress-induced mortality [8]. The first genetic work on piroplasms by Otiende et al., [9] has shown the existence of infection by piroplasm and the occurrence of three new haplotypes of *Theileria bicornis* circulating in both black and white rhinoceros in Kenya. The factors influencing piroplasms prevalence among Kenyan populations were previously unknown. Piroplasms have coevolved with rhinoceros and they coexist with the host without signs of clinical disease. However, stress induced by translocation has been linked to immune suppression and is a major cause of post translocation morbidity and/or fatality. Translocation is at the core of *in situ* management of rhinoceros metapopulation and yet it is incriminated as a disease inducer besides its inherent role in the spread of pathogens. The link between translocation and piroplasmosis is intricate because it is based on the modulatory effects of stress hormones on the immune system. Translocation elicits stress hormones, which allow uninhibited proliferation of piroplasms in the host resulting in disease and death. However, effects of stress hormones are not predictable or homogenous in the population as underlying individuals' conditions, such as injury, pregnancy, co-infection, vary and may elicit different immune response [10].

The goal of this study is to determine the epidemiology of *Theileria biconis* in Kenya. Specifically, we intended to (a) determine their prevalence in both species of rhinoceros and among sub-populations then (b) test the association of infection prevalence with host species, age, sex, location, season and population mix (black rhinoceros vs black and white rhinoceros populations). Information generated will be useful in guiding management and veterinary options such as translocation, differential diagnosis and chemotherapy.

Methods

Study area

Lake Nakuru National Park (*LNNP*) central coordinates are 0°22′S 36°05′E and is 4 km from Nakuru town center. The park covers an area of 188 km^2 completely fenced, of which 44 km^2 lies in the shallow alkaline soda lake, thereby leaving 144 km^2 for wildlife use. The area around the lake is flat bare lowland of 1200 m altitude surrounded by hills and gentle cliffs that rise to 1750 m above sea level. The park receives mean annual rainfall of 850 mm with rainfall in the months of April to May and again in October – November. The park consists of open grassland with elevated areas occupied by dry forests

of *Acacia xanthophloea*, *Olea capensis* sub sp. *Macrocarpa* and *Croton dichogamus*. Marshland along the river inflows and springs are covered by *Cyperus laevigatus and Typha spp*. Other striking plant species include the invasive *Tarchonanthus* spp. bush land, the deciduous (*Teclea & Olive*) forest and the *Euphorbia candelabrum* forest. The park has 33 white and 69 black rhinoceros that freely interact with other diverse species.

Nairobi National Park (*NNP*) central coordinates are 1°16′S, 36°49′E and is about 10 km from the city of Nairobi and covers an area of 117 km^2. A large section of the park is fenced with only 20 km left open for wildlife dispersal. Average annual rainfall is 800 mm with rainy season between April-May and October-November. The vegetation consists of mosaic grassland, thickets and Acacia and deciduous forests as well as woodlands especially along River Mbagathi that crosses it. The park has 77 black and 13 white rhinoceros besides many other wildlife species.

Ngulia rhino Sanctuary (*NgRS*) is within Tsavo West National Park occupying a fenced area of 90 km^2 at 3^0 01′S to 3^0 06′S and 38^0 06E to 38^0 10′E. Altitude ranges from 600 m of lowlands to 1800 m of craggy hills with average annual rainfall of 600 mm. Dry period is between December to March, while rains occur in the months of April to June and again in October and November. The vegetation is thickly wooded by *Commiphora-Acacia* woodland, dotted with baobab trees. This sanctuary contains 77 black rhinoceros without white rhinoceros, though other small-medium sized wildlife occurs in small density.

Meru Rhino Sanctuary (*MRS*) is 48Km^2 (central coordinates, N 00^0 15.125, E 038^{0}06.481) located within the Meru National Park has 44 black and 45 white rhinoceros. Altitude ranges from 1000 to 3400 m above the sea level. Average rainfall is 635-762 mm with the wet season occurring in late March to April, while the dry season begins from October. Major rivers such as Makutano, Kanjoo, Kathithi, Rujuwero and Kindani traverse MRS, which contributes to mosaic vegetation types that include thickets, bushland and grassland as well as a thick forest on its southern edge.

Solio and Mugie Rhino Sanctuaries are in the Laikipia-Samburu ecosystem, which is characterized by savannah-type grassland dominated by *Euclea divinorum*, *Acacia spp and Euphorbia* woodland while annual rainfall averages 300 to 700 mm. Rainfall level varies annually with intermittent patterns that peaks in April-May, July–August and October–November. The rest of the months are dry. Solio Sanctuary, 0°16′S 37°00′E / 0.27°S 37°E/ -0.27; 37, is 68.9 km^2 and has altitude of 1932 m, located at the base of the Aberdare ranges. The sanctuary holds 50 black and 110 white rhinoceros. Mugie rhino sanctuary (ceased to be a rhino sanctuary at the time of this study, as the entire population was translocated) was 90 km^2 with an altitude 1990 m.

Sampling design

This study was carried out between 2011 and 2012 in various sub populations of black and white rhinoceros in Kenya. Sampling was cross-sectional whereby samples were collected from apparently healthy rhinos immobilized for translocation or tagging. The biodata of each rhinoceros was obtained from the KWS rhinoceros database. Rhinoceros < 2 years of age were not immobilized for translocation. Juvenile rhinoceros are <3.5 years, sub-adults are (3.6 – 7 years) and adults are >7 years. Rhinoceros were immobilized using a combination of etorphine hydrochloride (M99®), Hyaluronidase (Kyron Laboratories, Benrose 2011, South Africa) and xylazine (Norvatis, [PTY] Ltd, South Africa). Venous blood was drawn from the front limb of the rhinoceros and then collected in EDTA tubes. Blood in EDTA tubes were gently mixed by turning the tubes up and down and then transferring aliquots in labeled cryovials followed by quick freezing in liquid nitrogen. The samples were transported in liquid nitrogen to Forensic and Genetics Laboratory of Kenya Wildlife Service in Nairobi for analysis.

DNA isolation and PCR amplification

Genomic DNA was extracted from blood using a genomic DNA extraction kit (DNeasy blood and Tissue Kit, QIAGEN, Southern Cross Biotechnologies, South Africa) following the manufacturers' protocol. A nested PCR amplification specific for the 18S rRNA gene of *Babesia* and *Theileria* was performed. A primary amplification was carried out in 50 µl reaction containing 3 µl of the genomic DNA, 45 µl of Platinum blue supermix, 1 µl (10 mM) each forward and reverse primers. The forward primer was ILO-9029, (5'-CGGTAATTCCAGCTCCAA TAGCGT-3') and reverse, ILO-9030 (5'-TTTCTCTC AAAGGTGCTGAAGGAGT-3') primer [11]. The amplification (Thermocycler, Veriti, ABI) was preceded by a 30 sec polymerase activation step at 95°C followed by 30 cycles of 1 min each at 94°C, annealing at 53°C for 30 sec, extension for 1 min at 72°C. Amplification was terminated by a final extension step 72°C for 9 min. The secondary amplification was in a 50 µl reaction containing 2 µl of the primary amplification product, 45 µl of Platinum blue supermix, 1.5 µl (10 mM) each of forward and reverse primers. The forward primer was MWG4/70, (5'-AGCTCGTAGTTGAATTTCTGCTGC-3') and the reverse was ILO-7782 (5'-AACTGACGACCTCCAAT CTCTAGTC-3') [11]. The secondary PCR (Thermocycler, Veriti, ABI) was initiated with an initial denaturation at 95°C for 30 sec, followed by 30 cycles of 1 min each at 94°C, annealing at 55°C for 30 s and extension at 72°C

for 1 min. The PCR was completed with a final extension step of 72°C for 9 min. PCR products showing successful amplification on agarose gel analysis were directly sequenced for both strands. PCR products were purified for direct sequencing by enzymatic treatment using exonuclease I and shrimp alkaline phosphatase (PCR Product Presequencing Kit, Amersham). All DNA sequencing was carried out by direct cycle sequencing on both strands of purified PCR DNA products from PCR amplification. Sequencing reactions were carried out with the ABI PRISM DigDye Terminator v3.1 cycle sequencing kit and analyzed on an ABI310 DNA sequencer (Applied Biosystems, CA).

Statistical analysis

Statistical analyses were performed using Fisher Exact test for count data and Chi Square test to determine the relationship between infection of rhinoceros with *Theileria* and the following variables: rhinoceros age, location, sex, and rhinoceros species. To confirm our results, we also used a Generalized Linear Model with a binomial error, and a complementary log-log link function. All possible interactions were included in the first model. As rhinoceros species are essentially clustered with locality (game park or sanctuary) a generalized linear mixed effect model was also applied, considering locality (game park or sanctuary) as random effect: *Theileria* Infection ~ Rhinos Species + (1 | Locality). Statistical significance was assessed at $p < 0.05$.

Ethic

The Committee of the Department of Veterinary and Capture Services of the Kenya Wildlife Service (KWS) approved the study including animal capture, translocation and sample collection. KWS guidelines on Wildlife Veterinary Practice-2006 were followed. All KWS veterinarians were guided by the Veterinary Surgeons Act Cap 366 Laws of Kenya that regulates veterinary practice in Kenya.

Results

A total of 114 blood samples of black ($n = 82$) and white rhinoceros ($n = 32$) were sampled from seven rhinoceros populations and molecularly examined for infection with *Babesia* and *Theileria*. We did not detect any infection with *Babesia* in the obtained sequences, while the overall *Theileria* prevalence was 49.1% (56/114). All *Theileria* sequences belonged to the three haplotypes already described by Otiende et al., [9]. The prevalence of *Theileria* infection was higher in white rhinoceros (66%) than in black rhinoceros (43%) (Table 1). We confirmed this result using a generalized linear model (b = −0.652, $p = 0.023$). The simplified glm model was *Theileria* Infection ~ Rhinos Species, family = binomial (cloglog):

Table 1 Proportion of rhinoceros infected as a function of age, location, sex and species evaluated using Fisher's exact test

Variable	Variable categories	% Negative	% Positive	N	p-value
AGE	Juvenile	58.8	41.2	17	0.764
	Sub-Adult	48.2	51.8	56	
	Adult	51.2	48.8	41	
LOCATION	LNNP	46.7	53.3	35	0.559
	Meru N. P.	50.0	50.0	12	
	Mugie	57.9	42.1	20	
	Ngulia	55.2	44.8	29	
	NNP	55.6	44.4	10	
	Solio	87.5	12.5	8	
SEX	Female	41.7	58.3	59	0.7026
	Male	30.0	70.0	55	
SPECIES	*C. simum*	34.4	65.6	32	**0.037**
	D. bicornis	57.3	42.7	82	

Theileria Infection ~ 0.0656 ± 0.2287 Rhinos Species - 0.6516 ± 0.2857. Since prevalence was higher in white rhinoceros, we tested whether presence of white rhinoceros together with black rhinoceros in the same locality was a risk factor for infection with *Theileria* in black rhinoceros. We found no significant association between infection of black rhinoceros with *Theileria* and the presence or absence of white rhinoceros in the same locality ($\chi^2 = 0321$; $p = 0.571$). The results were confirmed by applying a generalized lineal mixed effect model, considering locality (game park or sanctuary) as random effect. The last model in this case was *Theileria* Infection ~ Rhinos Species, family = binomial (logit): *Theileria* Infection ~ 0.0647 ± 0.3722 - 0.9414 ± 0.434 (Rhinos Species). Prevalence seemed to increase with age, but the infection by age-groups (juveniles, sub-adults and adults) was not statistically significant (Fisher test, $p = 0.764$, Table 1). Females of both species had higher prevalence 54% (29/54) than males 45% (27/60), this difference however was not statistically significant (Fisher test, $p = 0.702$, Table 1). Inter-population variations in prevalence (Figure 1) were not statistically different (Fisher test, $p = 0.681$, Table 1).

Discussion

The six sampled rhinoceros sub-populations in Kenya were infected with piroplasms but we molecularly detected only *Theileria* and not *Babesia* in all studied samples from black and white rhinoceros species.

Ticks and wildlife are the maintenance hosts of piroplasms but efficient transmission fundamentally requires presence of the protozoan, a competent tick species and the host.

Even with *B. bicornis* and *T. bicornis* originally identified from black rhinoceros [8] *T. bicornis* has now been detected in white rhinoceros, Nyala (*Tragelaphus angasii*) and Cattle [12-14]. This means that *T. bicornis* is a multi-host pathogen with possibility of having diverse tick species as vectors. Since *D. rhinocerinus* have been found in other animals such as cattle, sheep, donkey, elephant (*Loxodonta africana*), buffalo (*Syncerus caffer*) and eland (*Taurotragus oryx*) [15,16] this tick could be important in the cross-transmission of rhinocerotid piroplams. Pathogenicity of *T. bicornis* remains unresolved but *T. equi*, which is its close relative [8,17] and recently seen in white rhinoceros [13], has been reported to cause clinical piroplasmosis in translocated equids [18].

Translocation is intimately associated with flare up of latent infections that result in clinical state [18-20]. This is because translocation leads to elevation of glucocorticoids, whose effects are viewed to be obligatorily immunodepressant [10], yet in most cases, especially in transient acute stress, they prepare an animal to survive [10,21,22]. In the present study, sampling was carried out on asymptomatic individuals and despite underlying infection with *T. bicornis*, some of them were subjected to a longer period of stressor condition; during >1000 km road transportation to a new sanctuary in Ruma National Park. Nevertheless, for six months post-release monitoring of this population, they remained asymptomatic. This outcome may support the notion that *T. bicornis* is apathogenic or it may suggest that translocation-stress did not suppress immunity to induce clinical state. Theories behind disease induction by translocation-stress often focus on single parasite infections. However, in nature, wild animals are infected and infested simultaneously with a

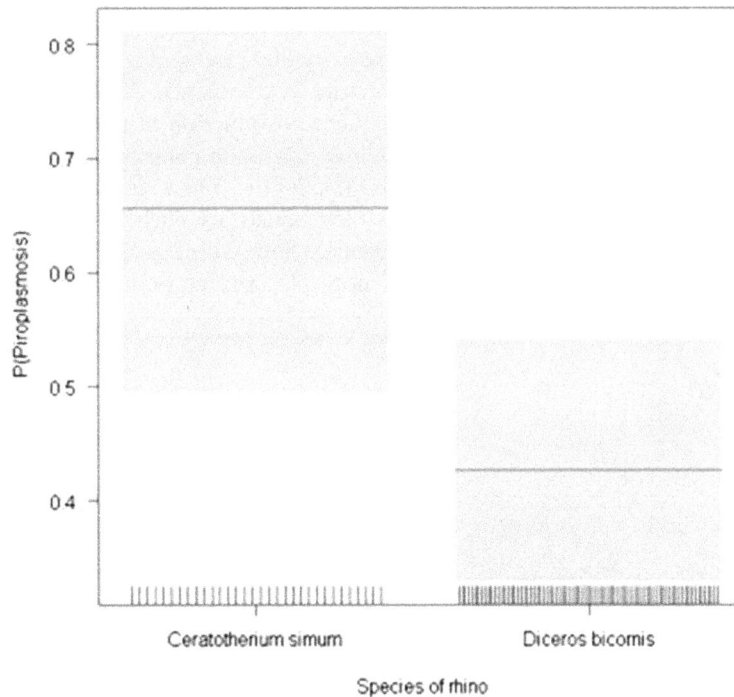

Figure 1 Variation of infection intensity of rhinoceros by species.

plethora of parasites that elicits complex immune response that may promote one parasite over the other. For instance, in concomitant infection involving African trypanosome superimposed with piroplasm leads to inhibition of the piroplasm in spite of the trypanosome immunodepressant effect [23]. In reference to fatal piroplasmosis [8], the deceased rhinoceros were subject to diverse and combined stressors; two black rhinoceros in Tanzania did not undergo prior capture and translocation event; the third fatal case involved high parasitemia, severe cold and injury while the fourth case was pregnant and developed translocation myopathy. This suggests that stressor factors that trigger clinical disease are many with maximum effect attained under synergistic state.

In the present study, the prevalence of *T. bicornis* was relatively high (49.1%) but clinical disease was absent in the metapopulation, a state that could mimics endemic stability [24]. This state, which was initially coined for bovine babesiosis and now widely applied in many diseases and hosts, is based on the premise that (1) severity of clinical disease increases with age and (2) that after one infection, the probability that subsequent infections result in disease is reduced [25].

We noted that higher prevalence of *T. bicornis* (odds ratio, 2.502) being detected in white rhinoceros than in black species (Table 1) indicating a species effect. However, we did not find significant effect associating species with prevalence, suggesting that white rhinoceros, even though more susceptible, is not a risk factor to black rhinoceros prevalence. Our result show that the Kenyan white rhino has higher prevalence of *T. bicornis* (66%) compared to 32.1% - 46.6% in the South African populations [13,26]. The high prevalence of *T. bicornis* in white rhinoceros suggests they are important hosts in the epidemiology of this piroplasm. On the contrary, according to a theory postulated by Schmidt & Ostfeld, [27] we suggest that white rhinoceros could benefit black rhinoceros by acting as 'sinks' for rhinocerotid piroplasms.

Further, our results show that prevalence among the age-groups of rhinoceros did not differ significantly (Table 1) contrary to the infection pattern in white rhinoceros population in South Africa in which female sub-adults had significantly higher prevalence [13]. Nevertheless, the age-associated inclination in our result is comparable with that of Govender *et al.*, [13] in that peak infections were observed among sub-adults (Table 1). It is postulated that sub-adult rhinoceros of both sexes are subject to numerous stress-related changes such as, reproductive maturity, courtship, mating and territorial fights [13,28] that may suppress immunity and enhance susceptibility [29,30].

Sex-biased prevalence is observed in many parasitic infections with males having higher prevalence and intensity of infections than their conspecific females [31]. In our results, there was no significant sex-biased difference in prevalence (Table 1) though females (56%) seemed to have higher prevalence than males (45%) an observation that concurs with that of Govender et al., [13]. Factors predisposing females to piroplasm are likely to be comparable with those affecting sub-adult rhinoceros.

The occurrence of *T. bicornis* in all the sampled rhinoceros sub-populations could have been facilitated by the regular translocations of individuals. Translocation assists spread of both tick vector and haemoparasites among habitat patches/populations. We observed apparent variations in prevalence among the sub-populations (Figure 2) but there was no significant difference (Table 1). This

means that local factors in these habitats, such as ecological and weather differences, mammalian diversity, sanctuary size, were not sufficient to cause significant disparity in prevalence. According to Lopez et al., [32], frequent introduction of parasites in to a patch/habitat via host migration contributes to local patch prevalence. This implies that rhino sanctuaries' that frequently receive new individuals are likely to harbor higher parasite prevalence. Okita-Ouma et al., [33] points out that LNNP is more of a source population that has supported 41

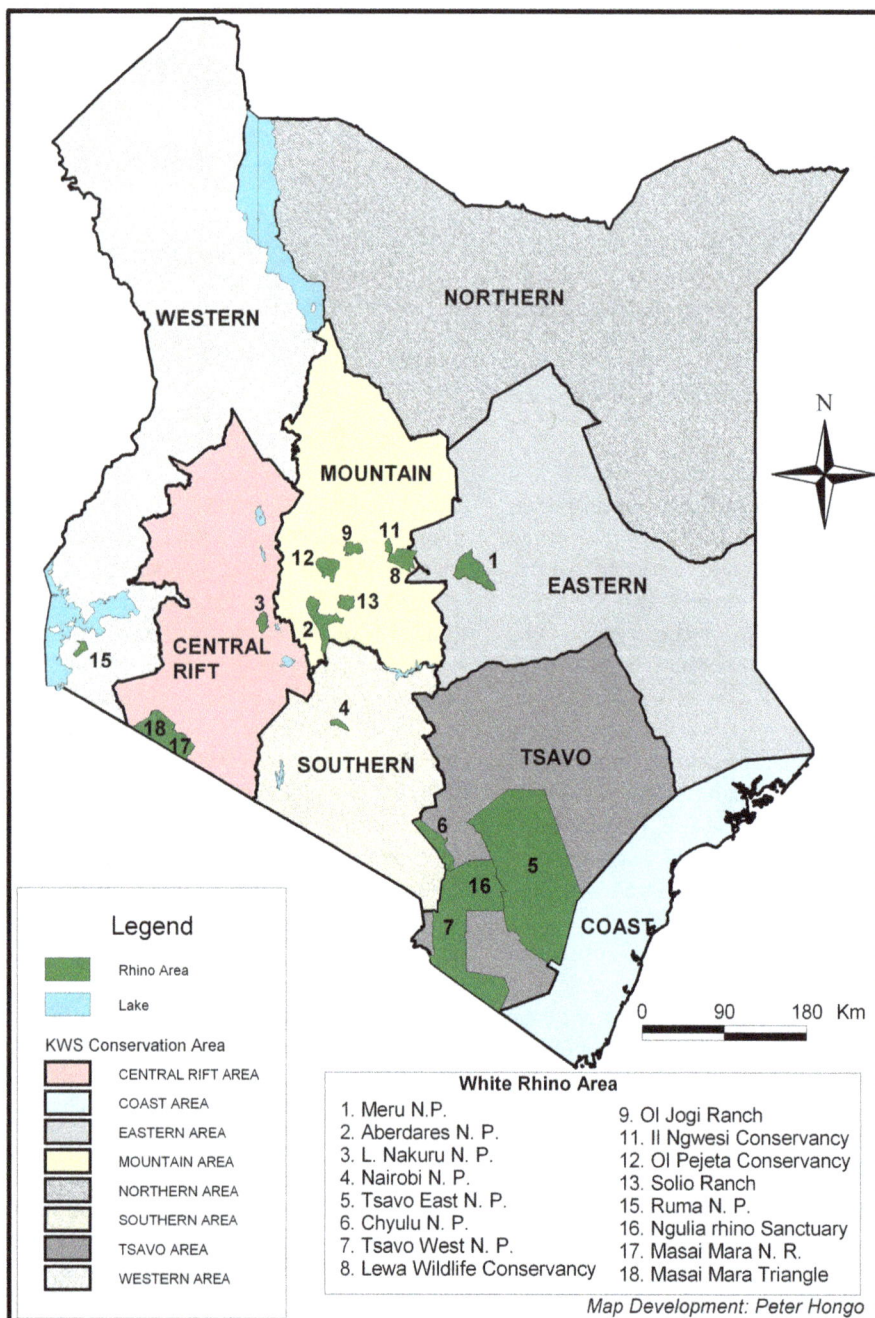

Figure 2 Locations of black rhinoceros conservation areas in Kenya.

outward translocations and received one inward translocation, whereas Ngulia RS is a recipient population having received 16 inward translocations and only one outward translocation. However, lack of significant association between location and prevalence (Table 1) does not concur with the postulation of Lopez et al., [32].

Conclusion

In the analyzed samples we did not detect the presence of *Babesia bicornis*, while *Theileria bicornis* was found to have 49.12% prevalence with white rhinoceros showing a higher prevalence than black rhinoceros. Other factors such as age, sex, location, and population mix were not found to play a significant role.

Competing interests

The authors declare no conflict of interest in this work.

Authors' contributions

Conceived and designed the experiments: MYO SA VO. Performed the experiments: MWK MNM JNM. Analyzed the data DO LK FG DM RCS. Contributed reagents/materials/analysis tools: RCS SA. Wrote the paper: MYO SA. All authors read and approved the final manuscript.

Author details

[1]Veterinary Services Department, Forensic and Genetics Laboratory Kenya Wildlife Service, P.O Box 40241–00100, Nairobi, Kenya. [2]Estación Biológica de Doñana, Consejo Superior de Investigaciones Científicas (CSIC), Avda. Américo Vespucio s/n 41092, Sevilla, Spain. [3]Institute of Evolutionary Biology and Environmental Studies (IEU), University of Zürich, Winterthurerstrasse 190, 8057 Zürich, Switzerland. [4]Department of Biochemistry and Biotechnology, Kenyatta University, P.O Box 43844–00100, Nairobi, Kenya.

References

1. Kelly JD, Blyde DJ, Denney IS. The importation of the black rhinoceros (*Diceros bicornis*) from Zimbabwe into Australia. Aus Vet J. 1995;72:369–74.
2. Altizer S, Harvell D, Friedle E. Rapid evolutionary dynamics and disease threats to biodiversity. Trends Ecol Evol. 2003;589:596.
3. Daszak P, Cunningham AA, Hyatt AD. Emerging Threats to Infectious Diseases Wildlife- Health Biodiversity and infectious. Adv Sci. 2000;287:443–9.
4. Wilcove DS, Rothstein D, Dubow J, Phillips A, Losos E. Quantifying Threats to Imperiled Species in the United States. Bioscience. 1998;48:607–15.
5. MucCullogh B, Achard PL. Mortalities associated with capture, translocation, trade and exhibition of black rhinoceroses. Int Zoo. 1960;9:184–95.
6. Brocklesby DW. A *Babesia* species of the black rhinoceros. Vet Rec. 1967;80:484.
7. Mugera GM, Wandera JG. Degenerative polymyopathies in East African domestic and wild animals. Vet Rec. 1967;80:410–3.
8. Nijhof AM, Penzhorn BL, Lynen G, Mollel JO, Morkel P, Bekker CPJ, et al. *Babesia bicornis* sp. nov. and *Theileria bicornis* sp. nov.: tick-borne parasites associated with mortality in the black rhinoceros (*Diceros bicornis*). J Clin Microbiol. 2003;41:2249–54.
9. Otiende MY, Kivata MW, Jowers MJ, Makumi JN, Runo S, Obanda V, et al. Three Novel Haplotypes of *Theileria bicornis* in Black and White Rhinoceros in Kenya. Transbound Emerg Dis. 2014; [Epub ahead of print].
10. Martin LB. Stress and immunity in wild vertebrates: Timing is everything. Gen Com Endocr. 2009;163:70–6.
11. Maamun JM, Suleman MA, Akinyi M, Ozwara H, Kariuki T, Carlsson H-E. Prevalence of Babesia microti in free-ranging baboons and African green monkeys. J Parasitol. 2011;97:63–7.
12. Muhanguzi D, Matovu E, Waiswa C. Prevalence and characterization of *Theileria* and *Babesia* species in cattle under different husbandry systems in western Uganda. Int J Anim Veter Adv. 2010;2:51–8.
13. Govender D, Oosthuisen MC, Penzhorn BL. Piroplasm parasites of white rhinoceroses (*Ceratotherium simum*) in the Kruger National Park, and their relation to anaemia. J S Afr Vet Assoc. 2011;82:36–40.
14. Pfitzer S, Oosthuizen MC, Bosman AM, Vorster I, Penzhorn BL. Tick-borne blood parasites in nyala (*Tragelaphus angasii*, Gray 1849) from KwaZulu-Natal, South Africa. Vet Parasitol. 2011;176:126–31.
15. Arthur DR. Ticks. A Monograph of the Ixodoidea. Part V. The Genera Dermacentor, Anocentor, Cosmiomma, Boophilus and Margaropus. London: Cambridge University Press; 1960.
16. Keirans JE. *Dermacentor rhinocerinus* (Denny 1843) (Acari: Ixodida: Ixodidae): redescription of the male, female and nymph and first description of the larva. J Vet Res. 1993;60:59–68.
17. Katzer F, McKellar S, Kirvar E, Shiels B. Phylogenetic analysis of *Theileria* and *Babesia equi* in relation to the establishment of parasite populations within novel host species and the development of diagnostic tests. Mol Biochem Parasit. 1998;95:33–44.
18. Dennig HK. The isolation of *Babesia* species from wild animals. P ICP Rome. 1965;24–26:262–3.
19. Nijhof AM, Pillay V, Steyl J, Prozesky L, Stoltsz WH, Lawrence A, et al. Molecular Characterization of *Theileria* Species Associated with Mortality in Four Species of African Antelopes Molecular Characterization of *Theileria* Species Associated with Mortality in Four Species of African Antelopes. J Clin Microbiol. 2005;43:5907–11.
20. Obanda V, Kagira JM, Chege S, Okita-Ouma B, Gakuya F. Trypanosomosis and other co-infections in translocated black (*Diceros bicornis michaeli*) and white (*Ceratotherium simum simum*) rhinoceroses in Kenya. Sci Parasitol. 2011;12:103–7.
21. Wingfield JC, Maney DL, Breuner CW, Jacobs JD, Lynn S, Ramenofsky M, et al. Ecological bases of hormone—behavior interactions: the "emergency life history stage.". Am Zool. 1998;38:191–206.
22. Dhabhar FS. Stress-induced augmentation of immune function- The role of stress hormones, leukocyte trafficking, and cytokines. Brain Behav Immun. 2000;16:785–98.
23. Millott SM, Cox FEG. Interactions between *Trypanosoma brucei* and *Babesia* spp. and Plasmodium spp. in mice. Parasitology. 1985;90:241–54.
24. Penzhorn BL, Oosthuizen MC, Bosman A-M, Kilian JW, Horak IG. Black rhinoceros (*Diceros bicornis*) populations in northwestern Namibia are apparently not infected with piroplasms. J Wildl Dis. 2008;44:1032–5.
25. Coleman PG, Perry BD, Woolhouse MEJ. Endemic stability—a veterinary idea applied to human public health. Lancet. 2001;357:1284.
26. Bigalke RD, Keep ME, Keep PJ, Schoeman JH. A large *Babesia* sp. and a *Theileria* like piroplasm of the square-lipped rhinoceros. J S Afr Vet Assoc. 1970;41:292–4.
27. Schmidt K, Ostfeld R. Biodiversity and the dilution effect in disease ecology. Ecology. 2001;82:609–19.
28. Brett R. Mortality factors and breeding performance of translocated black rhinos in Kenya: 1984–1995. Pachyderm. 1998;69:82.
29. Glaser R, Kiecolt-Glaser JK. Stress-induced immune dysfunction: implications for health. Nat Rev Immunol. 2005;5:243–51.
30. Muehlenbein MP. Intestinal parasite infections and fecal steroid levels in wild chimpanzees. Am J Phys Anthropol. 2006;130:546–50.
31. Klein SL. Hormonal and Immunological mechanisms mediating sex differences in parasite infection. Parasit Immunol. 2004;26:247–64.
32. Lopez J, Gallinot LP, Wade MJ. Spread of parasites in metapopulations: An experimental study of the effects of host migration rate and local host population size. Parasitology. 2005;130:323–32.
33. Okita-Ouma B, Amin R, Van Langevelde F, Leader-Williams N. Density dependence and population dynamics of black rhinos (*Diceros bicornis michaeli*) in Kenya's rhino sanctuaries. Afr J Ecol. 2010;48:791–9.

7

Transmission of border disease virus from a persistently infected calf to seronegative heifers in early pregnancy

Ueli Braun[1*], Monika Hilbe[2], Fredi Janett[1], Michael Hässig[1], Reto Zanoni[3,4], Sandra Frei[1] and Matthias Schweizer[3,4]

Abstract

Background: This study describes the transmission of border disease virus (BDV) from a persistently infected calf to seronegative heifers in early pregnancy, resulting in persistently infected fetuses. On day 50 of pregnancy (= day 0 of the infection phase), six heifers were co-housed in a free stall with a bull calf persistently infected with BDV (pi BVD) for 60 days. The heifers underwent daily clinical examination, and blood samples were collected regularly for detection of pestiviral RNA and anti-pestivirus antibodies. After day 60 (= day 110 of pregnancy), the heifers were slaughtered, and the fetuses and placentae underwent post-mortem and immunohistochemical examination and RT-PCR for viral RNA detection.

Results: Three heifers had mild viraemia from day 8 to day 14, and by day 40 all heifers had pestivirus antibodies identified as anti-BDV antibodies in the serum neutralisation test. The placenta of the three viraemic heifers had histological evidence of inflammation, and fetal organs from these heifers were positive for pestivirus antigen by immunohistochemical examination and for BD viral RNA by RT-PCR and sequencing. Thus, co-housing of heifers in early pregnancy with a pi-BDV calf led to seroconversion in all heifers and persistent fetal infection in three.

Conclusions: Considering that pi-BDV cattle can infect other cattle and lead to persistent infection of the fetus in pregnant cows, BDV should not be ignored in the context of the mandatory BVDV eradication and monitoring program. This strongly suggests that BDV should be taken into account in BVD eradication and control programs.

Keywords: Cattle, Border disease, Early pregnancy, Persistent infection, BVDV, Pestivirus

Background

It has long been known that Border disease virus (BDV) is transmissible from sheep to cattle under experimental as well as natural conditions [1-9], but whether BDV transmission is possible from cattle to cattle has not been investigated. There was a recent report of a Galloway bull persistently infected with BDV, and because all heifers co-pastured with this bull were seropositive for BDV, it was suggested that the bull was responsible for BDV infection in this herd [9]. Not only the mode of transmission among cattle but also the clinical picture of bovine BDV infection remains unclear. The infected bull was examined for BDV because of retarded growth and poor fertility [9]. In addition, two heifers with Border disease were described with clinical signs resembling bovine virus diarrhoea virus (BVDV) infection and mucosal disease [3]. The goal of this study was to investigate the transmissibility of BDV from a calf persistently infected with BDV (pi-BDV calf) to seronegative heifers in early pregnancy and whether the fetuses of the heifers become persistently infected. A pi-BDV bull calf was housed with six seronegative heifers in early pregnancy for 60 days, after which time the heifers were slaughtered and the uteri and fetuses examined.

Methods

pi-BDV bull calf

The Braunvieh × Limousine pi-BDV bull calf originated from a BVDV-free herd of 24 cows, which were co-housed with 20 sheep in the same barn. With the exception of this calf, ear punch biopsy samples [10,11] of all cattle in the herd were negative for BVDV in an antigen ELISA

---

* Correspondence: ubraun@vetclinics.uzh.ch
[1]Department of Farm Animals, Vetsuisse-Faculty, University of Zurich, Winterthurerstrasse 260, CH-8057 Zurich, Switzerland
Full list of author information is available at the end of the article

(IDEXX BVDV Ag/Serum Plus Test, IDEXX Switzerland AG, Bern-Liebefeld, Switzerland) as part of the national BVDV eradication program [12]. Immunohistochemical evaluation revealed that the bull calf was positive for the pestivirus-specific antibody C16 but not for the BVDV-specific antibody Ca3/34-C42. RT-PCR evaluation (see below) of a blood sample was positive for pestiviral RNA and the calf was considered persistently viraemic. Radiographic findings of the bones of the extremities of the calf were described separately [13], animal no. 3). RT-PCR testing of blood samples of all other cattle of the herd were negative. Because the cattle were in contact with sheep, virus sequencing was initiated by the official veterinarian to characterise the virus, and BDV (BDSwiss, R8540/ 11_ch149) [14] was identified. The calf was acquired by our clinic when it was 41 days old. It was kept in quarantine until the age of 195 days, at which time it was moved along with the pregnant heifers to an isolation barn, where it remained until the end of the study.

Heifers

Six open heifers of different breeds were acquired at the age of 382 to 748 days (means ± sd = 506 ± 126 days). Ear punch biopsy samples obtained from all the heifers had tested negative for pestivirus. The heifers were tested twice as seronegative by antibody ELISA as described below.

Acclimation phase

The entire study period was divided into an acclimation and an infection phase. During the acclimation phase, the heifers were kept in quarantine without the pi-BDV calf. After estrus synchronisation, they were artificially inseminated using sperm from a BVDV-negative bull. Pregnancy was diagnosed ultrasonographically 30 days after insemination. Four of the heifers returned to estrus but conceived after the second insemination. The acclimation phase lasted until day 50 of pregnancy in each heifer.

Infection phase

The infection phase was 60 days and lasted from day 50 (= day 0 of infection phase) to day 110 of pregnancy. During this phase the heifers were housed together with the pi-BDV calf in a separate free stall barn. Merging of the heifers with the calf was staggered because artificial insemination occurred on different days.

Clinical examination

The heifers underwent thorough clinical examination before and at the end of the acclimation phase. In addition, the demeanour, behaviour, appetite and fecal consistency were monitored daily during acclimation. During the infection phase, the demeanour, appetite,

circulatory, respiratory and digestive systems, mucous membranes and skin were assessed daily and the rectal temperature was recorded twice daily; the daily mean of the latter was calculated for each heifer. Ultrasonographic pregnancy examinations were carried out every ten days and the heifers were observed daily for signs of abortion.

Blood sampling

EDTA blood for pestivirus antigen testing was collected on day 0 and then every other day until day 20 of the infection phase. Whole blood for pestivirus antibody testing was collected on day 0 and then every ten days until day 60 of the infection phase.

Detection of viral RNA, pestivirus antibody and serum neutralisation test

RNA in the blood samples was isolated using a Bio-Robot-Universal-System (Qiagen AG, Hombrechtikon, Switzerland) and the QIAamp Virus BioRobot MDx Kit (Qiagen). RNA was detected according to the instructions of the Cador BVDV RT-PCR Kit (Qiagen) running as proposed for 45 cycles using a thermocycler ABI 7300 (Applied Biosystems, Rotkreuz, Switzerland). The primers and probes of this kit have a very high sensitivity for the detection of BVDV and BDV [15].

Following evaluation of the raw data, the amount of the viral RNA in the sample was expressed in Ct values; values of ≤30 were rated positive and values of >30 weakly positive. Blood samples were stored at 4°C, and weakly positive samples were re-tested after repeated RNA isolation.

An antibody ELISA developed at the Institute for Veterinary Virology, Vetsuisse Faculty, University of Bern [16], was used for pestivirus antibody detection in serum. After collection, the blood samples were stored at 4°C so that all samples from a heifer could be measured on the same day. The optical density (OD) was expressed as percentage of the OD of the standard serum; relative OD readings between 20% and 30% were considered indeterminate and those >30% were considered positive.

The serum neutralisation test (SNT) was used to identify the pestivirus species against which the antibody was directed [17]. The BDV type that was isolated from the bull calf (R8540/ 11_ch149) was used instead of the Moredun type. As cross reactions between BVDV and BDV are common based on their genetic relationship [18], only BDV titres at least four times higher than the BVDV titres were considered significantly higher [17].

Macroscopic, histologic and immunohistochemical examinations

The uterus, placenta and ovaries of the heifers and fetal organs (large and small intestines, brain, skin, heart, liver, lung, spleen, umbilicus, kidneys, thyroid gland, thymus, forestomachs, tongue) were examined macro-scopically and histologically. Tissues were fixed in for-malin, embedded in paraffin, sectioned and stained with H&E and examined using light microscopy.

Samples of the thyroid gland, tongue, aural skin and other fetal organs, and of placentomes were collected for immunohistochemistry. Pieces of thyroid gland, tongue and skin were snap frozen in liquid nitrogen, cryosec-tioned and processed with the antibodies Ca3/34-C42 and C16 [11,19,20]. Samples of placentomes and other organs such as fetal brain were fixed in formalin and embedded in paraffin, and sections were processed with the antibodies C42 and 15c5 [20]. The antibody CA3/34-C42 (dilution 1:100; Labor Dr. Bommeli AG, Bern, Switzerland) and C42 (dilution 1:400; Prof. Moennig, In-stitute for Virology, Hannover, Germany) are specific for BVDV. The mixture of the antibodies Ca3/34-C42 binds to glycoprotein E2, and C42 binds to glycoprotein gp48 (E^{rns}). The pestivirus-specific antibody C16 (dilution 1:100; Labor Dr. Bommeli AG) is directed against the nonstructural protein p125/80 (NS2-3/NS3), and the pestivirus-specific antibody 15C5 (dilution 1:10,000, E. Dubovi, New York State College of Veterinary Medicine, Cornell University, Ithaca, New York, USA) against the highly conserved glycoprotein gp48 (E^{rns}).

Virus detection in fetuses and placentae

Skin, thymus and small intestines from the fetuses and placentae were used for the detection of pestiviral RNA. Skin and thymus were disintegrated and homogenised mechanically using the Tissue Lyser (Qiagen) and small intestine and placenta enzymatically using the QIAamp Cador Pathogen Mini Kit according to manufacturer's instructions. RNA isolation and sequencing of the 5' terminal region (5'-UTR) of the pestiviral genome was done as described [21]. The same RNA was also used to detect the viral genome at the 5'-UTR using RT-PCR (Cador BVDV RT-PCR Kit, Qiagen) and traditional RT-PCR [20].

Statistical analysis

Data were recorded in Office Excel 2007 (Microsoft Inc.). Descriptive statistics were used to describe continuous data (IBM SPSS Statistics 20, IBM Switzerland AG, Zürich) and normality was tested using the Wilk-Shapiro test. Means ± standard deviations were calculated for normally distrib-uted data and medians, minimum and maximum values for data with non-normal distribution. The program STATA 12 (StataCorp., 2011, Stata Statistical Software, Texas, USA) was used to analyse OD values (antibody titres). A t-test, a general linear model and ANOVA were carried out to analyse differences in OD values as a function of day of the infection phase and presence of a pi fetus. The

underlying Stata model for the t-test was < by varx, sort: ttest vary, by (varx2)>, whereby varx = day variable, vary = OD value, varx2 = independent variable, for the general linear model it was < xtmixed vary varx2##varx || varx:> and for the ANOVA it was < vary varx3 c.varx2, repeated (varx) bse (varx4)>, whereby varx3 = heifer and varx4 = time point. A P-value ≤0.05 was considered significant.

Approval of the study by an ethical committee

The study was approved by an ethical committee of the canton of Zurich, Switzerland.

Results

Clinical findings

The pi-BDV calf was clinically healthy and afebrile but grew very little during the study period. Radiographic studies revealed a mild increase in radiopacity of the di-aphyses, which extended to the metaphyses, and mild osteopetrosis [13], animal no. 3. Except for week 4 of the infection phase, the six heifers were clinically healthy during the entire period; four heifers (nos. 1 to 4) had enzootic bronchopneumonia in week 4, which was most likely introduced by heifer 4. Heifers 5 and 6 were not in the infection phase at that time and were not affected. The details of the daily clinical examinations have been reported [22]. The rectal temperature varied from 37.9 to 40.1°C (median =38.5°C) during the infection phase. In three heifers, the rectal temperature exceeded 39.0°C on days 14, 29, 30 (heifer 1), day 22 (heifer 2) and days 6, 7, 10 and 60 (heifer 4). Heifer 4 was moved in with the first three heifers one week before the first increases in rectal temperature were noted; with two exceptions (heifer 1, day 14; heifer 4, day 60) all temperature spikes occurred in the fourth week of the infection phase and were attributed to enzootic bronchopneumonia. There were no cardiovascular system abnormalities, and the re-spiratory rate ranged from 20 to 52 breaths per minute (median =28 bpm). Four heifers had increased bronchial sounds on days 31 and 33 (heifer 1), 22 to 32 (heifer 2), 25 to 30 (heifer 3) and 7 to 17 (heifer 4). The heifers also had wheezes on days 22 to 32 (heifer 2) and day 27 (heifer 3). Abnormal lung sounds were accompanied by coughing, which persisted to day 60 in heifer 4. Abnor-malities of the skin and mucous membranes such as erythema and erosions were not seen. Ruminal motility, intestinal sounds and feces were normal and no abnor-mal vaginal discharge or signs of abortion were noticed. Pregnancy was confirmed and fetal heart beat observed ultrasonographically at each examination.

Virus detection in blood

Three heifers had weakly positive Ct values ranging from 37.8 to 42.5, indicative of pestiviral RNA and thus viraemia on day 10 (heifer 3), day 8 (heifer 4) and days 8 to 14 (heifer 5; Table 1). Re-examination of the weakly positive blood samples yielded positive results for heifers 4 and 5 on days 8 and 10, respectively, and negative results for the remaining samples.

Antibody detection in blood (ELISA)

All heifers were seronegative during the first ten days of the infection phase (Figure 1). In heifers 4, 5 and 6, the relative OD increased gradually between days 11 and 19, and in heifers 1, 2 and 3, it increased after day 20. On day 20, heifers 4 and 5 had an OD of 35% and 30%, respectively, which indicated seroconversion. Heifers 1 and 6 seroconverted by day 30 (OD 39%, 71%) and heifers 2 and 3 by day 40 (OD 61%, 104%). The relative OD increased in all heifers until day 60, at which time maximum relative OD values were measured in heifers 3 (274%), 4 (182%) and 5 (216%, Table 2). Heifers 1, 2 and 6 had values of 119%, 89% and 110%.

Serum neutralisation test

Serum samples collected on day 60 were positive for BDV in all heifers. Titres of specific neutralising BDV antibodies were high and varied from 152 to >512 (Table 2). In two heifers (1 and 2), the SNT was negative for BVDV and the remaining four heifers had very low titres between 8 and 27. The quotient of BDV and BVDV antibody titres was greater than 4 in all heifers and indicated antibody production in response to BDV infection.

Examination of uterus, placenta and fetus

All uteri, placentae and fetuses were macroscopically normal, and fetal organs were also histologically normal. The placentomes of heifers 3, 4 and 5 had multifocal to diffuse plasmacytic and lymphocytic infiltration and pronounced fibrosis, and those of heifers 4 and 5 also had moderate necrotic changes (Table 3). In heifers 3, 4 and 5, fetal organs and placentomes were positive for the pestivirus-specific antibodies C16 and 15C5 (Table 3) and negative for the BVDV-specific antibodies C42, CA3 and CA34. Notably, pestivirus-specific immunohistochemical staining was predominantly located in fetal cells of the placentomes and was scarce in maternal cells (Figure 2). Placentomes of heifers 1, 2 and 6 were negative when tested with pestivirus- and BVDV-specific antibodies.

Real-time and traditional PCR detected pestiviral RNA sequences in fetal organs and placentomes of heifers 3, 4 and 5 (Table 3). In heifers 3 and 5, the sequence of the 5' terminal region was identical to the sequence isolated from the pi-BDV calf. In all organs of heifer 4, there was a base-pair substitution of thymine for adenine at position 94. Pestivirus detection was limited to the small intestines of the fetus in heifer 1 but because the amount of RNA was too small for sequencing, contamination of the sample could not be ruled out. The placentomes of heifer 2 and skin and small intestine of her fetus yielded pestiviral RT-PCR products with sequences that were identical to the viral sequence of the pi-BDV calf, but the RT-PCR results of the fetal thyroid gland were not conclusive. The placentomes and small intestine of the fetus of heifer 6 also yielded several products corresponding to pestiviral RNA. The sequence of pestiviral PCR products from the placenta were identical to those from the pi-BDV calf and the products of the small intestine contained the same mutation as that described for the products from heifer 4.

Based on the unequivocally positive results of the immunohistochemical and virologic examination of all fetal organs, the fetuses from heifers 3, 4 and 5 were diagnosed as persistently infected with BDV, though we cannot predict whether these fetuses would have developed to full term and be born alive as persistently infected calves. The fetus of heifer 1 was classified as not infected with BDV because immunohistochemistry and RT-PCR did not allow reliable detection of the virus. Likewise, the fetuses of heifers 2 and 6 were not considered persistently infected although pestivirus was detected in some fetal organs; Real-time PCR was negative or the Ct values were greater than 30, the bands in the agarose gel following traditional PCR amplification were faint or absent and immunohistochemical analysis, which in most cases identifies only PI animals [20], was negative. This led to a tentative diagnosis of transient BDV infection.

Relationship between seroconversion and day of infection and presence of a persistently infected fetus

Analysis of the mean relative OD during the 60 days of the infection period (6 heifers × 7 measurements) with the generalised linear model revealed a significant effect

Table 1 Detection of viral RNA (Ct values) in EDTA blood from 3 heifers in early pregnancy on days 8 to 14 of the infection phase

DayTag	Assay	Ct value		
		Heifer 3	Heifer 4	Heifer 5
8	Primary	Negative	37.8	40.6
	Follow-up	Negative	39.7	Negative
10	Primary	40.7	Negative	39.6
	Follow-up	Negative	Negative	41.7
12	Primary	Negative	Negative	42.5
	Follow-up	Negative	Negative	Negative
14	Primary	Negative	Negative	40.8
	Follow-up	Negative	Negative	Negative

Ct values of >30 were considered weakly positive.
Viral RNA was not isolated from heifers 1, 2 and 6.
Viral RNA was not isolated from heifers 3, 4 and 5 on days 0 to 6 and 16 to 20.

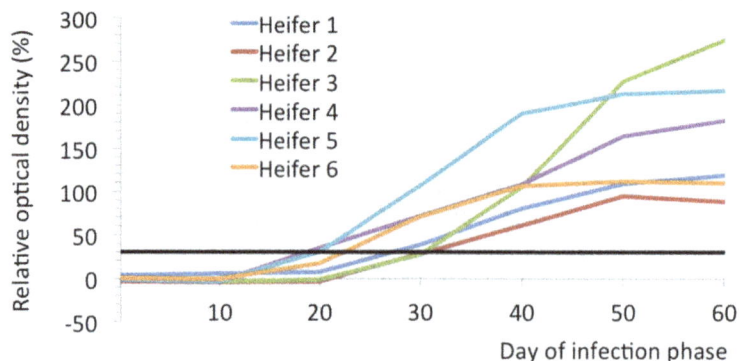

Figure 1 Relative optical density from day 0 to day 60 of the infection phase. Relative optical density (OD) expressed as percentage of the optical density of a standard serum in six heifers in early pregnancy from day 0 to day 60 of the infection phase. Relative OD values >30% (black line) are defined as positive.

of day of infection phase and status of fetal infection (infected or not infected) on relative OD. The *t*-test revealed significant differences between heifers with a persistently infected fetus and those without with respect to mean relative OD values on days 50 and 60 (Figure 3). Based on the generalised linear model, heifers with a persistently infected fetus had significantly higher mean relative OD than heifers without a persistently infected fetus from as early as day 40. The 90%-confidence intervals of the relative OD overlapped slightly on day 40 but clearly diverged on days 50 and 60. There was no temporal relationship between day of seroconversion and respective clinical findings.

Discussion

Pestiviral RNA was isolated from three heifers (3, 4, 5) on several occasions between days 8 and 14. Re-examination of the samples confirmed infection in two heifers (4, 5) but not in the third, which had only been weakly positive once on day 10. These findings support pestiviral viraemia, albeit at a low level. The time frame of the viraemia was similar to that observed in calves (8 to 21 days) [23,24], sheep (2 to 21 days) [25], and lambs (4 to 9 days) [26] infected with BDV. The observation that pestiviral RNA was only isolated from heifers with a persistently infected fetus

and that, at the same time, display the highest antibody titres, supports the presence of true viraemia. This is therefore the first report of BDV viraemia in cattle after contact with a persistently infected animal of the same species. Calves and heifers co-housed with sheep persistently infected with BDV seroconverted but did not become viraemic [5,7,24,27]. On the other hand, viral RNA could be isolated from blood of calves orally infected with BDV [13,24].

Two heifers seroconverted as early as day 20, and the remaining heifers seroconverted by day 40. This variability may have been the result of differences in susceptibility to BDV, viral dose and time of exposure to the virus, but was similar to the variability in pregnant heifers that seroconverted 23 to 38 days after first contact with sheep persistently infected with BDV [27]. Heifers with a persistently infected fetus had significantly higher titres from day 40 than heifers without an infected fetus, and there was a significant effect of duration of viraemia in the heifers and infectious status of the fetus on mean relative OD over the entire study period. The effect of a persistently infected fetus on antibody titre has not been described for BDV infection but has been known for BVDV infection; cows carrying a fetus persistently infected with BVDV had antibody titres at day 180 of pregnancy that were on average ten times higher than in cows with a non-infected fetus [28]. Similarly, the comparison of cows with and without a fetus persistently infected with BVDV showed that OD values were significantly related to duration of pregnancy, time of sampling and fetal infectious status [29,30]. Antibody titres rose much faster when the fetus was persistently infected, and after day 135 of pregnancy, OD differed significantly between the two groups of cows [30].

Serum neutralisation testing indicated that all heifers had high titres of specific antibodies against BDV at the end of the infection phase. Four heifers also had low antibody titres against BVDV, which was thought to be

Table 2 Relative OD values, SNT titres and quotients of BDV and BVDV SNT titres of 6 heifers in early pregnancy on day 60 of the infection phase

Heifer	OD value (%)	SNT BDV	SNT BVDV	Quotient of BDV and BVDV titres
1	119	152	≤ 4	≥ 38
2	89	215	≤ 4	≥ 53
3	274	304	8	38
4	182	431	27	16
5	216	> 512	16	> 32
6	110	> 512	8	> 64

Table 3 Histological, immunohistochemical (IHC) and virologic (RT-PCR) findings of the placentomes from 6 heifers in early pregnancy and fetal organs

| Heifer | | Finding | | | Fetal infectious status |
		Histology	IHC	RT-PCR	
1	Heifer	Negative	Negative	Negative	NA
	Fetus	Negative	Negative	One organ weakly positive	Not infected
2	Heifer	Negative	Negative	Positive	NA
	Fetus	Negative	Negative	Partially positive	Transiently infected
3	Heifer	I, F	Positive	Positive	NA
	Fetus	Negative	Positive	Positive	Persistently infected
4	Heifer	I, F, N	Positive	Positive	NA
	Fetus	Negative	Positive	Positive	Persistently infected
5	Heifer	I, F, N	Positive	Positive	NA
	Fetus	Negative	Positive	Positive	Persistently infected
6	Heifer	Negative	Negative	Partially positive	NA
	Fetus	Negative	Negative	Partially positive	Transiently infected

IHC immunohistochemical staining with antibody C16/15C5.
I inflammation, F fibrosis, N necrosis.
NA Not applicable.

due to slight cross-neutralisation within the pestivirus genus. Nonetheless, titres against BDV were 16 to 64 times higher than the titres against BVDV, indicating that the heifers were infected with BDV as a BDV titre at least four times higher than a BVDV titre is considered to be specific [31].

All uteri, placentae and fetuses were macroscopically normal and the fetal organs were also histologically normal. There was histological evidence of inflammation in the placentomes of the three heifers carrying an infected fetus, similar to lesions seen in BDV-infected pregnant sheep [32] and cows [27,33] and in BVDV-

infected pregnant cows [32]. It can be assumed that the fetal infection originated from the placenta.

Immunohistochemical examination of tongue, skin, thyroid gland and placenta is an established and sensitive method for the detection of persistent fetal pestivirus infection [19]. Three of the six fetuses and placentae were positive for the pestivirus-specific antibodies C16 and 15C5 but negative for the BVDV-specific antibodies C42, CA3 and CA34, and it is therefore most likely that these three fetuses were persistently infected with BDV. Interestingly, staining was all but limited to the fetal part of the placentome. Heifers 3, 4 and 5 had high titres against

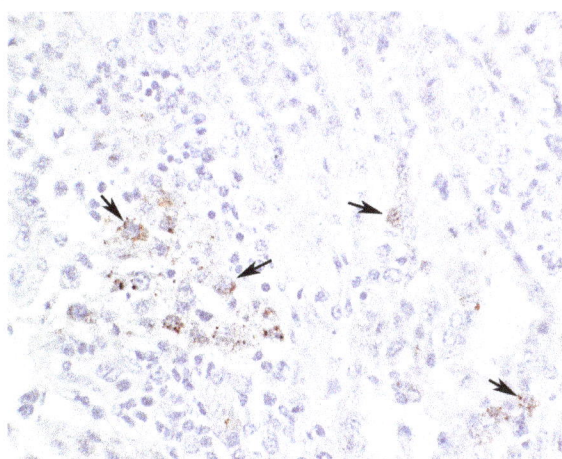

Figure 2 Immunohistochemical staining of a placentome.
Immunohistochemical staining of a placentome from heifer 5 (Dako EnVision staining system, antibody 15C5, hemalaun counterstain). The cytoplasm of pestivirus-positive fetal cells is stained red (arrows).

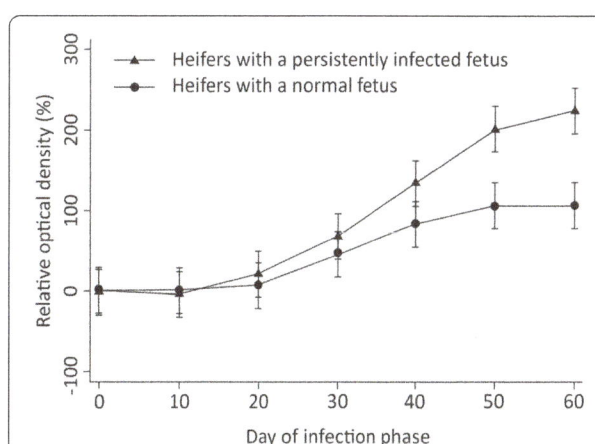

Figure 3 Mean relative OD of the pestivirus antibody ELISA for heifers with a persistently infected fetus and heifers with a normal fetus. Mean relative OD of the pestivirus antibody ELISA and 95% confidence intervals for 3 heifers with a persistently infected fetus (▲) and 3 heifers with a normal fetus (●). * P ≤0.05.

BDV from days 20 to 40, which could have neutralised the viral antigen in the maternal circulation. Because the passage of molecules across the epitheliochorial bovine placental barrier is highly selective [34], BDV antibodies may have been prevented from entering the fetal circulation, thus allowing infection of the fetus to occur.

Reverse transcriptase PCR allowed confirmation of BDV infection of the fetuses from heifers 3, 4 and 5. The RNA sequence isolated from heifers 3 and 5 was identical to the sequence isolated from the pi-BDV calf. The base-pair substitution of thymine for adenine at position 94 might be based on a RNA-virus specific characteristic whereby viruses produced within an infected cell are not always identical but may vary because of mutation and recombination within the viral genome [35]. Similar changes in amino acid sequences over time and the generation of variant viruses were observed in two pi-BVDV calves [36]. Isolation of pestiviral RNA from fetal organs and placentomes of heifers 2 and 6 could possibly have been based on true infection or on contamination of the sample. Assuming that persistent BDV and BVDV infections have similar underlying mechanisms, immunohistochemical examination of fetuses persistently infected with BDV should have yielded positive results for viral antigen. In bovine fetuses persistently infected with BVDV, immunohistochemical staining of fetal organs was as sensitive as virus isolation [19,37] and RT-PCR [20]. Therefore, we suspect that the fetuses of heifers 2 and 6 were transiently infected, which is supported by the fact that the isolation of RNA from organs of calves transiently infected with BVDV has been reported [20,38]. Isolation of pestiviral RNA from the fetus and placentome of heifer 1 was not conclusive but based on the seroconversion similar to heifers 2 and 6, it has to be assumed that heifer 1 became infected after contact with the pi-BDV calf.

Conclusion
Considering that pi-BDV cattle can infect other cattle and lead to persistent infection of the fetus in pregnant cows, BDV should not be ignored in the context of the mandatory BVDV eradication and monitoring programs such as the one instituted in Switzeland. In Switzerland and other countries, sheep and cattle are commonly kept in the same barn or co-pastured on alpine summer pastures, and it is therefore likely that BDV is transmitted from sheep to cattle and subsequently from the infected cattle to other cattle. For this reason, testing for BDV should be included in BVD eradication and control programs. It is doubtful whether pestiviruses in cattle can be eradicated without differentiating BVDV and BDV infection and the inclusion of other susceptible species such as sheep in the Swiss control program. It is therefore possible that pestivirus in cattle can not be eradicated without differentiating BVDV and BDV infection and the inclusion of other susceptible species such as sheep in the Swiss control program.

Competing interests
The authors declare that they have no competing interests.

Authors' contributions
UB initiated, planned and supervised the study and co-authored the manuscript with the other authors; SF completed the clinical part of the study as part of her dissertation [22] and collated the findings; MHi conducted the post-mortem examination of the uterus and histological and immunohistochemical examinations; MS planned the virologic and serologic examinations, analysed the data and together with RZ coordinated and supervised blood sample and fetal organ examination, which was carried out by laboratory technicians; FJ procured the seronegative heifers and was responsible for estrus synchronisation, artificial insemination and pregnancy examination; and MHä conducted the statistical analysis. All authors contributed equally to this study. All authors read and approved the final manuscript.

Acknowledgements
We thank Dr. Josef Risi and Dr. Toni Linggi, Veterinary Office of the primordial cantons for provision of the pi-BDV calf, the laboratory technicians of the Institutes for Veterinary Pathology and Veterinary Virology for the examination of the samples and Hanspeter Müller for taking care of the animals.

Sources of funding
This study was financed by the University of Zurich, Switzerland.

Author details
[1]Department of Farm Animals, Vetsuisse-Faculty, University of Zurich, Winterthurerstrasse 260, CH-8057 Zurich, Switzerland. [2]Institute of Veterinary Pathology, Vetsuisse-Faculty, University of Zurich, Winterthurerstrasse 260, CH-8057 Zurich, Switzerland. [3]Institute of Veterinary Virology, Vetsuisse-Faculty, University of Bern, Länggass-Strasse 122, 3001 Bern, Switzerland. [4]New Name: Institute of Virology and Immunology, Federal Food Safety and Veterinary Office, University of Bern, Länggass-Strasse 122, CH-3001 Bern, Switzerland.

References
1. Carlsson U, Belák K: Border disease virus transmitted to sheep and cattle by a persistently infected ewe: epidemiology and control. Acta Vet Scand 1994, 35:79–88.
2. Becher P, Orlich M, Shannon AD, Horner G, König M, Thiel HJ: Phylogenetic analysis of pestiviruses from domestic and wild ruminants. J Gen Virol 1997, 78:1357–1366.
3. Cranwell MP, Otter A, Errington J, Hogg RA, Wakeley P, Sandvik T: Detection of border disease virus in cattle. Vet Rec 2007, 161:211–212.
4. Krametter-Frötscher R, Schmitz C, Benetka V, Bagó Z, Möstl K, Vanek E, Baumgartner W: First descriptive study of an outbreak of border disease in a sheep flock in Austria – a high risk factor for bovine viral diarrhea virus free cattle herds: a case report. Vet Med (Praha) 2008, 53:625–628.
5. Krametter-Frötscher R, Benetka V, Möstl K, Baumgartner W: Transmission of border disease virus from sheep to calves – a possible risk factor for the Austrian BVD eradication programme in cattle? Wien Tierärztl Mschr 2008, 95:200–203.
6. Hornberg A, Fernández SR, Vogl C, Vilček S, Matt M, Fink M, Köfer J, Schöpf K: Genetic diversity of pestivirus isolates in cattle from Western Austria. Vet Microbiol 2009, 135:205–213.
7. Reichle SF: Untersuchungen bei Kälbern, die mit Border-Disease infizierten Lämmern zusammengehalten werden. Dr Med Vet Thesis. Zurich: University of Zurich; 2009.
8. Strong R, La Rocca SA, Ibata G, Sandvik T: Antigenic and genetic characterisation of border disease viruses isolated from UK cattle. Vet Microbiol 2010, 141:208–215.

9. McFadden AMJ, Tisdall DJ, Hill FI, Otterson P, Pulford D, Peake J, Finnegan CJ, La Rocca SA, Kok-Mun T, Weir AM: **The first case of a bull persistently infected with border disease virus in New Zealand.** *N Z Vet J* 2012, **60**:290–296.

10. Thür B, Zlinszky K, Ehrensperger F: **Immunohistochemical detection of bovine viral diarrhea virus in skin biopsies: A reliable and fast diagnostic tool.** *J Vet Med B* 1996, **43**:163–166.

11. Hilbe M, Arquint A, Schaller P, Zlinszky K, Braun U, Peterhans E, Ehrensperger F: **Immunohistochemical diagnosis of persistent infection with bovine viral diarrhea virus (BVDV) on skin biopsies.** *Schweiz Arch Tierheilk* 2007, **149**:337–344.

12. Bachofen C, Stalder HP, Vogt HR, Wegmüller M, Schweizer M, Zanoni R, Peterhans E: **Bovine Virusdiarrhöe (BVD): von der Biologie zur Bekämpfung.** *Berl Münch Tierärztl Wschr* 2013, **126**:452–461.

13. Frei S, Braun U, Dennler M, Hilbe M, Stalder HP, Schweizer M, Nuss K: **Border disease in persistently infected calves: radiological and pathological findings.** *Vet Rec* 2014, **174**:170. doi:10.1136/vr.102095.

14. Peterhans E, Bachofen C, Stalder HP, Schweizer M: **Cytopathic bovine viral diarrhea viruses (BVDV): emerging pestiviruses doomed to extinction.** *Vet Res* 2010, **41**:44.

15. Braun U, Bachofen C, Büchi R, Hässig M, Peterhans E: **Infection of cattle with border disease virus by sheep on communal alpine pastures.** *Schweiz Arch Tierheilk* 2013, **155**:123–128.

16. Canal CW, Strasser M, Hertig C, Masuda A, Peterhans E: **Detection of antibodies to bovine viral diarrhoea virus (BVDV) and characterization of genomes of BVDV from Brazil.** *Vet Microbiol* 1998, **63**:85–97.

17. Danuser R, Vogt HR, Kaufmann T, Peterhans E, Zanoni R: **Seroprevalence and characterization of pestivirus infections in small ruminants and new world camelids in Switzerland.** *Schweiz Arch Tierheilk* 2009, **151**:109–117.

18. Becher P, Avalos Ramirez R, Orlich M, Cedillo Rosales S, König M, Schweizer M, Stalder H, Schirrmeier H, Thiel HJ: **Genetic and antigenetic characterization of novel pestivirus genotypes: implications for classification.** *Virology* 2003, **311**:96–104.

19. Thür B, Hilbe M, Strasser M, Ehrensperger F: **Immunohistochemical diagnosis of pestivirus infection associated with bovine and ovine abortion and perinatal death.** *Am J Vet Res* 1997, **58**:1371–1375.

20. Hilbe M, Stalder H, Peterhans E, Haessig M, Nussbaumer M, Egli C, Schelp C, Zlinszky K, Ehrensperger F: **Comparison of five diagnostic methods for detecting bovine viral diarrhea virus infection in calves.** *J Vet Diagn Invest* 2007, **19**:28–34.

21. Bachofen C, Stalder HP, Braun U, Hilbe M, Ehrensperger F, Peterhans E: **Co-existence of genetically and antigenically diverse bovine viral diarrhoea viruses in an endemic situation.** *Vet Microbiol* 2008, **131**:93–102.

22. Frei S: **Übertragung des Border-Disease-Virus von einem persistent infizierten Rind auf seronegative Rinder durch Kontaktinfektion und virushaltiges Sperma.** In *Dr Med Vet Thesis.* Zurich: University of Zurich; 2014.

23. Reichert C: Infektion von Kälbern, Schafen und Ziegen mit Border-Disease-Virus. Dr Med Vet Thesis, University of Zurich, 2009

24. Braun U, Reichle SF, Reichert C, Hässig M, Stalder HP, Bachofen C, Peterhans E: **Sheep persistently infected with Border disease readily transmit virus to calves seronegative to BVD virus.** *Vet Microbiol* 2014, **168**:98–104.

25. Hurtado A, Sanchez I, Bastida F, Minguijón E, Juste RA, García-Pérez AL: **Detection and quantification of pestivirus in experimentally infected pregnant ewes and their progeny.** *Virol J* 2009, **6**:189.

26. Thabti F, Fronzaroli L, Dlissi E, Guibert JM, Hammami S, Pepin M, Russo P: **Experimental model of border disease virus infection in lambs: comparative pathogenicity of pestiviruses isolated in France and Tunisia.** *Vet Res* 2002, **33**:35–45.

27. Krametter-Frötscher R, Mason N, Rötzel J, Benetka V, Bagó Z, Möstl K, Baumgartner W: **Effects of border disease virus (genotype 3) naturally transmitted by persistently infected sheep to pregnant heifers and their progeny.** *Vet Med (Praha)* 2010, **55**:145–153.

28. Brownlie J, Hooper LB, Thompson I, Collins ME: **Maternal recognition of foetal infection with bovine virus diarrhoea virus (BVDV) – the bovine pestivirus.** *Clin Diagn Virol* 1998, **10**:141–150.

29. Lindberg A, Groenendaal H, Alenius S, Emanuelson U: **Validation of a test for dams carrying foetuses persistently infected with bovine viral diarrhoea virus based on determination of antibody levels in late pregnancy.** *Prev Vet Med* 2001, **51**:199–214.

30. Stokstad M, Niskanen R, Lindberg A, Thorén P, Belák S, Alenius S, Løken T: **Experimental infection of cows with bovine viral diarrhoea virus in early pregnancy – findings in serum and foetal fluids.** *J Vet Med B* 2003, **50**:424–429.

31. Braun U, Bachofen C, Schenk B, Hässig M, Peterhans E: **Investigation of border disease and bovine virus diarrhoea in sheep from 76 mixed cattle and sheep farms in eastern Switzerland.** *Schweiz Arch Tierheilk* 2013, **155**:293–298.

32. Osburn BI, Castrucci G: **Diaplacental infections with ruminant pestiviruses.** *Arch Virol Suppl* 1991, **3**:71–78.

33. Gibbons DF, Winkler CE, Shaw IG, Terlecki S, Richardson C, Done JT: **Pathogenicity of the border disease agent for the bovine foetus.** *Br Vet J* 1974, **130**:357–360.

34. Rüsse I, Grunert E: **Die normale Gravidität.** In *J Richter, R Götze Tiergeburtshilfe.* Edited by Grunert E, Arbeiter K. Berlin, Hamburg: Paul Parey; 1993:29–82.

35. Domingo E, Sheldon J, Perales C: **Viral quasispecies evolution.** *Microbiol Mol Biol Rev* 2012, **76**:159–216.

36. Collins ME, Desport M, Brownlie J: **Bovine viral diarrhea virus quasispecies during persistent infection.** *Virology* 1999, **259**:85–98.

37. Njaa BL, Clark EG, Janzen E, Ellis JA, Haines DM: **Diagnosis of persistent bovine viral diarrhea virus infection by immunhistochemical staining of formalin-fixed skin biopsy specimens.** *J Vet Diagn Invest* 2000, **12**:393–399.

38. Hansen TR, Smirnova NP, Van Campen H, Shoemaker ML, Ptitsyn AA, Bielefeldt-Ohmann H: **Maternal and fetal response to fetal persistent infection with bovine viral diarrhea virus.** *Am J Reprod Immunol* 2010, **64**:295–306.

8

Characterisation of recent foot-and-mouth disease viruses from African buffalo (*Syncerus caffer*) and cattle in Kenya is consistent with independent virus populations

Sabenzia Nabalayo Wekesa[1,2], Abraham Kiprotich Sangula[1], Graham J Belsham[3], Kirsten Tjornehoj[3], Vincent B Muwanika[2], Francis Gakuya[4], Dominic Mijele[4] and Hans Redlef Siegismund[5*]

Abstract

Background: Understanding the epidemiology of foot-and-mouth disease (FMD), including roles played by different hosts, is essential for improving disease control. The African buffalo (*Syncerus caffer*) is a reservoir for the SAT serotypes of FMD virus (FMDV). Large buffalo populations commonly intermingle with livestock in Kenya, yet earlier studies have focused on FMD in the domestic livestock, hence the contribution of buffalo to disease in livestock is largely unknown. This study analysed 47 epithelia collected from FMD outbreaks in Kenyan cattle between 2008 and 2012, and 102 probang and serum samples collected from buffalo in three different Kenyan ecosystems; Maasai-Mara (MME) (*n* = 40), Tsavo (TSE) (*n* = 33), and Meru (ME) (*n* = 29).

Results: Antibodies against FMDV non-structural proteins were found in 65 of 102 (64%) sera from buffalo with 44/102 and 53/102 also having neutralising antibodies directed against FMDV SAT 1 and SAT 2, respectively. FMDV RNA was detected in 42% of the buffalo probang samples by RT-qPCR (Cycle Threshold (Ct) ≤32). Two buffalo probang samples were positive by VI and were identified as FMDV SAT 1 and SAT 2 by Ag-ELISA, while the latter assay detected serotypes O (1), A (20), SAT 1 (7) and SAT 2 (19) in the 47 cattle epithelia. VP1 coding sequences were generated for two buffalo and 21 cattle samples. Phylogenetic analyses revealed SAT 1 and SAT 2 virus lineages within buffalo that were distinct from those detected in cattle.

Conclusions: We found that FMDV serotypes O, A, SAT 1 and SAT 2 were circulating among cattle in Kenya and cause disease, but only SAT 1 and SAT 2 viruses were successfully isolated from clinically normal buffalo. The buffalo isolates were genetically distinct from isolates obtained from cattle. Control efforts should focus primarily on reducing FMDV circulation among livestock and limiting interaction with buffalo. Comprehensive studies incorporating additional buffalo viruses are recommended.

Keywords: African buffalo, Cattle, Control, Epidemiology, Foot-and-mouth disease, Lineages

* Correspondence: hsiegismund@bio.ku.dk
[5]Department of Biology, University of Copenhagen, Ole Maaløes Vej 5, DK-2200 Copenhagen, Denmark
Full list of author information is available at the end of the article

Background

Numerous species of cloven-hoofed wildlife and livestock, including buffalo, impala, cattle, sheep, goats and pigs are affected by foot-and-mouth disease (FMD) [1]. The disease is clinically characterised by fever, lameness and vesicular lesions on the tongue, feet, snout/muzzle and teats of various susceptible species [2]. Globally, the disease causing agent, FMD virus (FMDV), exists in seven different serotypes (O, A, C, Asia 1, SAT 1, SAT 2 and SAT 3) and vaccination against (or infection with) one serotype does not cross-protect against other serotypes, hence the need for constant surveillance of circulating strains for appropriate vaccine selection [3].

In the eastern Africa region, including Kenya, four of the seven serotypes (O, A, SAT 1 and SAT 2) were previously known to circulate [4], but recently in 2013, SAT 3 was isolated from an apparently healthy long-horned Ankole calf in Uganda [5]. This multiplicity of serotypes, combined with the co-existence of a number of different wild and domestic hosts within large geographical areas, makes our understanding of the epidemiology and control of this disease complicated [6]. In eastern Africa, existing policies largely comprise vaccination and livestock movement control. Infection by the virus may result in substantial economic losses; these include production losses (e.g. reduced milk yields, lameness in draught animals, loss of weight, abortions, delayed conception, peri-natal mortality) as well as effects from restrictions on sales and exports of livestock and livestock products [7].

The severity of FMD varies from host to host, e.g. cattle commonly suffer acute, clinically apparant infections [2], while in the African buffalo (*Syncerus caffer*) the disease is usually subclinical [8,9] and hence is not easy to detect. It has been reported that within wildlife, the African buffalo are reservoirs for the SAT serotypes [8,10] and may play a role in the maintenance and spread of these serotypes to livestock [9] as reported in southern Africa. Moreover, this buffalo species is capable of harbouring the virus for as long as 5 years within an individual animal and for 24 years within a single herd [11]. Animals with these long-term infections are referred to as persistently infected animals or carriers, and are defined as animals in which the virus can be detected from the oesophago-pharyngeal scrapings (OP/probang sample) at 28 days or more after infection [12,13]. Unlike in southern Africa, the role of the African buffalo in the epidemiology of FMD is still unclear in eastern Africa [14,15], yet buffalo interact with livestock, grazing together in the vast and numerous un-fenced wildlife ecosystems.

It has been argued that wildlife might act as a source of sporadic disease occurrence in livestock with negative impacts on the harmonious co-existence of these species

[16,17]. On the one hand, there is experimental evidence that FMD may spread from buffalo to cattle, while on the other hand, there is a lack of adequate supportive scientific evidence for the role of wildlife in the epidemiology of FMD in livestock [18]. Indeed, some studies have argued that FMD may be predominantly a disease of livestock [17,19] and that the spread of FMDV among livestock may be more associated with human activities than with wildlife [20]. Moreover, the importance of enhancing our understanding of disease spread at the wildlife-livestock interface and the need to balance biodiversity management with livestock production have been emphasized previously [16,21]. It is therefore necessary to study the disease spread at this interface to ensure that appropriate policies and control measures are implemented. This should help to protect the wildlife heritage and concurrently promote harmonious, profitable and sustainable livestock-wildlife interaction.

According to unpublished Kenya Wildlife Service (KWS) records, Kenya has an estimated total population of 26,325 buffalo distributed among numerous parks, reserves, sanctuaries and ranches found within several major ecosystems including Tsavo, Meru, Laikipia/Samburu, Amboseli, Nakuru and Maasai-Mara. This buffalo population and other less susceptible wildlife species complements the numerous domestic FMDV-susceptible hosts in Kenya, including 17.5 million cattle, 27.7 million goats, 17.1 million sheep and 300,000 domestic pigs recorded during the 2009 national animal census [22]. Records at the national Foot-and-Mouth Disease Laboratory (FMDL), Embakasi, show that previous studies on FMD in Kenya have been mainly focused on cattle and not other susceptible domestic species such as pigs [23] and only to a minor extent on wildlife. However, in 1979, a field survey isolated SAT 1 and SAT 2 FMDVs from buffalo populations in the southern part of Kenya [24], while a more recent study (1994-2002) established a higher seroprevalence of antibodies against FMDV in buffalo than in other susceptible wildlife species, but also highlighted some limitations of the specificity of the serological tests that were used [25].

Elsewhere in the east African region, studies of buffalo within neighbouring Uganda's Queen Elizabeth National Park isolated SAT 3 virus in 1997 [26], reported antibodies against FMDV serotypes O, SAT 1, SAT 2 and SAT 3 in sera collected during 2001-2003 [15], and successfully isolated and genetically characterized SAT 1 and SAT 2 viruses in 2005-2008 [27].

This study, aimed at determining the presence of antibodies against different serotypes of FMDV within buffalo populations in selected wildlife ecosystems in Kenya and at comparing FMDV isolates from these buffalo populations with the FMDVs found in cattle within this country and elsewhere in Africa. The study endevoured to contribute towards generating reliable information regarding FMDV circulation in eastern Africa.

Methods

Ethical approval

This study was ethically approved by the Kenya Wildlife Services (permit no. KWS/BRM/5001) and undertaken in collaboration with the Department of Veterinary Services (DVS) of the Ministry of Livestock Development in Kenya under the Transboundary Animal Diseases in East Africa (TADEA) project, DFC no. 10-006KU.

Samples from buffalo

The buffalo sampling was carried out between March and July 2012. The study was designed as a cross-sectional study targeting buffalo populations interacting with domestic animals regardless of their age. The buffalo were clustered into three major buffalo ecosystems located within four out of the eight major administrative regions/provinces of Kenya (North-Eastern, Eastern, Rift Valley and Coast) (Figure 1). These include the Meru ecosystem (ME), represented by Meru National Park, the Maasai-Mara ecosystem (MME), represented by Maasai-Mara National Reserve and the Tsavo ecosystem (TSE), represented by Tsavo East National Park. These ecosystems have estimated populations of 4069, 3030 and 7281 buffalo, respectively, according to the KWS records. Within these ecosystems, there is a high level of interaction between livestock and wildlife. MME and TSE have open savannah-type vegetation, which eases the capture and handling of the animals, while ME has patches of wooded grassland vegetation.

Two groups of veterinarians and technicians in two separate vehicles carried out the buffalo sampling; one identified the herds and chemically immobilized the animals as described by [28], while the other traced, marked and sampled the immobilized animals, taking records of geographical location, age by dentition [29], sex, clinical signs, body condition and estimated herd size. Two or three animals per herd were randomly selected to enable sampling of as many herds as possible.

In total 102 serum and corresponding probang samples were collected from buffalo; these comprised samples from MME ($n = 40$), TSE ($n = 33$) and ME ($n = 29$) with approximate animal ages ranging between 8 months and 19 years. The probang samples were diluted 1:1 in phosphate buffered saline (PBS) (pH 7.2) supplemented with 0.01% bovine serum albumin (BSA), 0.002% phenol red and 0.25% antibiotics (Pen-Strep-Neo, Sigma-Aldrich, St. Louis, MO, USA), stored in liquid nitrogen and transported to FMDL, Embakasi, where they were stored at −80°C.

Samples from cattle

Taking into consideration the time of sampling, quality of material and the geographical source with a focus on districts around ecosystems of interest for this study and the sampling period (2008-2012), cattle epithelial samples were selected from the repository of all Kenyan field samples at the FMDL, Embakasi (Figure 1 and Table 1).

Testing strategy

This study compared evidence of infection by FMDV in buffalo and cattle using serological and virological assays as recommended by the OIE terrestrial manual [30]. All serological tests (except VNT for antibodies against SAT 3) were performed at FMDL, Embakasi, while all tests on epithelia from cattle and probang samples from buffalo, including sequencing were performed at the National Veterinary Institute, Lindholm, Denmark.

Buffalo sera were screened for antibodies against FMDV non-structural proteins (NSPs) as an indicator of prior infection with FMDV. Serotype-specific antibody titres were initially determined using liquid phase blocking ELISAs (LPBEs) (for antibodies against all FMDV serotypes except Asia 1). Thereafter (due to expected cross-reactivity among ELISAs [31-33]), VNTs, which exhibit lower level of cross-reactivity [31,32], were performed for neutralizing antibodies against six serotypes of FMDV (all except Asia 1).

All buffalo probang samples were tested using the 3D coding region-targeted real time RT-PCR (3D RT-qPCR) assay and virus isolation (VI) was attempted. Harvests of samples that induced cytopathic effect (CPE) in primary bovine thyroid (BTY) cells were tested in antigen ELISA (Ag-ELISA) and in 5'UTR-targeted real time RT-PCR (5'UTR RT-qPCR). Harvests positive in Ag-ELISA and with sufficient FMDV RNA to generate an amplicon corresponding to the VP1 coding sequence were characterized by sequencing. Cattle epithelia were tested directly in the Ag-ELISA and using the 5'UTR RT-qPCR assay and when amplicons could be generated directly were sequenced.

Laboratory methods

Detection of antibodies against FMDV non-structural proteins (NSPs) in buffalo sera

All 102 buffalo sera were screened using the Prio-CHECK® FMDV NS kit (Prionics AG, Switzerland) to detect antibodies against the NSPs of FMDV. The assay was performed according to the manufacturer's instructions. Sera were tested using a 1:5 dilution and optical density (OD) measured at wavelength 450 nm (OD_{450} test sample). The results were expressed as Percentage Inhibition (PI) relative to the negative control (OD_{450} max) as follows: $PI = 100 - [OD_{450}$ test sample/OD_{450} max$] \times 100$. Sera with PI <50 were considered negative and sera with PI ≥50% positive.

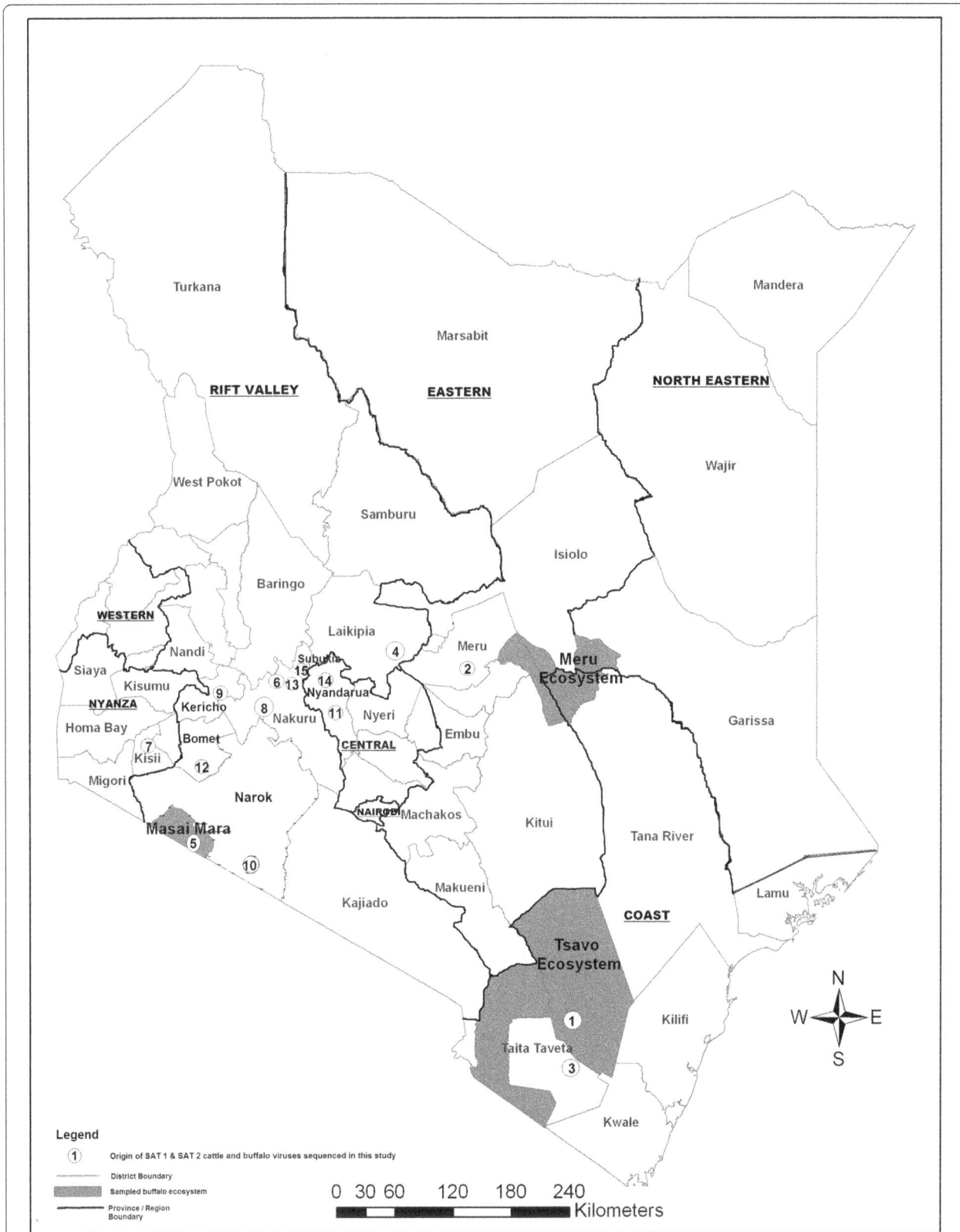

Figure 1 Map of Kenya showing sampled wildlife ecosystems (shaded), administrative regions (underlined) and districts. Circles with numbers indicate geographic origins of the 15 SAT 1 and SAT 2 foot-and-mouth disease viruses (FMDVs) isolated from buffalo and cattle sample analysed in this study. The numbers correspond to the serial numbers in Table 1. The map was created using ArcGIS (ArcMap v 9.3) copyright 2008 ESRI.

Table 1 List of the 49 FMD viruses analysed in this study

*Serial no.	**Sample reference no.	Date of collection	Host species	District of origin	Province	Serotype on Ag ELISA	Ct value on RT-qPCR	Serotype on VP1 sequencing	Accession no.
1	Ken/TSE1/2012	31/07/2012	Buffalo	Taita	Coast	SAT 1	17.19[a]	SAT 1	KP263443
2	K159/2012	19/12/2012	Cattle	Meru	Eastern	SAT 1	24.1[b]	SAT 1	KP263444
3	K127/2011	01/12/2011	Cattle	Taita-Taveta	Coast	SAT 1	9.96	SAT 1	KP263445
4	K56/2010	24/03/2010	Cattle	Laikipia	Rift Valley	SAT 1	24.48	SAT 1	KP263446
5	KenMMB37/2012	25/02/2012	Buffalo	Narok	Rift Valley	SAT 2	25.12	SAT 2	KP263447
6	K146/2012	31/10/2012	Cattle	Nakuru North	Rift Valley	SAT 2	14.66	SAT 2	KP263448
7	K125/2012	05/09/2012	Cattle	Kisii	Nyanza	SAT 2	14.6	SAT 2	KP263449
8	K126/2012	09/10/2012	Cattle	Nakuru	Rift Valley	SAT 2	15.64	SAT 2	KP263450
9	K53/2012	25/05/2012	Cattle	Kericho	Rift Valley	SAT 2	17.79	SAT 2	KP263451
10	K26/2012	21/02/2012	Cattle	Narok South	Rift Valley	SAT 2	10.44	SAT 2	KP263452
11	K28/2012	25/02/2012	Cattle	Nyandarua	Central	SAT 2	13.57	SAT 2	KP263453
12	K10/2012	20/01/2012	Cattle	Bomet	Rift Valley	SAT 2	23.11	SAT 2	KP263454
13	K46/2012	27/04/2012	Cattle	Nakuru North	Rift Valley	SAT 2	15.7	SAT 2	KP263455
14	K128/2011	01/12/2011	Cattle	Nyandarua	Central	SAT 2	19.37	SAT 2	KP263456
15	K30/2012	28/02/2012	Cattle	Subukia	Rift Valley	SAT 2	14.03	SAT 2	KP263457
16	K138/2012	05/10/2012	Cattle	Gilgil	Rift Valley	A	11.31	A	KJ440872
17	K143/2012	19/10/2012	Cattle	Naivasha	Rift Valley	A	24.13	A	KJ440873
18	K148/2012	13/11/2012	Cattle	Nakuru North	Rift Valley	A	19.29	A	KJ440874
19	K154/2012	03/12/2012	Cattle	Koibatek	Rift Valley	A	23.5	A	KJ440875
20	K3/2013	09/01/2013	Cattle	Thika East	Central	A	22.56	A	KJ440876
21	K63/2009	31/03/2009	Cattle	Narok South	Rift Valley	A	25.75	A	KJ440871
22	K73/2008	23/08/2008	Cattle	Loitokitok	Rift Valley	A	23.17	A	KJ440870
23	K33/2010	01/12/2010	Cattle	Ijara	North Eastern	O	25.75	O	KP765607
24	K10/2009	26/01/2009	Cattle	Machakos	Eastern	A	28.65	N/A	N/A
25	K14/2013	28/01/2013	Cattle	Sotik	Rift Valley	A	No Ct	N/A	N/A
26	K140/2012	12/10/2012	Cattle	Koibatek	Rift Valley	A	30.12	N/A	N/A
27	K144/2012	25/10/2012	Cattle	Sotik	Rift Valley	A	29.44	N/A	N/A
28	K151/2012	26/11/2012	Cattle	Subukia	Rift Valley	A	26.69	N/A	N/A
29	K152/2010	07/12/2010	Cattle	Transmara	Rift Valley	A	25.4	N/A	N/A
30	K160/2012	28/12/2012	Cattle	Rongai	Rift Valley	A	27.41	N/A	N/A
31	K18/2013	31/01/2013	Cattle	Rongai	Rift Valley	A	16.74	N/A	N/A
32	K2/2013	09/01/2013	Cattle	Mogotio	Rift Valley	A	16.43	N/A	N/A
33	K5/2013	10/01/2013	Cattle	Murang'a	Central	A	18.38	N/A	N/A
34	K64/2010	04/06/2010	Cattle	Narok	Rift Valley	A	36.78	N/A	N/A
35	K7/2013	16/01/2013	Cattle	Nakuru	Rift Valley	A	27.58	N/A	N/A
36	K88/2010	14/05/2010	Cattle	Githunguri	Central	A	31.86	N/A	N/A
37	K43/2011	19/03/2011	Cattle	Suba	Nyanza	SAT 1	29.12	N/A	N/A
38	K78/2011	26/08/2011	Cattle	Lamu West	Coast	SAT 1	28.21	N/A	N/A
39	K8/2011	01/07/2011	Cattle	Nyeri South	Central	SAT 1	23.64	N/A	N/A
40	K84/2012	07/03/2012	Cattle	Kathonzweni	Eastern	SAT 1	13.77	N/A	N/A
41	K113/2012	09/08/2012	Cattle	Mathioya	Central	SAT 2	25.69	N/A	N/A
42	K122/2011	23/11/2011	Cattle	Njoro	Rift Valley	SAT 2	25.65	N/A	N/A
43	K127/2012	12/09/2012	Cattle	Kisumu East	Nyanza	SAT 2	24.62	N/A	N/A

Table 1 List of the 49 FMD viruses analysed in this study *(Continued)*

44	K33/2012	01/03/2012	Cattle	Njoro	Rift Valley	SAT 2	24.06	N/A	N/A
45	K39/2012	16/03/2012	Cattle	Kenyanya	Nyanza	SAT 2	28.08	N/A	N/A
46	K54/2012	31/05/2012	Cattle	Mashuru	Rift Valley	SAT 2	21.16	N/A	N/A
47	K55/2012	04/06/2012	Cattle	Koibatek	Rift Valley	SAT 2	28.86	N/A	N/A
48	K78/2012	28/06/2012	Cattle	Naivasha	Rift Valley	SAT 2	22.07	N/A	N/A
49	K98/2012	22/07/2012	Cattle	Nyandarua West	Central	SAT 2	9.9	N/A	N/A

*No. 1-15 correspond to the numbers in Figure 1 showing the geographic origin of the 15 SAT 1 and SAT 2 cattle and buffalo FMD viruses sequenced and compared in this study, while No. 1-23 indicate all the 23 FMD viruses that were successfully sequenced in the entire study.
N/A - Not applicable since the sequence was not determined.
**Sample reference number: the letter (K) indicates the first letter of the name of the country of origin (Kenya), followed by the serial number of the isolate and the year of sampling.
[a]Ct value for buffalo samples based on 3D RT-qPCR assay.
[b]Ct value for all cattle samples based on 5'UTR RT-qPCR assay.

Assay for antibodies against FMDV using serotype-specific liquid phase blocking ELISA (LPBE) in buffalo sera

The LPBE assay was performed on all 102 buffalo serum samples using a commercial kit (BDSL, Scotland, UK), in accordance with the OIE manual [30]. The antigens used for this assay were: O_1 Manisa, A_{22} IRQ 24/64, C PHI 7/84, SAT 1 (105), SAT 2 Eritrea, SAT 3 (309), and Asia 1 Shamir as contained in the kit. The sera were tested in two-fold dilution series from 1/32 to 1/256. The results were expressed as the reciprocal of the last positive dilution (the titre); samples with titres ≥90 were considered positive in accordance with instructions in the OIE manual.

Assay for neutralising antibodies against FMDV in buffalo sera

VNTs were performed to detect neutralizing antibodies against six serotypes (all except Asia 1) on all the 102 buffalo sera to confirm the LPBE results and to clarify possible cross-reactions as described in the OIE manual [30]. Briefly, quadruplicate two-fold dilution series of serum samples were incubated for 1 hr in flat-bottomed tissue culture grade microtitre plates with about 100 $TCID_{50}$ of each of the Kenyan FMDV vaccine strains (O K77/78, A K5/80, C K267/67, SAT 1 T155/71, SAT 2 K52/84) and a Zimbabwean SAT 3 isolate (SAT 3 ZIM 4/81). The use of these old isolates was based on previous experience [23] and their satisfactory performance during the annual World Reference Laboratory (WRL) proficiency tests. Subsequently, a suspension of baby hamster kidney (BHK) cells was added to the samples followed by incubation for 2 days at 37°C. For SAT 3, incubation was in primary swine kidney (SK) cells for 3 days at 37°C. The controls included titration of a standard positive serum, cell control and a ten-fold titration of the virus suspension. The final end point titres were calculated as described previously [34] and titres ≥45 were considered positive, 16-44 doubtful and <16 negative [30].

Serological data recording and statistical analysis

Serological results were recorded and descriptive statistics calculated in MS Excel 2007 (Microsoft Corporation). Analyses of estimated prevalences and Confidence Intervals were performed using the Survey toolbox software [35].

Epithelial and probang sample processing and virus isolation (VI)

All epithelia and probang samples were thawed at room temperature and processed as recommended in the OIE manual [30]. Epithelial samples from cattle were ground in Eagles minimum essential media supplemented with protein hydrolysate, 2% fetal calf serum and antibiotics (2 million I.U. benzyl-penicillin, 1 g dihydrostreptomycin sulphate, 0.5 g neomycin sulphate, 1 g streptomycin and 8.5 μg amphotericin per litre) using sterile sand, mortar and pestle to make a 10% (w/v) suspension. These lysates were tested directly in the Ag-ELISA and used for RNA extraction, RT-qPCR and sequencing (see below). Probang suspensions from buffalo were inoculated onto BTY cells for 1 hour at 37°C followed by a change of media and continued incubation. The cultures were examined after 24 and 48 hours and harvested when CPE developed. The CPE negative samples were harvested by freeze-thawing and inoculated onto fresh cells for another 48 hours. CPE positive samples were harvested, while cultures negative after 2 passages were discarded. Positive harvests were tested in the Ag-ELISA and tested in the 5'UTR RT-qPCR assay (see below).

Detection of FMDV RNA using quantitative real time RT-PCR (RT-qPCR)

Quantitative RT-qPCR assays targeting the FMDV 3D coding sequence of the FMDV RNA were performed on buffalo probang samples as described previously [36] using a Superscript III/Platinum Taq one-step RT-qPCR kit (PE Biosystems, Life Technologies, Carlsbad, California, USA) with 3D probe (5′-FAM-TCCTTTGCACGCCGTGGGAC-

TAMRA 3'), forward primer (5'-ACTGGTTTTACAAA CCTGTGA-3') and reverse primer (5'-GCGAGTCCTGC CACGGA-3'). In addition, RT-qPCR assays targeting the FMDV 5' UTR were performed on all the 47 cattle epithelia and CPE positive buffalo harvests using TaqMan® Universal 2X PCR Master Mix (PE Biosystems, Life Technologies, Carlsbad, California, USA). The PCR was run, as described previously [37], using the FMDV MultiII IRES primers (FMDV Multi II forward primer and FMDV Multi II reverse primer) and FMDV Multi II-288 probe (FAM-labelled).

Antigen detection ELISA (Ag-ELISA)

Ag-ELISA to detect the presence of FMDV was performed as described in the OIE manual [30] and by [38], and, when positive, to determine the serotype. Samples with an OD difference between sample and negative control of >0.2 were considered positive, while those between 0.1 and 0.2 were considered inconclusive and repeated.

Sequencing of the FMDV VP1 coding region

Viral RNA was extracted from Ag-ELISA positive harvests of cell culture generated using buffalo probang samples and cattle epithelia samples. This was achieved by using the QIAmp® RNA blood mini kit (Qiagen, Hamburg, Germany) following the protocol for extraction of total RNA as described by the manufacturer. The RNA was eluted using 60 µl of RNase-free water and stored at -80°C. It was tested using the 5'UTR RT-qPCR assay. For selected RNAs the Ready-To-Go You-Prime First-Strand beads (GE Healthcare Life Sciences, Uppsala, Sweden) were used to synthesize new cDNA with random hexamer primers (pdN6).

The FMDV cDNA sequences were amplified using the reverse primer 1.0 PN 15 (NK-72) [39] and forward primers 1.0-U PN E (AKS-2) [40] or 13-KPN 100 or 13-KPN 101 (Table 2). The latter two primers were designed from the sequences of the Kenyan SAT 1 (K127/2011) and SAT 2 (K10/2012) cattle samples from this study, respectively. The PCRs were performed as described previously [41] and the products (≈840 bp) were analysed by electrophoresis on 1.5 % agarose gels (Seakem GTG agarose in 1 X TAE - low EDTA buffer) at 120 volts for 30 min. in parallel with a 1 kb DNA ladder GeneRuler® (Fermentas, Vilnius, Lithuania).

PCR products were purified using SigmaSpin® Sequencing Reaction Clean-Up Columns (Sigma-Aldrich, St. Louis, MO, USA) following the manufacturer's instructions. Quantification of products and cycle sequencing were performed as previously described [41]. Cycle sequencing in both directions was achieved using the same forward and reverse primers as for the RT-PCRs.

Sequence assembly, alignment and analysis

The nucleotide sequences were assembled and edited using SeqMan Pro software (DNAstar, Inc., Madison, WI, USA). Serotype identification of the sequences was achieved by comparison with Genbank data using the Basic Local Alignment Search Tool (BLAST) [42].

The buffalo and cattle VP1 coding sequences generated in this study were compared to selected FMDV SAT 1 and SAT 2 sequences from Kenyan cattle determined in previous studies, from the WRLFMD [43] and from Genbank (see list in Additional file 1: Table S1 and Additional file 2: Table S2). Sequence alignment was achieved using MUSCLE [44] incorporated in MEGA software version 5.2 [45] and trimmed to 639 nucleotides encompassing the complete VP1 coding region of the viral RNA genome. Substitution models were also determined in MEGA5.2 as earlier described [41], briefly, Maximum Likelihood fits of 24 different nucleotide substitution models were estimated and Akaike Information Criterion (AIC) was used. Non-uniformity evolution rates were modelled using discrete gamma distribution (G) and the Tamura Nei substitution model with gamma distribution and invariable rates (I) (TN93 + G + I) was chosen [45]. The evolutionary history was inferred using the neighbor-joining method [45] and a bootstrap consensus tree estimated from 1000 replicates [46]. Percentage nucleotide differences among taxa in the data sets were calculated using MEGA5.2 [45] and genetic distances compared using the P-distance.

Results

None of the 102 buffalo sampled in this study had clinical signs suggestive of FMDV infections during the sampling, while all the 47 cattle samples analysed were from animals with apparent clinical signs of FMD (data not shown).

Table 2 Primers used for amplification of FMDV VP1 cDNA in this study

Primer name	Sequence (5'-3')	Isolate of origin	Reference
1.0 PN 15 (NK-72) (reverse)	GAAGGGCCCAGGGTTGGACTC	Accession no. AJ 539141	Mason et al., 2003 [35].
13-KPN 100 (forward)	GGGTGGBBGTSTWMCAGRTSACMGACAC	K127/2011	This study
13-KPN 101(forward)	CACTGCTAYCAYKCNGARTGGGA	K10/2012	This study
1.0-U PN E (AKS-2) (forward)	TTAACTACCACTTCATGTACACXG	Accession no AY593849	Sangula et al., 2010 [36].

V = A,C,G; H = A,C,T; B = C,G,T; S = C,G; W = A,T; M = A,C; R = A,G; Y = C,T; K = G,T; N = Any; X = Inosine.

Antibodies against FMDV non-structural proteins (NSP) in buffalo sera

Out of 102 buffalo sera tested, 65 (64%) had antibodies against FMDV NSPs; these were distributed between the three different ecosystems as follows: MME 36/40 (90%: CI = 84–100%); ME 17/29 (59%: CI = 51–71%) and TSE 12/33 (36%: CI = 22–40%) (Table 3).

Serotype-specific antibodies against FMDV in buffalo sera detected by LPBE

Generally, antibodies were detected by the LPBE against each of the six FMDV serotypes tested for (O, A, C, SAT 1, SAT 2 and SAT 3). Only three of the 102 buffalo samples were negative (with titres ≤90) for antibodies against all six serotypes tested for by LPBE, while 15, 15, 10, 19, 19 and 21 samples were positive for antibodies against all six, five, four, three, two and one serotype, respectively (data not shown). Moreover, high antibody titres (≥256) against serotypes O, A, SAT 1, SAT 2 and SAT 3 were found in 33, 20, 37, 39 and 29 sera, respectively (data not shown). The positive samples were distributed in the three ecosystems in different proportions as indicated in Table 3, i.e. SAT 2 dominating in MME, O/SAT 3 in ME and SAT 1/O in TSE.

Detection of neutralising antibodies against FMDV by VNT in buffalo sera

The buffalo sera were also tested in VNT assays. In contrast to the LPBE results, there was no evidence for the presence of neutralising antibodies against FMDV serotypes C and SAT 3 among the 102 buffalo in the three ecosystems. Only one and two sera had neutralizing antibodies against serotypes O and A, respectively; moreover, these three sera had higher or equal titres against SAT 1 and/or SAT 2 and thus the apparent presence of anti-O and anti-A antibodies may result from cross reactivity in the assays. In contrast, neutralising antibodies against serotypes SAT 1 and SAT 2 were detected in 44/102 (43%) and 53/102 (52%) samples, respectively. Thirty of these samples were positive for antibodies against both serotypes and generally had higher titres against SAT 2 than against SAT 1, while 14 and 23 samples only

had antibodies against SAT 1 or SAT 2, respectively (Table 3). Altogether 67 sera had neutralising antibodies against FMDV, including 41 of the 65 sera with antibodies against NSP, meaning that 24 and 26 sera only were positive in one of these test systems (data not shown). The distribution of the positive sera between the three ecosystems is shown in Table 3. MME and ME had higher levels of neutralising antibodies against SAT 2 than against SAT 1, while TSE predominantly had SAT 1 neutralising antibodies.

Presence of FMDV and FMDV RNA in buffalo probang samples

Among the buffalo probang samples, 43/102 (42%) had evidence of FMDV RNA as detected by the 3D RT-qPCR assay on the original, non-passaged samples (Table 3) with Ct values ≤32 and were distributed as follows: MME (22/40), ME (6/29) and TSE (15/33). Twenty seven of these 43 (63%) positive samples came from buffalo with neutralising antibodies against FMDV SAT 1 and/or SAT 2.

The 43 buffalo probang samples that were positive in the 3D RT-qPCRs were inoculated onto BTY cells. Thirty three of these samples induced CPE, but only two of the cell harvests tested positive in the FMDV Ag-ELISA and were identified as SAT 1 and SAT 2, respectively (data not shown). Moreover, only these same two cell culture harvests (from MME and TSE) contained significant levels of FMDV RNA (Ct values of 17.19 and 25.12, Table 1) in the 5′UTR RT-qPCR assay and were used for VP1 sequencing following RT-PCR.

Presence of FMDV antigen and RNA in cattle epithelia

All the 47 cattle epithelium samples (directly tested without virus isolation) were positive on Ag-ELISA, and their distribution between the serotypes was as follows: O (1); A (20); SAT 1 (7) and SAT 2 (19) (Table 1). All but two of the 47 cattle epithelial samples had Ct values <32 and amplicons corresponding to the VP1 coding sequence were successfully generated and sequenced from 21 of them (Table 1).

Table 3 Detection of FMDV RNA and antibodies against FMDV in buffalo from selected wildlife ecosystems in Kenya

Ecosystem	Total no. sampled	Sampling period in 2012	Real time 3D RT-qPCR	NS ELISA	LPBE per serotype (titres ≥90)						dVNT per serotype		
					O	A	C	SAT 1	SAT 2	SAT 3	SAT 1 only	SAT 2 only	eSAT 1 & SAT 2
aMME	40	Feb.	22	36	16	10	5	15	34	12	11	18	8
bME	29	March	6	17	25	16	3	10	16	19	4	14	3
cTSE	33	Aug.	15	12	29	27	11	32	24	19	29	21	19
Total	102		43	65	70	53	19	57	74	50	44	53	30

aMaasai-Mara Ecosystem; bMeru Ecosystem; cTsavo Ecosystem; dVNT assay did not detect any antibodies against FMDV serotypes O, A, C and SAT 3. ePositive for both SAT 1 and SAT 2.

Determination of VP1 coding region sequences

A total of 23 FMDV VP1 coding region sequences were successfully generated in this study (Table 1). These comprised two buffalo sequences (generated after VI) and 21 cattle sequences (directly sequenced from epithelial suspensions without VI). The buffalo sequences were identified as FMDV SAT 1 and SAT 2 originating from TSE and MME, respectively, while the 21 cattle sequences were identified as O (1), A (7), SAT 1 (3) or SAT 2 (10). The serotype identification, based on the sequence comparison (using BLAST), of samples from both species corresponded to the Ag-ELISA results. The cattle viruses originated from various parts of the country and for the purpose of this study, only the 3 serotype SAT 1 and the 10 SAT 2 cattle sequences were included in the phylogenetic analysis presented here, while the serotype O and A sequences were analysed elsewhere [41,47] (Table 1).

Statistical analysis and interpretation of FMDV prevalences in buffalo

The overall prevalence of antibodies against FMDV in buffalo as determined from the NSP assays was 64%, and the detection of FMDV RNA in probang samples by 3D RT-qPCR was 42%. Thirty seven of the 43 (86%) animals with FMDV RNA in the pharynx also had antibodies against FMDV NSPs, while six buffalo had FMDV RNA in their pharynx without being antibody positive and 28 buffalo had antibodies against NSP without FMDV RNA in the pharynx (data not shown). The two positive buffalo isolates came from animals that had RNA in the pharynx, had antibodies against NSPs and were sero-positive (on VNT assay) for the same serotypes (SAT 1 and SAT 2) of virus.

VP1 coding sequence analysis in this study

A total of 73 FMDV SAT 1 and 75 SAT 2 VP1 coding sequences (including the 15 SAT 1 and SAT 2 FMDV sequences generated in this study) were analysed in combination with sequences derived from other FMDVs originating in Kenya, other countries in eastern Africa and also other regions of Africa that were available from Genbank and WRLFMD (see Additional file 1: Table S1 and Additional file 2: Table S2). The estimated phylogenetic trees, using the Neighbor-Joining method, for the SAT 1 and SAT 2 virus sequences are shown in Figures 2 and 3 respectively.

The four SAT 1 VP1 coding sequences generated in this study comprised one (KenTSE1/2012) that was collected from a buffalo in TSE in Taita district, coast province, and three that were collected from cattle in different areas, namely Taita-Taveta (K127/2011), Laikipia in Rift Valley province (K56/2010) and Meru in Eastern Province (K159/2012) (Table 1, Figures 1 and 2). The

2012 buffalo isolate (KenTSE1/2012) clustered within the same topotype (I-NWZ) as both recent and older FMDV cattle isolates from Kenya but belonged to a separate, independently evolving lineage, from the cattle isolates (Figure 2). However, it shared a recent common ancestor with some recent Kenyan cattle viruses including K159/2012, K56/2010 and some of the 2009 group of viruses. Within the VP1 coding sequences, the buffalo KenTSE1/2012 isolate had 11%, 10% and 9% nt difference from these recent Kenyan cattle virus sequences, respectively. In addition, KenTSE1/2012 had 10% and 13% nt difference from the isolate found in cattle in the same district (Taita) (K127/2011) and from the current vaccine strain (T155/1971), respectively. This buffalo isolate also had >10% nt difference from the other cattle viruses collected in 2010-2011 from various districts in various regions of the country (data not shown). It is also noteworthy that these recent SAT 1 cattle sequences clustered within a separate lineage from the current vaccine strain. When compared to other African buffalo derived FMDV sequences, it was apparent that the KenTSE1/2012 belonged to a separate topotype (I-NWZ) (Figure 2). This isolate had 27% nt difference from the 2007 buffalo isolate from neighbouring Uganda (UGA/1/2007), 23% nt difference from the 1990 buffalo isolates from Zimbabwe (ZIM/3/1990 and ZIM/13/1990) and 24% nt difference from those collected in Kruger National Park (KNP/148/1991 and KNP/41/1995) in South Africa (data not shown).

The SAT 2 VP1 coding sequences included 11 sequences generated in this study (Table 1). These comprised 10 cattle sequences from various regions of the country and one buffalo sequence (KenMMB37/2012) from MME in Narok district of the Rift Valley province. The buffalo isolate grouped within the same topotype (IV) as some Tanzanian cattle viruses from 2004 and the Kenyan cattle viruses, including the viruses from 2004-2005 and 2007-2008, but has evolved as an independent lineage (Figure 3). Moreover, this Kenyan buffalo isolate also belonged to a different lineage from the current vaccine strain (SAT 2 K52/1984) (Figure 3) with 14% nt difference (data not shown) in this part of the genome. Comparisons of this buffalo isolate with the recent 2011-2012 cattle viruses showed >13% nt difference. It was also notable that, these recent SAT 2 cattle isolates clustered within a separate lineage (within topotype IV) than the current vaccine strain (Figure 3). Compared to the other buffalo sequences in eastern Africa, KenMMB 37/2012 belonged to a different topotype (IV) and had on average >21% nt difference from the recent buffalo SAT 2 Ugandan viruses (UGA/1/2007 and UGA/2/2007) that grouped within East Africa topotype X (Figure 3). Similarly, this Kenyan buffalo SAT 2 virus belonged to a different topotype from the 1998 viruses from Botswana

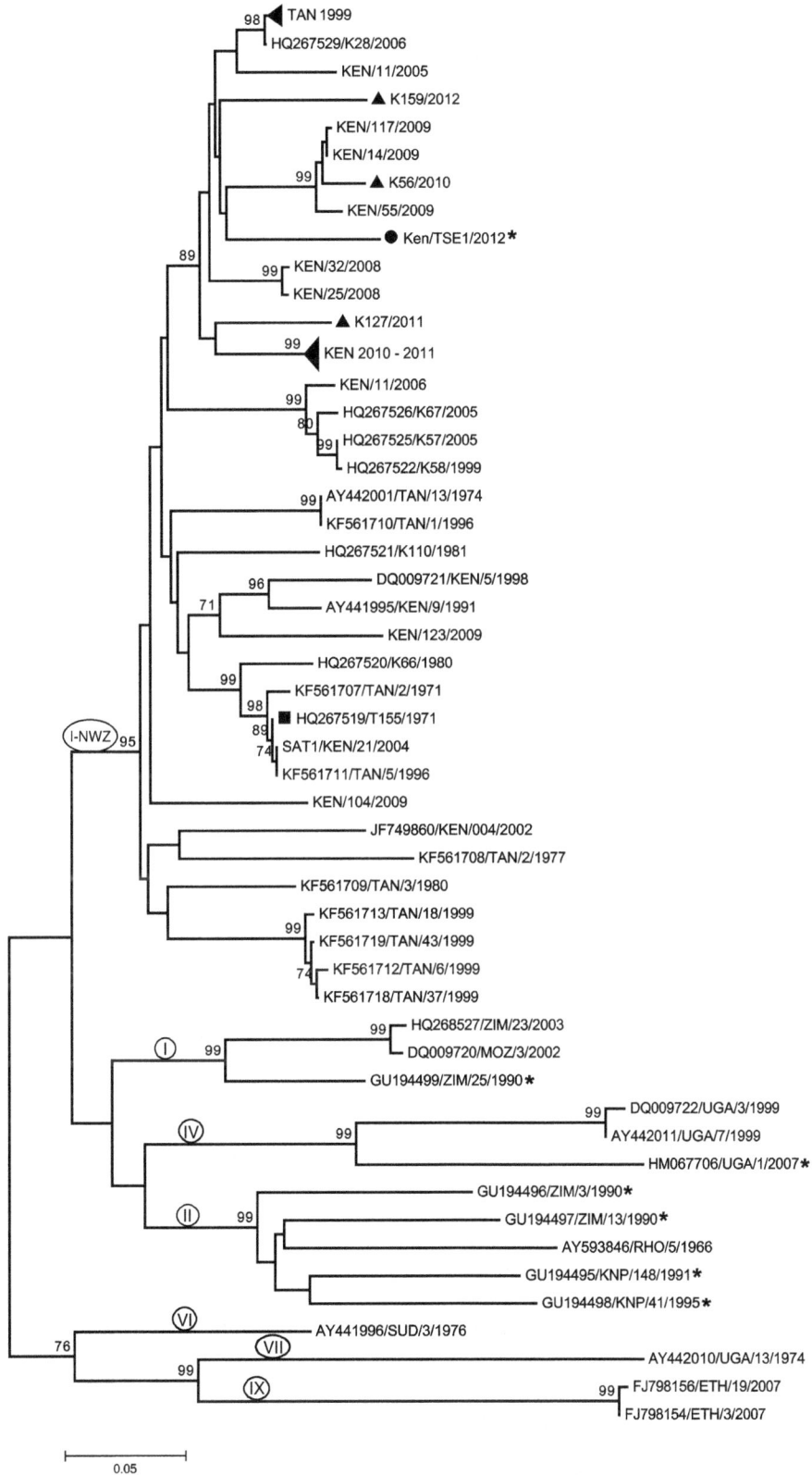

Figure 2 (See legend on next page.)

(See figure on previous page.)
Figure 2 Neighbor-Joining tree depicting one Kenyan foot-and-mouth disease virus (FMDV) SAT 1 buffalo sequence from this study (•) compared to recent SAT 1 Kenyan cattle sequences from this study (▲) and from World Reference Laboratory for FMD (WRLFMD) (◄); recent Ugandan buffalo sequence (UGA/1/2007); the current Kenyan vaccine strain (■); older Kenyan cattle sequences from WRLFMD (with prefix "KEN") and Genbank; and selected cattle and buffalo sequences from eastern and southern Africa obtained from GenBank and listed in the Additional file 1: Table S1. Sequences from buffalo species are marked with an asterisk (*). Only Bootstrap test values above 70 are shown on the branches. Topotypes are indicated on the branches by the prefix I-NWZ for one topotype and by Roman numbers for the rest.

and the 1991-1995 South African (KNP) group of viruses and had on average, 20-30% nt differences from these viruses (data not shown).

Discussion

This study has characterised and compared FMDVs that have recently infected buffalo and cattle in Kenya using a combination of assays. The PrioCHECK® FMDV NS ELISA demonstrated an overall seroprevalence of antibodies against FMDV NSPs of 64% in the studied Kenyan buffalo populations, which is comparable to the 68 % recorded by [25] in buffalo in eastern Africa but lower than the 74% and 85% reported in Ugandan buffalo in 2001-2003 and 2005-2008, respectively [15,27]. For comparison, the seroprevalence in Kenyan cattle in 2010 was 52.5% [48]. The NSP antibody seroprevalence varied between the three investigated ecosystems, with the highest recorded in MME followed by ME and lastly TSE; this is comparable to the reported variation in buffalo NSP antibody seroprevalence between Ugandan national parks [15,27].

Serotype-specific LPBE identified high titres (≥90) of antibodies against each of the six FMDV serotypes tested for, however, essentially only the antibodies against FMDV SAT 1 and SAT 2 were confirmed by VNT, suggesting high levels of cross-reactions in the commercial LPBE assay that was used. Such cross-reactions have been experienced using other serotype-specific antibody ELISAs in buffalo populations in Uganda [15,27] and in eastern Africa [25], as well as with sera from FMDV infected cattle with fresh or healing lesions (1-14 days after infection) [41,49]. However, clearer results have been obtained using SPBE in domestic ruminants sampled 2-4 months after infection [38,49] and in pigs sampled during an outbreak of SAT 1 in Kenya [23]. Moreover, since individual buffalo and buffalo herds are known to carry and maintain FMDV infections for a long time [11], it is likely that they are continuously exposed to FMDVs, resulting in the existence of animals with multiple previous infections by the virus. Therefore, high levels of cross-reactivity are to be expected due to boosting of antibodies against shared epitopes between the serotypes [50]. Consequently, the serotype-specific ELISAs may not be expected to give clear results in free-ranging African

buffalo, underpinning the necessity of collecting and sequencing the circulating FMDVs from this species [26,41].

It is noteworthy that none of the sampled buffalo in this study had clinical signs suggestive of FMD, despite the fact that 42% (based on Ct ≤32) of the probang samples were positive for FMDV RNA by RT-qPCR. Furthermore, SAT 1 and SAT 2 FMDVs were each isolated from buffalo probang samples. This is not surprising because infection in African buffalo with FMDV has been known to be largely sub-clinical [8]; thus our results concur with previous studies in the region [15,27] and with three experimental infection studies in buffalo [51-53].

In this study, we isolated and characterised two FMD viruses, one SAT 1 and one SAT 2, from buffalo probang samples, while serotypes O (1), A (7), SAT 1 (3) and SAT 2 (10) FMDVs, respectively, were characterised directly from epithelial samples from acutely infected cattle from different regions of Kenya. These findings agree with previous reports that have found these four serotypes in circulation in Kenyan cattle [4] and confirm the continued presence of multiple serotypes of FMDV in Kenya since FMD was first diagnosed in 1932 [43]. In addition, the study also found that the recent SAT 1 and SAT 2 FMDVs in cattle and buffalo were divergent from the current vaccine strains, consistent with findings for serotypes O and A [41,47]. This finding raises concerns regarding the effectiveness of currently available vaccine strains against circulating viruses, suggesting the need for vaccine matching.

Among the SAT serotypes, the occurrence of SAT 3 FMDV has been mainly associated with buffalo and neutralising antibodies against SAT 3 have previously been demonstrated (albeit in lower proportions than the other SATs) in buffalo populations in Kenya [25], while in neighbouring Uganda both antibodies [15,26,27] and virus [26] have been reported in buffalo. Furthermore, the presence of SAT 3 virus in a long horned Ankole calf in Uganda has recently been reported for the first time [5]. Interestingly, the current study did not find SAT 3 FMDV or neutralising antibodies against SAT 3 (by VNT), neither among cattle nor within the buffalo populations in the three ecosystems studied within Kenya. These findings are consistent with reports from the WRLFMD [43] and records at the FMDL, Embakasi, that FMDV SAT 3 has

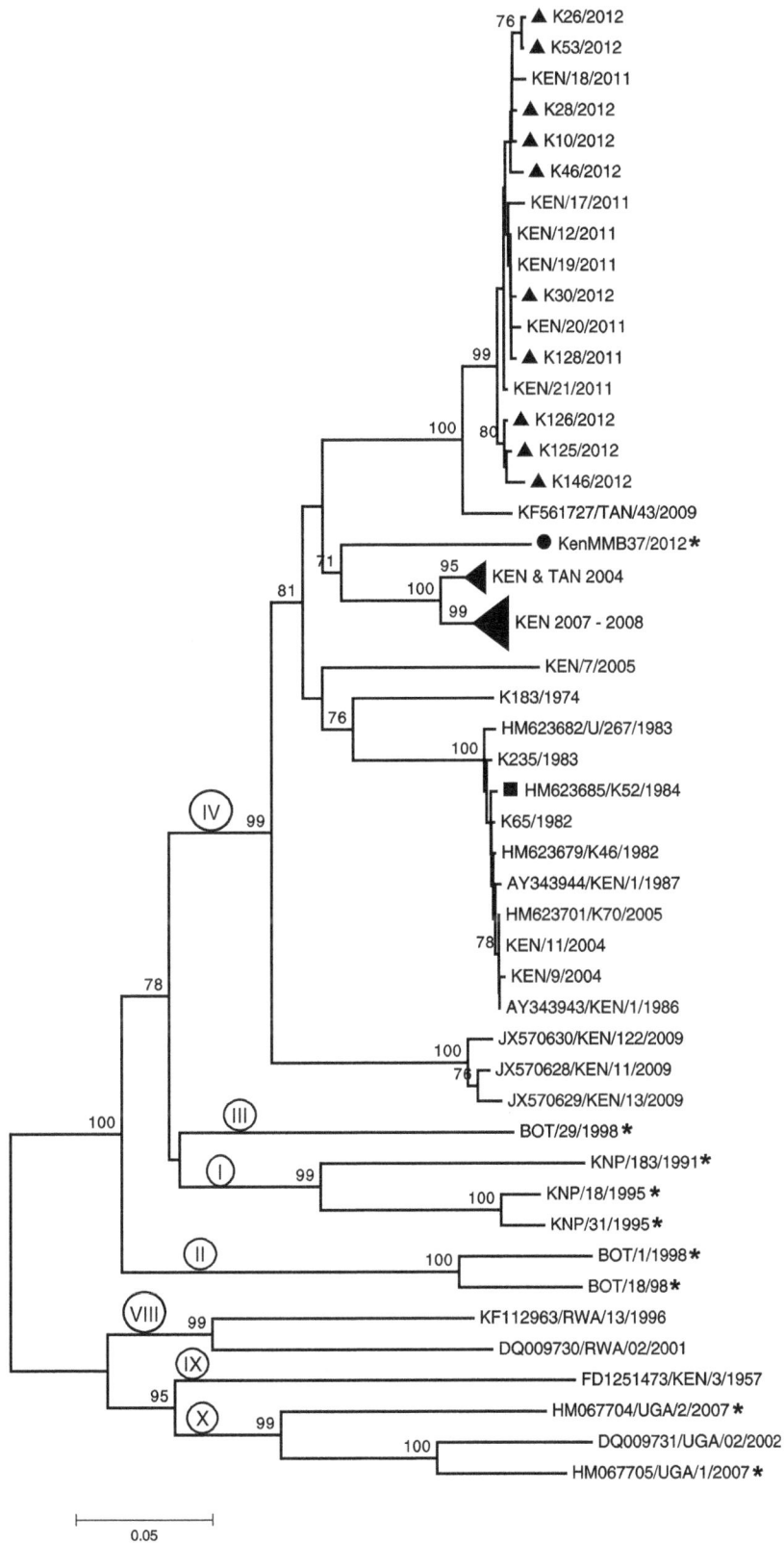

Figure 3 (See legend on next page.)

(See figure on previous page.)
Figure 3 Neighbor-Joining tree showing one Kenyan foot-and-mouth disease virus (FMDV) SAT 2 buffalo sequence from this study (●) compared to recent SAT 2 Kenyan cattle sequences obtained in this study (▲) and from World Reference Laboratory for FMD (WRLFMD) (With the prefix "KEN"); recent buffalo sequences from Uganda (UGA/1/2007 and UGA/2/2007); the current Kenyan vaccine strain (■); older Kenyan cattle sequences from WRLFMD (◄) and from Genbank; and cattle and buffalo sequences from eastern Africa and southern Africa obtained from GenBank and listed in the Additional file 2: Table S2. Sequences from buffalo species are marked with an asterisk (*). Only Bootstrap test values above 70 are shown on the branches. Topotypes are indicated by Roman numbers on the branches.

never been detected in Kenya. Similarly, there was no evidence for the presence of serotype C in either buffalo or cattle. This serotype has not been isolated in Kenya since 2004 [54], although some serological evidence (subject to the caveats about antibody ELISA cross-reactivity) for exposure to this serotype has been found recently among cattle in Kenya [55], buffalo in neighbouring Uganda [27] and regionally among cattle in Eritrea [56] and Ethiopia [57]. There is a need for wider and more comprehensive studies among all FMDV susceptible species to verify the absence of these two serotypes in the country, considering the widespread movement of livestock and wildlife within and across national borders.

FMDV isolation, antigen detection ELISA and sequencing have been commonly performed on cattle samples in Kenya but rarely in other susceptible species (wildlife included) as is evident from the records of the FMDL, Embakasi, the WRLFMD [43] and from a recent study [23]. In the present study, the antigen ELISA and sequencing were fully consistent with each other. Taken together with the serological data, this study provided evidence that FMDV serotypes SAT 1 and SAT 2 are in circulation within the three buffalo ecosystems studied. This finding is consistent with an earlier field survey in 1979 among buffalo in MME and cattle around this ecosystem which isolated FMDV SAT 1 and SAT 2 from buffalo [24].

Guided by the principles published for SAT viruses that nt differences >20% define separate topotypes [58], this study found that although the SAT 1 buffalo virus identified in this study clustered within the same topotype (I-NWZ) as both recent and older FMDV isolates from Kenya, it belonged to a separate independently evolving lineage. Interestingly, even one virus (K127/2011) from cattle in the same district (Taita-Taveta) as the SAT 1 buffalo isolate did not group within the same lineage. However, the phylogenetic tree also showed that although this buffalo virus has been evolving independently from the cattle viruses, they originated from a common ancestor (Figure 2), suggestive of an ancestral species jump [10]. A similar trend was observed with the SAT 2 buffalo isolate KenMMB37/2012 collected from MME that belonged to the same topotype (IV) as both recent and earlier SAT 2 Kenyan cattle viruses but had ≥13% nt difference from them, including a recent

virus from Narok district (K126/2012) in which MME is located (Figure 3).

These findings (albeit with a very small number of buffalo viruses) are consistent with the idea that there may be largely independent cycles of FMDV circulations in Kenya; one that occurs within buffalo populations and another within livestock populations, concurring with earlier observations indicating that eastern Africa may be experiencing these separate FMDV cycles [59]. This idea is also consistent with the absence of evidence from the current study of other serotypes circulating among buffalo populations either from virological or serological assays, yet serotypes O and A were frequently found in cattle.

The findings in this study contribute to the debate of whether FMD is mainly a disease of livestock in endemic Africa [17]. On the one hand, natural transmission from buffalo to livestock has been demonstrated in Zimbabwe [60,61] and South Africa [9], on the other hand, the real risks posed by carrier animals to susceptible hosts have not been adequately quantified [62]. However, the results presented here indicate that although other serotypes (O and A), together with SAT 1 and SAT 2 FMDVs are constantly circulating in Kenyan cattle, buffalo mainly harbour SAT serotypes. The current Kenyan findings are in agreement with previous studies in eastern Africa [24,25,27] and consistent with wildlife playing a limited role in the epidemiology of FMD in cattle in eastern Africa. However, owing to the limited number of buffalo viruses in our data set, it is not possible to draw firm conclusions.

Conclusions

This study found that four serotypes of FMDV (O, A, SAT 1 and SAT 2) circulate among cattle in different regions of Kenya. Buffalo species were found to harbour SAT 1 and SAT 2 serotypes with no virological or serological evidence for other serotypes. Moreover, there was no evidence for the recent occurrence of serotypes C and SAT 3 in cattle or buffalo. The identified African buffalo virus lineages in the wild have apparently evolved separately from lineages found in livestock in Kenya and in the region. Hence, FMD control in Kenya should primarily focus on reducing the high virus burden among livestock and subsequently limit the association of livestock with wildlife. However, due to the limited data in this study, there is need for more comprehensive research incorporating a larger number of buffalo viruses and deeper analysis including evolutionary tracking of the origins of the viruses to determine the role of buffalo in the epidemiology of this disease.

Additional files

Additional file 1: Table S1. List of 73 foot-and-mouth disease virus (FMDV) SAT 1 sequences included in the phylogenetic tree in Figure 2 of this study.

Additional file 2: Table S2. List of 75 foot-and-mouth disease viruse (FMDV) SAT 2 sequences included in the phylogenetic tree in Figure 3 of this study.

Competing interests
The authors declare that they have no competing interests.

Authors' contributions
SNW, AKS, HRS, GJB, VBM, KT conceived and designed the study. SNW, AKS, FG and DM planned and carried out the sampling. AKS, GJB and KT supervised the laboratory work. SNW was responsible for laboratory analyses, data analysis, manuscript preparation, revisions and submission. AKS, HRS, GJB, VM, KT, FG oversaw the data analysis and critically reviewed the manuscript. All authors read and approved the final manuscript.

Acknowledgements
This work was funded by the Danish International Development Agency (DANIDA) under the TADEA project, DFC no. 10-006KU. We thank the Directors of Veterinary Services Kenya and the Kenya Wildlife Services for enabling the acquisition of samples. We are grateful to Drs Mathew Mutinda and Jeremiah Poghon and to Vincent Obanda of KWS for their professional assistance in the capture and sampling of buffalo. Great appreciation also goes to Drs Kenneth Ketter and Eunice Chepkwony and to Teresia Kenduiywo, William Birgen, Joseph Kabugi and Salim Kiarie of FMDL, Embakasi, for their support in sample collection, transportation and preservation. Preben Normann, Inge Nielsen, Jane Borch and Jane Christiansen of DTU-VET Lindholm are thanked for their technical assistance. Special appreciation also goes to Drs Sheila Balinda, Alice Namatovu and Moses Dhikusooka for their support.

Author details
[1]Foot-and-Mouth Disease Laboratory, Embakasi, P. O. Box 18021 00500 Nairobi, Kenya. [2]Department of Environmental Management, College of Agricultural and Environmental Sciences, Makerere University, P. O. Box 7062/7298, Kampala, Uganda. [3]National Veterinary Institute, Technical University of Denmark, Lindholm DK-4771 Kalvehave, Denmark. [4]Kenya Wildlife Service, Veterinary Services Department, P.O Box 40241 (00100), Nairobi, Kenya. [5]Department of Biology, University of Copenhagen, Ole Maaløes Vej 5, DK-2200 Copenhagen, Denmark.

References
1. Alexandersen S, Mowat N. Foot-and-mouth disease: host range and pathogenesis. Curr Top Microbiol Immunol. 2005;288:9–42.
2. Kitching RP. Clinical variation in foot and mouth disease: cattle. Rev Sci Tech. 2002;21(3):499–504.
3. Paton DJ, Valarcher JF, Bergmann I, Matlho OG, Zakharov VM, Palma EL, et al. Selection of foot and mouth disease vaccine strains–a review. Rev Sci Tech. 2005;24(3):981–93.
4. FAO. OIE/FAO World Reference Laboratories Network annual report 2012. Found at http://www.fao.org/fileadmin/user_upload/eufmd/docs/Pirbright_reports/OIE-FAO_FMD_Reference_Laboratory_Network_report_2012__.pdf. Accessed 19th January 2015.
5. Dhikusooka MT, Tjørnehøj K, Ayebazibwe C, Namatovu A, Ruhweza S, Siegismund HR, et al. Foot-and-mouth disease virus serotype SAT 3 in long-horned Ankole calf, Uganda. Emerg Infect Dis. 2015;21(1):111–4.
6. Rweyemamu M, Roeder P, MacKay D, Sumption K, Brownlie J, Leforban Y. Planning for the progressive control of foot-and-mouth disease worldwide. Transbound Emerg Dis. 2008;55(1):73–87.
7. James AD, Rushton J. The economics of foot and mouth disease. Rev Sci Tech. 2002;21(3):637–44.
8. Thomson GR, Vosloo W, Bastos AD. Foot and mouth disease in wildlife. Virus Res. 2003;91(1):145–61.
9. Vosloo W, de Klerk LM, Boshoff CI, Botha B, Dwarka RM, Keet D, et al. Characterisation of a SAT-1 outbreak of foot-and-mouth disease in captive African buffalo (Syncerus caffer): clinical symptoms, genetic characterisation and phylogenetic comparison of outbreak isolates. Vet Microbiol. 2007;120(3–4):226–40.
10. Hall MD, Knowles NJ, Wadsworth J, Rambaut A, Woolhouse MEJ. Reconstructing geographical movements and host species transitions of foot-and-mouth disease virus serotype SAT 2 2013; mBio 4(5):e00591-13. doi:10.1128/mBio.00591-13
11. Condy JB, Hedger RS, Hamblin C, Barnett IT. The duration of the foot-and-mouth disease virus carrier state in African buffalo (i) in the individual animal and (ii) in a free-living herd. Comp Immunol Microbiol Infect Dis. 1985;8(3–4):259–65.
12. Zhang ZD, Kitching RP. The localization of persistent foot and mouth disease virus in the epithelial cells of the soft palate and pharynx. J Comp Pathol. 2001;124(2–3):89–94.
13. Thomson GR, Bastos ADS. Foot-and-mouth disease. In: Coetzer JAW, Tustin RC, editors. Infectious diseases of livestock. 2nd ed. South Africa: Oxford University Press; 2004. p. 1324–65.
14. Hedger R. Foot-and-mouth disease in wildlife with particular reference to the African buffalo (Syncerus caffer). London, England: Plenum Press; 1976.
15. Ayebazibwe C, Mwiine FN, Balinda SN, Tjornehoj K, Masembe C, Muwanika VB, et al. Antibodies against foot-and-mouth disease (FMD) virus in African buffalos (Syncerus caffer) in selected National Parks in Uganda (2001-2003). Transbound Emerg Dis. 2010;57(4):286–92.
16. Thomson GR, Penrith ML, Atkinson MW, Atkinson SJ, Cassidy D, Osofsky SA. Balancing livestock production and wildlife conservation in and around southern Africa's transfrontier conservation areas. Transbound Emerg Dis. 2013;60(6):492–506.
17. Weaver GV, Domenech J, Thiermann AR, Karesh WB. Foot and Mouth Disease: A look from the wild side. J Wild Dis. 2013;49(4):759–85.
18. Roeder PL. Opportunities and constraints posed by wildlife in the diagnosis and epidemiological analysis of foot and mouth disease virus infection. In: Proceedings from the first OIE/FAO Global Conference on foot-and-mouth disease: The way towards global control 24–26 June 2009; Asuncion, Paraguay, 24–26 June. Found at; http://www.oie.int/fileadmin/Home/fr/Conferences_Events/sites/F_FMD_2009/FMD_presentation/Session%202_2/2_2_5_Roeder.pdf. Accessed 17th February 2014.
19. Blench R (ed.). Can wildlife and livestock co-exist? An interdisciplinary approach. London: Overseas Development Institute. Found at http://www.academia.edu/3738307. Accessed 3rd Sept. 2013.
20. Picado A, Speybroeck N, Kivaria F, Mosha RM, Sumaye RD, Casal J, et al. Foot-and-mouth disease in Tanzania from 2001 to 2006. Transbound Emerg Dis. 2011;58(1):44–52.
21. Vosloo W, Thomson GR. Natural habitats in which foot-and-mouth disease virus is maintained. In: Domingo FSE, editor. "Foot-and-mouth disease, Current perspectives". Norfolk, UK: Horizon Bioscience; 2004. p. 383–410.
22. Anonymous. Livestock population by type and district: 2009 Kenya population and housing census. Kenya National Bureau of Statistics (KNBS) wwwknbsorke Accessed 28/11/2011.
23. Wekesa SN, Namatovu A, Sangula AK, Dhikusooka MT, Muwanika VB, Tjørnehøj K. A serological survey for foot-and-mouth disease (FMD) in domestic pigs during outbreaks in Kenya. Trop Anim Health Prod. 2014;46(3):575–81.
24. Anderson EC, Doughty WJ, Anderson J, Paling R. The pathogenesis of foot-and-mouth disease in the African buffalo (Syncerus caffer) and the role of this species in the epidemiology of the disease in Kenya. J Comp Pathol. 1979;89(4):541–9.
25. Bronsvoort BM, Parida S, Handel I, McFarland S, Fleming L, Hamblin P, et al. Serological survey for foot-and-mouth disease virus in wildlife in eastern Africa and estimation of test parameters of a nonstructural protein enzyme-

linked immunosorbent assay for buffalo. Clin Vaccine Immunol. 2008;15(6):1003–11.

26. Kalema-Zikusoka G, Bengis RG, Michel AL, Woodford MH. A preliminary investigation of tuberculosis and other diseases in African buffalo (*Syncerus caffer*) in Queen Elizabeth National Park, Uganda. Onderstepoort J Vet Res. 2005;72(2):145–51.

27. Ayebazibwe C, Mwiine FN, Tjornehoj K, Balinda SN, Muwanika VB, Ademun Okurut AR, et al. The role of African buffalos (*Syncerus caffer*) in the maintenance of foot-and-mouth disease in Uganda. BMC Vet Res. 2010;6:54.

28. Harthoorn A. The chemical capture of Animals. A guide to the chemical restraint of wild and captive animals. London: Tindall BA; 1976. p. 416.

29. How to age sheep, goats, cattle and buffalo: Found at http://www.fao.org/docrep/T0690E/t0690e05.htm#unit9. Accessed 6th Sept. 2013.

30. Anonymous. Foot and mouth disease. Chapter 2.1.5 in: OIE manual of diagnostic tests and vaccines for terrestrial animals. http://www.oie.int/fileadmin/Home/eng/Health_standards/tahm/2.01.05_FMD.pdf. Accessed 16 Feb 2015.

31. Hamblin C, Barnett IT, Hedger RS. A new enzyme-linked immunosorbent assay (ELISA) for the detection of antibodies against foot-and-mouth disease virus. I. Development and method of ELISA. J Immunol Methods. 1986;93(1):115–21.

32. Hamblin C, Barnett IT, Crowther JR. A new enzyme-linked immunosorbent assay (ELISA) for the detection of antibodies against foot-and-mouth disease virus. II. Application. J Immunol Methods. 1986;93(1):123–9.

33. Mackay DK, Bulut AN, Rendle T, Davidson F, Ferris NP. A solid-phase competition ELISA for measuring antibody to foot-and-mouth disease virus. J Virol Methods. 2001;97(1–2):33–48.

34. Reed LJ, Muench H. A simple method of estimating fifty per cent endpoints. Am J Epidemiol. 1938;27(3):493–7.

35. Cameron A. Survey Toolbox for Livestock Diseases – A Practical Manual and Software Package for Active Surveillance in Developing Countries. Canberra: Australian Centre for International Agricultural Research Monograph No. 54; 1999.

36. Callahan JD, Brown F, Osorio FA, Sur JH, Kramer E, Long GW, et al. Use of a portable real-time reverse transcriptase-polymerase chain reaction assay for rapid detection of foot-and-mouth disease virus. J Am Vet Med Assoc. 2002;220(11):1636–42.

37. Reid SM, Ferris NP, Hutchings GH, Zhang Z, Belsham GJ, Alexandersen S. Detection of all seven serotypes of foot-and-mouth disease virus by real-time, fluorogenic reverse transcription polymerase chain reaction assay. J Virol Methods. 2002;105:67–80.

38. Namatovu A, Belsham GJ, Ayebazibwe C, Dhikusooka MT, Wekesa SN, Siegismund HR, Muwanika VB, Tjørnehøj K. Challenges for serology-based characterization of foot-and-mouth disease outbreaks in endemic areas; Identification of two separate lineages of serotype O FMDV in Uganda in 2011. Transbound Emerg Dis DOI: 101111/tbed12170.

39. Mason PW, Pacheco JM, Zhao QZ, Knowles NJ. Comparisons of the complete genomes of Asian, African and European isolates of a recent foot-and-mouth disease virus type O pandemic strain (PanAsia). J Gen Virol. 2003;84(Pt 6):1583–93.

40. Sangula AK, Belsham GJ, Muwanika VB, Heller R, Balinda SN, Siegismund HR. Co-circulation of two extremely divergent serotype SAT 2 lineages in Kenya highlights challenges to foot-and-mouth disease control. Arch Virol. 2010;155(10):1625–30.

41. Wekesa SN, Muwanika VB, Siegismund HR, Sangula AK, Namatovu A, Dhikusooka MT, Tjørnehøj K, et al. Analysis of recent serotype O foot-and-mouth disease viruses from livestock in Kenya: evidence of four independently evolving lineages. Transbound Emerg Dis. 2013. doi:10.1111/tbed.12152.

42. Altschul SF, Gish W, Miller W, Myers EW, Lipman DJ. Basic local alignment search tool. J Mol Biol. 1990;215:403–10.

43. ME reports. 2013. World Reference Laboratory for Foot-and-Mouth Disease. Genotyping report for Africa [http://www.wrlfmd.org/fmd_genotyping/africa.html. Accessed 10th August 2013].

44. Edgar RC. MUSCLE: a multiple sequence alignment method with reduced time and space complexity. BMC Bioinformatics 2004, 5:113 doi:10.1186/1471-2105-5-113

45. Tamura KPD. Peterson N., Stecher G., Nei M., S. K: MEGA5: Molecular evolutionary genetics analysis using maximum likelihood, evolutionary distance, and maximum parsimony methods. Mol Biol Evol. 2011;28(10):2731–9.

46. Felsenstein J. Confidence limits on phylogenies: An approach using the bootstrap. Evolution. 1985;39:783–91.

47. Wekesa SN, Sangula AK, Belsham GJ, Muwanika VB, Heller R, Balinda SN, et al. Genetic diversity of serotype A foot-and-mouth disease viruses in Kenya from 1964 to 2013; implications for control strategies in eastern Africa. Infect Genet Evol. 2014;21:408–17.

48. Kibore B, Gitao CG, Sangula A, Kitala P. Foot and mouth disease sero-prevalence in cattle in Kenya. J Vet Med Anim Health. 2013;5(9):262–8.

49. Mwiine FN, Ayebazibwe C, Olaho-Mukani W, Alexandersen S, Balinda SN, Masembe C, et al. Serotype specificity of antibodies against foot-and-mouth disease virus in cattle in selected districts in Uganda. Transbound Emerg Dis. 2010;57(5):365–74.

50. Hedger RS, Barnett ITR, Gradwell DV, Travassos Dias P. Serological tests for foot-and-mouth disease in bovine serum samples. Problems of interpretation. Rev sci tech Off int Epiz. 1982;1(2):387–93.

51. Ferris NP, Condy JB, Barnett IT, Armstrong RM. Experimental infection of eland (*Taurotrages oryx*), sable antelope (*Ozanna grandicomis*) and buffalo (*Syncerus caffer*) with foot-and-mouth disease virus. J Comp Pathol. 1989;101(3):307–16.

52. Dawe PS, Sorensen K, Ferris NP, Barnett IT, Armstrong RM, Knowles NJ. Experimental transmission of foot-and-mouth disease virus from carrier African buffalo (*Syncerus caffer*) to cattle in Zimbabwe. Vet Rec. 1994;134(9):211–5.

53. Vosloo W, Bastos AD, Kirkbride E, Esterhuysen JJ, van Rensburg DJ, Bengis RG, et al. Persistent infection of African buffalo (*Syncerus caffer*) with SAT-type foot-and-mouth disease viruses: rate of fixation of mutations, antigenic change and interspecies transmission. J Gen Virol. 1996;77(Pt 7):1457–67.

54. Sangula AK, Siegismund HR, Belsham GJ, Balinda SN, Masembe C, Muwanika VB. Low diversity of foot-and-mouth disease serotype C virus in Kenya: evidence for probable vaccine strain re-introductions in the field. Epidemiol Infect. 2011;139(2):189–96.

55. Chepkwony EC, Gitao CG, Muchemi GM. Seroprevalence of foot-and-mouth disease in the Somali eco-system in Kenya. J Anim Vet Adv. 2012;4(3):198–203.

56. Tekleghiorghis T, Moormann RJ, Weerdmeester K, Dekker A. Serological evidence indicates that foot-and-mouth disease virus serotype O, C and SAT1 are most dominant in Eritrea Transbound Emerg Dis. doi:10.1111/tbed12065.

57. Rufael T, Catley A, Bogale A, Sahle M, Shiferaw Y. Foot and mouth disease in the Borana pastoral system, southern Ethiopia and implications for livelihoods and international trade. Trop Anim Health Prod. 2008;40(1):29–38.

58. Knowles NJ, Samuel AR. Molecular epidemiology of foot-and-mouth disease virus. Virus Res. 2003;91(1):65–80.

59. Vosloo W, Bastos AD, Sahle M, Sangare O, Dwarka RM. Virus topotypes and the role of wildlife in foot and mouth disease in Africa. In: Osofsky SA CS, Karesh WB, Kock MD, Nyhus PJ, Starr L, Yang A, editors. Conservation and development interventions at the wildlife/livestock interface: Implications for wildlife, livestock and human health. Gland, Switzerland and Cambridge, UK: IUCN; 2005. p. 67–80.

60. Dawe PS, Flanagan FO, Madekurozwa RL, Sorensen KJ, Anderson EC, Foggin CM, et al. Natural transmission of foot-and-mouth disease virus from African buffalo (*Syncerus caffer*) to cattle in a wildlife area of Zimbabwe. Vet Rec. 1994;134(10):230–2.

61. Miguel E, Grosbois V, Caron A, Boulinier T, Fritz H, Cornélis D, et al. Contacts and foot and mouth disease transmission from wild to domestic bovines in Africa. Ecosphere. 2013;4(4):51. http://www.esajournals.org/doi/pdf/10.1890/ES12-00239.1.

62. Tenzin, Dekker A, Vernooij H, Bouma A, Stegeman A. Rate of foot-and-mouth disease virus transmission by carriers quantified from experimental data. Risk Anal. 2008;28(2):303–9.

9

Effects of ribavirin on the replication and genetic stability of porcine reproductive and respiratory syndrome virus

Amina Khatun[1], Nadeem Shabir[1], Kyoung-Jin Yoon[2] and Won-Il Kim[1*]

Abstract

Background: Although modified live virus (MLV) vaccines are commonly used for porcine reproductive and respiratory syndrome virus (PRRSV) control, there have been safety concerns due to the quick reversion of MLV to virulence during replication in pigs. Previous studies have demonstrated that mutant viruses emerged from lethal mutagenesis driven by antiviral mutagens and that those viruses had higher genetic stability compared to their parental strains because they acquired resistance to random mutation. Thus, this strategy was explored to stabilize the PRRSV genome in the current study.

Results: Four antiviral mutagens (ribavirin, 5-fluorouracil, 5-azacytidine, and amiloride) were evaluated for their antiviral effects against VR2332, a prototype of type 2 PRRSV. Among the mutagens, ribavirin and 5-fluorouracil had significant antiviral effects against VR2332. Consequently, VR2332 was serially passaged in MARC-145 cells in the presence of ribavirin at several concentrations to facilitate the emergence of ribavirin-resistant mutants. Two ribavirin-resistant mutants, RVRp13 and RVRp22, emerged from serial passages in the presence of 0.1 and 0.2 mM ribavirin, respectively. The genetic stability of these resistant mutants was evaluated in MARC-145 cells and compared with VR2332. As expected, the ribavirin-resistant mutants exhibited higher genetic stability compared to their parental virus.

Conclusions: In summary, ribavirin and 5-fluorouracil effectively suppressed PRRSV replication in MARC-145 cells. However, ribavirin-resistant mutants emerged when treated with low concentrations ($\leq$0.2 mM) of ribavirin, and those mutants were genetically more stable during serial passages in cell culture.

Keywords: PRRS, Ribavirin, 5-Fluorouracil, 5-Azacytidine and Amiloride

Background

Porcine Reproductive and Respiratory Syndrome (PRRS) is one of the most economically important infectious diseases of swine worldwide. The annual loss associated with PRRS to the United States swine industry has been estimated to be approximately 664 million USD [1]. PRRS virus (PRRSV), the etiological agent of PRRS, is classified as a member of the *Arteriviridae* virus family, along with equine arteritis virus (EAV), lactate dehydrogenase-elevating virus (LDV) of mice, and simian hemorrhagic fever virus (SHFV), and belongs to the order *Nidovirales* [2,3]. PRRSV is a small, enveloped virus that contains a single-stranded, non-segmented, positive-sense RNA genome approximately 15 kb in length. The PRRSV genome encodes at least ten open reading frames (ORFs) designated as ORF1a, ORF1b, ORF2a, ORF2b, ORF3, ORF4, ORF5a, ORF5, ORF6, and ORF7 [4-8]. Because PRRSV evolves very quickly [9,10], there is a great deal of genetic variability among PRRSV strains. In general, PRRSV strains are grouped into European (type 1) and North American (type 2) genotypes [11-13], but high levels of genetic variability still exist among viruses, even within the same genotype [10,14,15], which results in suboptimal cross-protection between different PRRSV strains and becomes a significant impediment to the development of effective vaccines. Modified live virus (MLV) vaccines have been most commonly used to control PRRSV because they confer better protection against homologous virus strains compared to inactivated or recombinant vaccines [16]. However, there have been

* Correspondence: kwi0621@jbnu.ac.kr
[1]College of Veterinary Medicine, Chonbuk National University Jeonju, Korea, 664-14 Deokjin-Dong 1 Ga, Jeonju, Jeonbuk 561-756, Republic of Korea
Full list of author information is available at the end of the article

serious safety concerns about using these MLV vaccines because they quickly revert to virulence during serial passages in pigs [17-21]. Therefore, it is important to develop a new strategy to stabilize the PRRSV genome during virus replication for the purpose of vaccine safety.

Previously, a number of nucleoside analogs, including ribavirin (guanosine analog) [22,23], 5-fluorouracil (pyrimidine analog) [24], and 5-azacytidine (cytidine analog) [25], have been shown to be mutagenic, antiviral compounds that are effective against various RNA viruses, such as foot-and-mouth disease virus (FMDV), poliovirus, and hepatitis C virus (HCV). These mutagens increase the mutation frequency of RNA viruses above a tolerable error threshold during replication, ultimately driving viral infection into extinction [26-35]. Amiloride hydrochloride hydrate (hereafter "amiloride") is another antiviral drug with efficacy against many RNA viruses, including rhinovirus, coxsackievirus B3 (CVB3), coronaviruses, flaviviruses, and retroviruses [36-40]. Moreover, it has been demonstrated that amiloride increases the mutation frequency of RNA viruses, in addition to its other antiviral activities [41]. It has also been demonstrated that mutant viruses that emerged following sequential passages of HCV, CVB3, poliovirus, and FMDV [41-44] in the presence of ribavirin had higher genetic stability than wild-type viruses. Therefore, this strategy was employed to select a mutagen-resistant strain of PRRSV that would have higher genetic stability. In the current study, the effects of four mutagens (ribavirin, 5-fluorouracil, 5-azacytidine, and amiloride) on PRRSV replication in MARC-145 cells were evaluated to select the mutagen that is most effective against PRRSV. Then, mutagen-resistant viruses were rescued after sequential passages in the presence of the mutagen and were evaluated for their genetic stability during additional sequential passages in cell culture systems.

Methods
Antiviral mutagens
Ribavirin (Sigma-Aldrich, St. Louis, MO, USA), 5-fluorouracil (Sigma-Aldrich), 5-azacytidine (Sigma-Aldrich), and amiloride (Sigma-Aldrich) were used in this study. All of these mutagens were dissolved in RPMI-1640 medium (Sigma-Aldrich) at stock concentrations of 15 mM (ribavirin) and 20 mM (5-fluorouracil, 5-azacytidine, and amiloride), sterile-filtered using a 0.22-μm syringe filter, aliquoted, and stored at –20°C until use.

Virus and cell culture
VR2332, a prototype strain of PRRSV type 2, was used in the study. MARC-145, an African Green Monkey kidney cell line highly permissive to PRRSV infection, was used for PRRSV propagation and antiviral assays. MARC-145 cells were maintained in RPMI-1640

medium supplemented with heat-inactivated 10% fetal bovine serum (FBS, Invitrogen, Carlsbad, CA, USA), 2 mM L-glutamine, and 100× antibiotic-antimycotic solution [Anti-anti, Invitrogen; 1× solution contains 100 IU/ml penicillin, 100 μg/ml streptomycin, and 0.25 μg/ml Fungizone® (amphotericin B)] (hereafter referred to as "RPMI growth medium") at 37°C in a humidified 5% CO_2 atmosphere.

Evaluation of effects of mutagens on PRRSV replication
Confluent monolayers of MARC-145 cells were prepared in 25-cm^2 flasks and were inoculated with VR2332 at a multiplicity of infection (MOI) of 0.01. After incubation for 1 hour in a humidified 5% CO_2 incubator at 37°C, the virus inoculum was removed, and the cell monolayer was replenished with RPMI growth medium containing one of the antiviral mutagens. Ribavirin, 5-fluorouracil, and amiloride were evaluated at six different concentrations (0, 0.2, 0.4, 0.6, 0.8, and 1 mM), while 5-azacytidine was evaluated at ten different concentrations (0, 0.0001, 0.001, 0.01, 0.1, 0.2, 0.4, 0.6, 0.8, and 1 mM), based on previous reports [45,46]. The treated flasks were then incubated for four more days under the same culture conditions described above, during which time cell culture medium was collected from each flask every 24 hours, centrifuged, and stored at –80°C until analysis.

Virus titration assay
Progeny virus titers were determined using a microtitration infectivity assay [47]. In brief, up to 8, 10-fold serial dilutions of samples were prepared. Confluent monolayers of MARC-145 cells prepared in 96-well plates were inoculated in quadruplicate with 100 μl of each sample and were incubated for 1 hour under the same culture conditions described above. After incubation, the inoculum was discarded, and the cell monolayer was replenished with RPMI growth medium. The plates were then incubated for an additional six days and monitored for cytopathic effects (CPE) daily. The titer of each virus sample was calculated based on CPE and was expressed as a 50% tissue culture infective dose $(TCID_{50})$/ml [48].

Cytotoxicity assay
A commercially available cytotoxicity assay kit (CytoTox-Glo™, Promega, Fitchburg, Wisconsin, USA) was used to assess the cytotoxic effects of the four antiviral mutagens in MARC-145 cells. In short, the CytoTox-Glo™ assay measures a distinct protease (dead-cell protease) activity associated with cytotoxicity [49]. The assay uses a luminogenic peptide substrate (alanyl-alanylphenylalanyl-aminoluciferin; AAF-Glo™ substrate) to measure the activity of dead-cell protease released from cells that have lost membrane integrity. To determine the cytotoxicities of the mutagens, confluent monolayers of

MARC-145 cells were prepared in 25-cm^2 flasks. After rinsing, the cells were replenished with RPMI growth medium containing one of the mutagens at one of four different concentrations (0, 0.5, 1, and 1.5 mM) and further incubated under the culture conditions described above. Supernatants were collected from each flask every 12 hours for up to 48 hours, and the levels of luminescence (RLU) generated from the cleavage of luminogenic AAF-Glo™ substrate by protease in the collected supernatants were measured to determine the cytotoxicity levels induced by each mutagen according to the manufacturer's instructions.

Serial passages of PRRSV in MARC-145 cells in the presence of ribavirin

VR2332 was serially passaged in cell culture in the presence of 0, 0.05, 0.1, 0.2, 0.3, 0.5, or 0.7 mM ribavirin to study the emergence of ribavirin-resistant PRRSV mutants. Confluent monolayers of MARC-145 cells were prepared in 6-well plates and pre-treated with RPMI growth medium containing ribavirin for 7 hours prior to infection at 37°C. After the pre-treatment incubation, cells were inoculated with VR2332 at an MOI of 0.01. After incubation for 1 hour, virus inoculum was removed, and cells were replenished with RPMI growth medium containing the same concentrations of ribavirin as described above for post-treatment. The infection was then allowed to proceed for 24 hours, after which the cell culture fluid was collected from each well, centrifuged, and stored at −80°C until use. The supernatant from each passage became the inoculum for the next passage. This procedure was repeated a total of 22 times.

Assessment of growth kinetics for ribavirin-resistant mutants in the presence of ribavirin at several concentrations using multi-step growth curve analysis

The growth competencies of two ribavirin-resistant candidate mutants (RVRp13 and RVRp22) were assessed in MARC-145 cells in the presence of ribavirin, compared to VR2332 in the presence of ribavirin. Confluent monolayers of MARC-145 cells were prepared in 25-cm^2 flasks, inoculated with each virus at an MOI of 0.01, and incubated for 1 hour under the same conditions described above. After incubation, the inoculum was discarded, and cells were replenished with RPMI-1640 growth medium containing several concentrations (0, 0.1, 0.2, 0.3, 0.4, and 0.5 mM) of ribavirin. The treated flasks were then incubated for 4 more days. Supernatants were collected from each flask every 24 hours, and the virus in these supernatants was titered.

Assessment of genetic stability of ribavirin-resistant mutants during passages in MARC-145 cells

To assess the genetic stability of the ribavirin-resistant mutants (RVRp13 and RVRp22) that arose from

sequential passages of VR2332 in the presence of ribavirin as described above, the mutant viruses were passaged 10 more times, along with VR2332. Plaque purification was performed using each strain to achieve a highly homogenous virus clone, as described previously [17]. For each passage, confluent MARC-145 cell monolayer prepared in 6-well plates were inoculated with each virus strain and incubated for 1 hour. After incubation, the cells were replenished with RPMI growth medium and incubated for 24 hours. Then, supernatants were collected and used for the next passage of cells. This procedure was repeated 10 times.

Plaque purification was conducted on the supernatants collected after 10 passages to isolate 15 plaque clones per viral strain. Viral RNA was extracted from each virus clone using a commercial kit (Ribo_spin vRD™, GeneAll, Seoul, South Korea) according to the manufacturer's instructions. nsp2 and ORF5, which are known to be the most variable regions in the PRRSV genome [12,14,50-54], were amplified with a one-step RT-PCR kit (Takara Bio Inc., Otsu, Shiga, Japan) and were submitted for sequencing (Macrogen Inc., South Korea). PCR amplification and sequencing primers are shown in Table 1.

Data analysis

The effects of the four mutagens on PRRSV replication were analyzed by repeated measures analysis of variance (ANOVA). The Wilcoxon signed-rank test was used to compare the mutation rates of the ribavirin-resistant mutants with that of their parental virus strain. Nucleotide sequences were aligned and analyzed using Lasergene® MagAlign software (DNASTAR Inc., Madison, WI, USA).

Results

Effects of antiviral mutagens on in vitro PRRSV replication

The effects of the four antiviral mutagens studied on PRRSV replication are summarized in Figure 1. The rate of VR2332 replication in MARC-145 cells decreased more than 100-fold in the presence of 0.2 mM ribavirin and was completely suppressed at concentrations of ribavirin higher than 0.2 mM. Despite the efficient antiviral effect of ribavirin at low concentrations, no significant cytotoxicity was observed, even at the highest concentration (1.5 mM) of ribavirin studied, up to 48 hours post-treatment {Figure 1 (A and B)}. Similarly, 5-fluorouracil suppressed VR2332 replication in a dose-dependent manner: the rate of VR2332 replication decreased approximately 100-fold or more than 1000-fold in the presence of 0.2 or 1 mM 5-fluorouracil, respectively. No significant cytotoxicity was observed with up to 1.5 mM 5-fluorouracil {Figure 1 (C and D)}. However, significant levels of cytotoxicity were observed with 1 and 1.5 mM azacytidine at 48 hours post-treatment,

Table 1 Sequences of primers used for PCR amplification and sequencing of the nsp2 and ORF5 regions in the VR2332 genome

Sequenced region	Primer name	Nucleotide location[a]	Sequences (5'-3')	Sequenced length (bp)
nsp2	[p]nsp2F	1249-1268	CCTCCTCAGAATAAGGGTTG	3588
	[p]nsp2R	5120-5138	TGTCAAGGGCAGGGTAAG	
	1a 1481R	1463-1481	GGGAGTAGTGTTTGAGGTG	
	1a 1366F	1366-1383	CTCTTGTGCGACTGCTAC	
	1a 2115R	2097-2115	TACAGGTCAATCTTTGCTG	
	1a 2058F	2058-2075	CCCAGAACAAAACCAACC	
	1a 2867R	2850-2867	ATTGCGGTGAGGACACAA	
	1a 2771F	2771-2788	TGGGAAGATTTGGCTGTT	
	1a 3581R	3563-3581	CAATGGTAAGGTCGCTCTC	
	1a 3511F	3511-3529	TCCGTGTGAGTTTGTGATG	
	1a 4276R	4258-4276	CAGTAACCTGCCAAGAATG	
	1a 4141F	4141-4158	CGCTGCTTGTGAGTTTGA	
ORF5	[p]P5F[r]	13716-13734	CCTGAGACCATGAGGTGGG	603
	[p]P5R[r]	14457-14479	TTTAGGGCATATATCATCACTGG	

a: Location of primers in the full-length VR2332 genome (GenBank accession [AY150564]). p: primers used for PCR amplification and sequencing. The remaining primers were used only for sequencing. r: reference primers used in a previous study [17].

although VR2332 replication was significantly suppressed when at least 0.1 mM 5-azacytidine was included in the culture medium {Figure 1 (E and F)}. No significant antiviral activity against VR2332 was measured at low concentrations (<0.1 mM) of 5-azacytidine (data not shown). Similarly, high concentrations (1 and 1.5 mM) of amiloride also caused significant cytotoxicity in MARC-145 cells after 36 hours post-treatment {Figure 1 (H)}; however, VR2332 replication was suppressed by amiloride in a dose-dependent manner and was completely suppressed by more than 0.6 mM amiloride {Figure 1 (G)}. Based on these results, ribavirin was selected for further experiments because it was most effective at suppressing PRRSV replication without causing significant cytotoxicity in MARC-145 cells.

Emergence of ribavirin-resistant mutants after serial passage of PRRSV in MARC-145 cells in the presence of ribavirin

VR2332 was serially passaged in MARC-145 cells in the presence of ribavirin at concentrations of 0, 0.05, 0.1, 0.2, 0.3, 0.5, and 0.7 mM. Although 0.05 mM ribavirin failed to mediate significant suppression of VR2332 replication, concentrations of 0.1 and 0.2 mM ribavirin were able to suppress virus replication to undetectable levels based on a virus titration assay at passage 2. However, virus replication started to resume at passages 5 and 17 in the presence of 0.1 and 0.2 mM ribavirin, respectively. The reemerging viruses maintained increasing progeny virus production in successive passages, and two virus strains, RVRp13 and RVRp22, were recovered at passages 13 and 22 in the presence of 0.1 and 0.2 mM

ribavirin, respectively. Ribavirin doses greater than or equal to 0.3 mM completely suppressed the replication of VR2332 below the detection limit of the virus titration assay for all 22 passages (Figure 2).

Growth kinetics of ribavirin-resistant mutants in the presence of ribavirin at several concentrations

RVRp13 and RVRp22 were evaluated for their resistance to ribavirin by assessing their growth competence in MARC-145 cells in the presence of several concentrations (0, 0.1, 0.2, 0.3, 0.4, and 0.5 mM) of ribavirin, compared to the growth competence of the parental virus, VR2332. Both mutant virus strains exhibited higher replication efficiency than did VR2332 in the presence of ribavirin (Figure 3); RVRp13 and RVRp22 both replicated over 10- or 100-times more efficiently than VR2332 in the presence of 0.1 or 0.2 mM ribavirin, respectively. Moreover, VR2332 was unable to replicate in the presence of ribavirin at concentrations of 0.2 mM or higher, whereas RVRp13 and RVRp22 were able to grow to a moderate extent in the presence of ribavirin at concentrations as high as 0.5 mM.

Higher genetic stability of ribavirin-resistant mutants after serial passages in MARC-145 cells

The ribavirin-resistant mutants, RVRp13 and RVRp22, and VR2332 were plaque-purified and designated as RVRp13-p, RVRp22-p, and VR2332-p, respectively. The plaque-purified viruses were then serially passaged 10 times in MARC-145 cells without ribavirin. After 10 passages, 15 virus clones were rescued from each supernatant by plaque purification for each virus strain, and

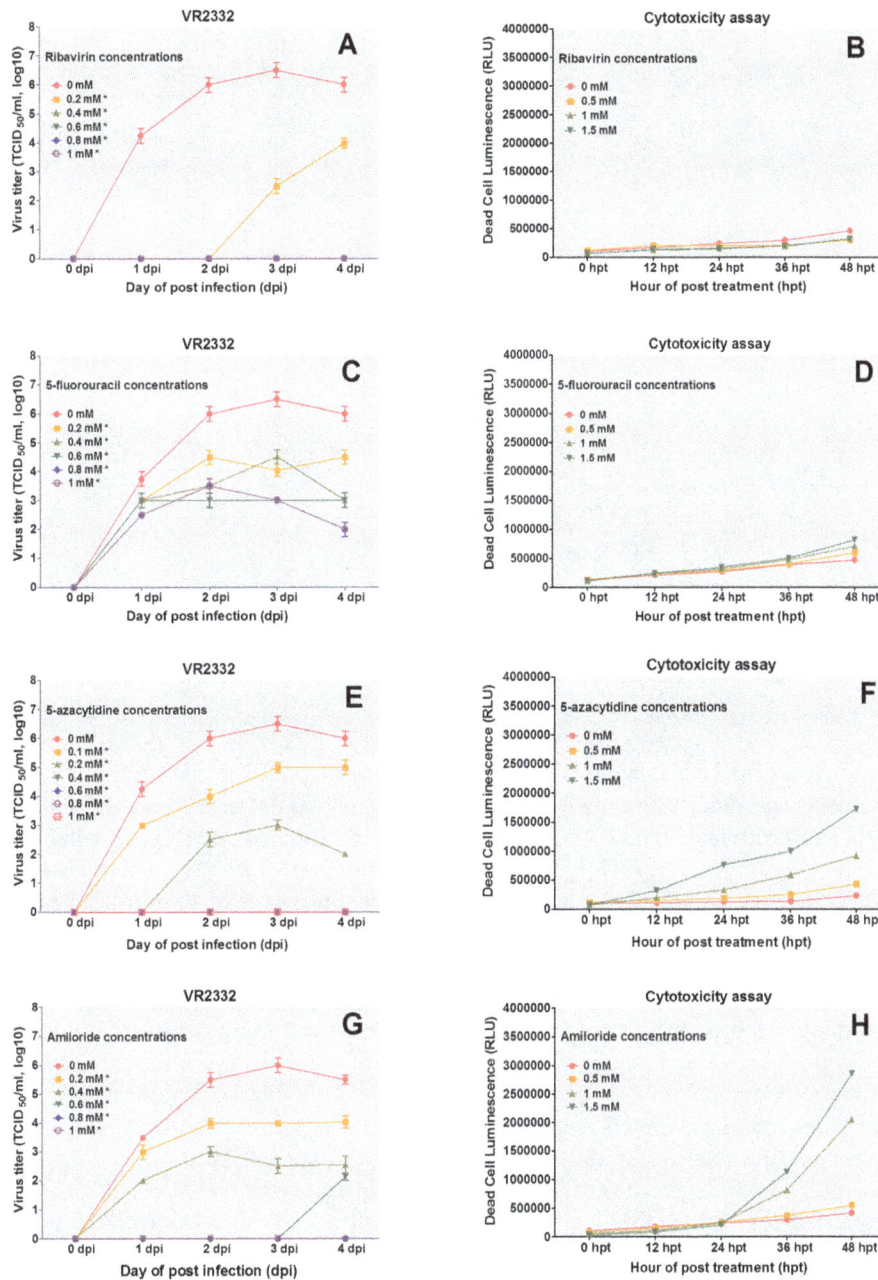

Figure 1 Evaluation of the effects of four antiviral mutagens on PRRSV replication. The effects of different concentrations of ribavirin (**A**), 5-fluorouracil (**C**), 5-azacytidine (**E**), and amiloride (**G**) in RPMI-1640 medium on the replication of the PRRSV isolate VR2332 in MARC-145 cells were evaluated, as determined by the production of progeny viruses (TCID$_{50}$/ml) over time. Cytotoxicity assays were performed using cell culture fluids collected from MARC-145 cells every 12 hours after being incubated with the following mutagens: ribavirin (**B**), 5-fluorouracil (**D**), 5-azacytidine (**F**), and amiloride (**H**), as indicated in the panel. The results are expressed as the luminescence (RLU) from dead-cell protease activity. Asterisks represent a significant difference ($p < 0.05$) in virus replication after mutagen treatment compared to that after vehicle treatment.

the hypervariable regions (nsp2 and ORF5) of the 15 virus clones were amplified for sequencing. As summarized in Table 2 and Figure 4, RVRp13-p and RVRp22-p exhibited lower mutation frequencies than VR2332-p after 10 sequential passages in MARC-145 cells: 175 nucleotide and 96 amino acid substitutions were identified in the nsp2 region of VR2332-p, whereas RVRp13-p had

98 nucleotide ($p < 0.05$) and 70 amino acid substitutions ($p < 0.05$) and RVRp22-p had 51 nucleotide ($p < 0.001$) and 24 amino acid substitutions ($p < 0.001$) in the same region {Figure 4 (A)}. In ORF5, both RVRp13-p and VR23323-p had similar mutation frequencies, with 57 nucleotide and 29 amino acid substitutions for RVRp13-p and 51 nucleotide and 32 amino acid substitutions for

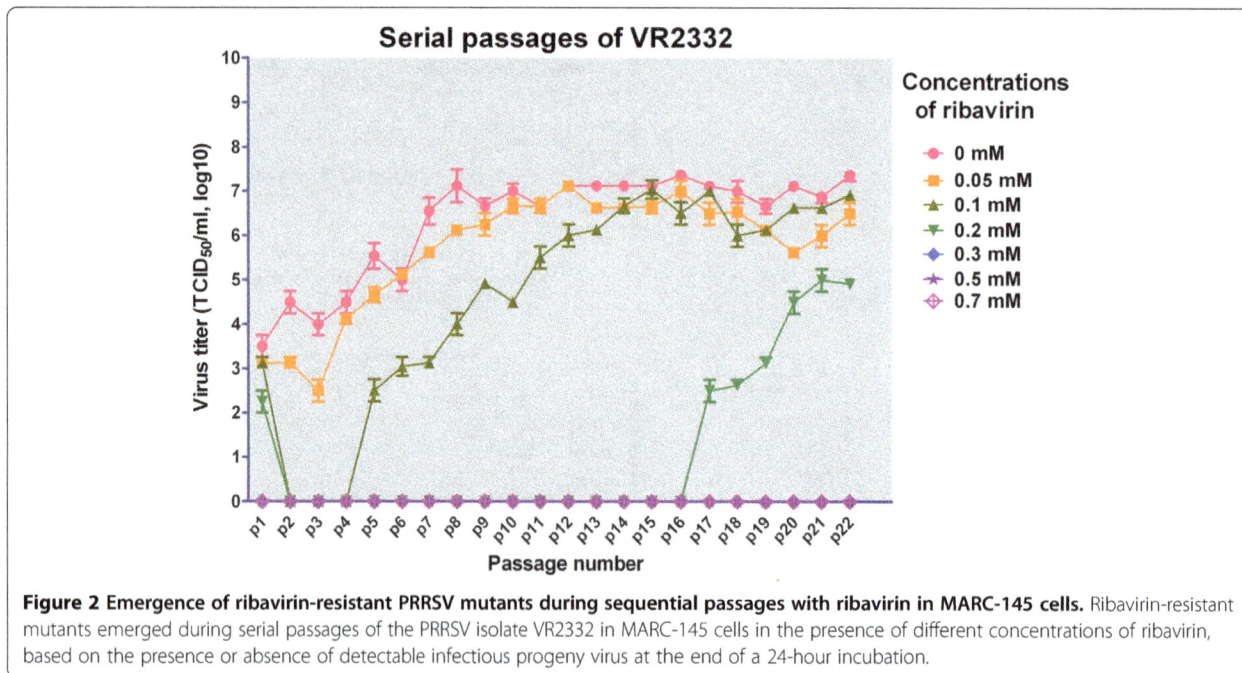

Figure 2 Emergence of ribavirin-resistant PRRSV mutants during sequential passages with ribavirin in MARC-145 cells. Ribavirin-resistant mutants emerged during serial passages of the PRRSV isolate VR2332 in MARC-145 cells in the presence of different concentrations of ribavirin, based on the presence or absence of detectable infectious progeny virus at the end of a 24-hour incubation.

VR23323-p. In contrast, RVRp22-p had a much lower ($p < 0.001$) mutation frequency, accumulating only 6 nucleotide and 4 amino acid substitutions {Figure 4 (B)}.

Discussion

In the current study, the possibility of rescuing a genetically stable PRRSV mutant during sequential passages in MARC-145 cells in the presence of mutagens was explored on the basis of previous reports that showed that mutant viruses that emerged from lethal mutagenesis driven by antiviral mutagens exhibited higher genetic stability than wild-type viruses [35,41,43]. To choose the most appropriate mutagen for the study, four different antiviral mutagens (ribavirin, 5-fluorouracil, 5-azacytidine, and amiloride) were evaluated for their antiviral effects against PRRSV and for their cytotoxicity in MARC-145 cells. In the presence of ribavirin at concentrations higher than 0.2 mM, the replication of VR2332 was completely suppressed, whereas even at the highest concentration, 1.5 mM, ribavirin did not cause significant cytotoxicity in MARC-145 cells {Figure 1 (A and B)}. This result is in good agreement with previous studies conducted to evaluate the antiviral effects of ribavirin on several RNA viruses, including HCV, respiratory syncytial virus (RSV), poliovirus, FMDV, and Influenza A and B viruses [28,30,32,33,42,55-57]. Recently, ribavirin was reported as a potential antiviral drug against PRRSV because it reduced virus replication approximately 100 times in PAM-pCD163 cells when added at a concentration of 0.05 mM, which was the highest

concentration applied in the study [58]. However, in the current study, 0.05 mM ribavirin failed to suppress PRRSV replication in MARC-145 cells, and concentrations higher than 0.2 mM ribavirin were required for complete suppression of PRRSV replication (Figure 2). Unlike the results observed in PAM-pCD163 cells, no significant cytotoxicity was observed in MARC-145 cells, even when treated with 1.5 mM ribavirin. Thus, ribavirin-resistant mutant viruses were rescued in the presence of ribavirin at concentrations as high as 0.1 and 0.2 mM. Similarly, 5-fluorouracil effectively suppressed VR2332 replication in MARC-145 cells at concentrations ranging from 0.2 to 1 mM without causing significant cytotoxicity {Figure 1 (C and D)}. The effective antiviral activity of 5-fluorouracil has also been reported for rift valley fever virus, vesicular stomatitis virus, poliovirus, and FMDV [26,59-63]. In contrast, 5-azacytidine or amiloride at concentrations between 1 and 1.5 mM induced significant cytotoxicity in MARC-145 cells, although concentrations of 5-azacytidine or amiloride lower than 1 mM showed substantial antiviral efficacy against PRRSV {Figure 1 (E and F) and Figure 1 (G and H)}. A previous study reported that 1 mM 5-azacytidine caused significant cytotoxicity in 293 T and U373-MAGI$_{CXCR4}$ cells 24 hours after treatment [46] although a significant level of antiviral activity against HIV-1 was reported with 5-azacytidine at concentrations between 1 μM and 100 μM [45,46]. However, low concentrations (<0.1 mM) of 5-azacytidine did not result in significant antiviral activity against PRRSV in the

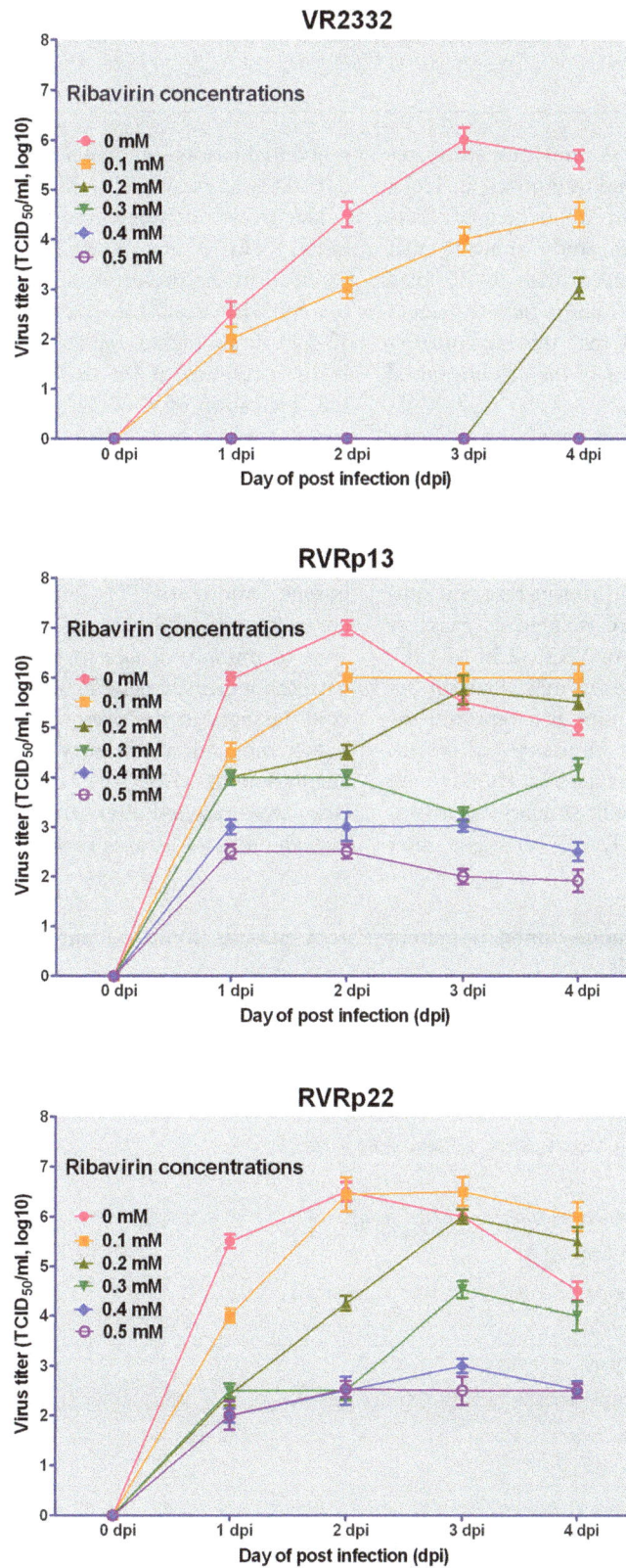

Figure 3 (See legend on next page.)

(See figure on previous page.)
Figure 3 Assessment of the growth kinetics of ribavirin-resistant mutants in the presence of ribavirin. The growth kinetics of two ribavirin-resistant PRRSV mutants (RVRp13 and RVRp22) were evaluated in MARC-145 cells in the presence of several concentrations of ribavirin compared to their parental strain VR2332.

current study (data not shown). A previous study reported that 1 mM amiloride was non-cytotoxic in HeLa T cells for 48 hours post-treatment [38], which conflicts with the results observed in this study showing that substantial cytotoxicity was observed with 1–1.5 mM amiloride in MARC-145 cells at 36 hours post-treatment {Figure 1 (H)}. It was speculated that this dissimilarity might be due to the different origins of the cell lines used in the studies.

Based on the initial assessment of antiviral mutagens, ribavirin was selected for further study to evaluate the possible emergence of ribavirin-resistant mutants because it showed the greatest effect on PRRSV replication without causing significant cytotoxicity even at the highest concentration (1.5 mM). Two ribavirin-resistant mutants (RVRp13 and RVRp22) were isolated at passages 13 and 22 during serial passages of VR2332 in MARC-145 cells in the presence of 0.1 and 0.2 mM ribavirin, respectively (Figure 2). Previous studies also reported the emergence of ribavirin-resistant mutants: ribavirin-resistant HCV emerged after 7 passages in Huh7D cells cultured with 0.25 mM ribavirin [42]. Similarly, ribavirin-resistant CVB3, poliovirus, and FMDV emerged after

sequential passages in HeLa or BHK-21 cells cultured with 0.05-0.8 mM ribavirin [41,43,44].

The growth competence of the ribavirin-resistant mutants RVRp13 and RVRp22 in MARC-145 cells was assessed in the presence or absence of ribavirin. Both of the ribavirin-resistant mutants showed approximately 10-100-times higher replication efficiency than VR2332 in the presence of 0.1 or 0.2 mM ribavirin. Moreover, the replication of VR2332 was completely suppressed at concentrations higher than 0.2 mM ribavirin, while both mutants were able to generate infectious progeny viruses, reaching titers close to 10^3 $TCID_{50}$/ml in the presence of 0.5 mM ribavirin (Figure 3). As reported in many previous studies conducted with poliovirus [43], human enterovirus 71 (HEV71) [64], FMDV [65,66], coxsackie virus B3 [41] and HCV [42], enhanced resistance of mutant viruses to ribavirin might be associated with the increased genetic fidelity that is acquired during viral passages in the presence of ribavirin. However, the higher replication efficiency might also result from virus adaptation to MARC-145 cells because the mutant viruses were rescued after 13 or 22 sequential passages. In fact, the mutant viruses replicated more efficiently in the

Table 2 Mutation frequencies of plaque-cloned, ribavirin-resistant mutants (RVRp13-P and RVRp22-P) and VR2332-p after 10 passages in MARC-145 cells

Sequenced region		VR2332-p	RVRp13-p	RVRp22-p
	Total no. of clones sequenced[a]	15	15	15
	Total no. of nucleotides sequenced(3588 nt per clone)	53820	53820	53820
	Total no. of mutations	175	98	51
	Total no. of nucleotide deletionsin sequenced length	63	0	6
nsp2	Mutation rate/10^3 nt	3.25	1.82[*]	0.94[**]
	Total no. of amino acids sequenced(1196 aa per clone)	17940	17940	17940
	Total no. of mutations	96	70	24
	Total no. of amino acid deletionsin sequenced length	21	0	2
	Mutation rate/10^3 aa	5.35	3.90[*]	1.33[**]
	Total no. of clones sequenced	15	15	15
	Total no. of nucleotides sequenced(603 nt per clone)	9045	9045	9045
	Total no. of mutations	51	57	6
ORF5	Mutation rate/10^3 nt	5.64	6.30	0.66[**]
	Total no. of amino acids sequenced(201 aa per clone)	3015	3015	3015
	Total no. of mutations	32	29	4
	Mutation rate/10^3 aa	10.61	9.61	1.32[**]

a: The numbers of nucleotide mutations and amino acid substitutions were determined by sequencing 15 plaque-purified virus clones from cell culture fluids collected at the completion of 10 passages of each virus and comparing those samples to the original viruses not submitted to sequential cell passages.
nt: nucleotide, aa: amino acid, significance levels when comparing a drug-resistant strain with VR2332 are indicated by asterisks: *$p < 0.05$, **$p < 0.001$.

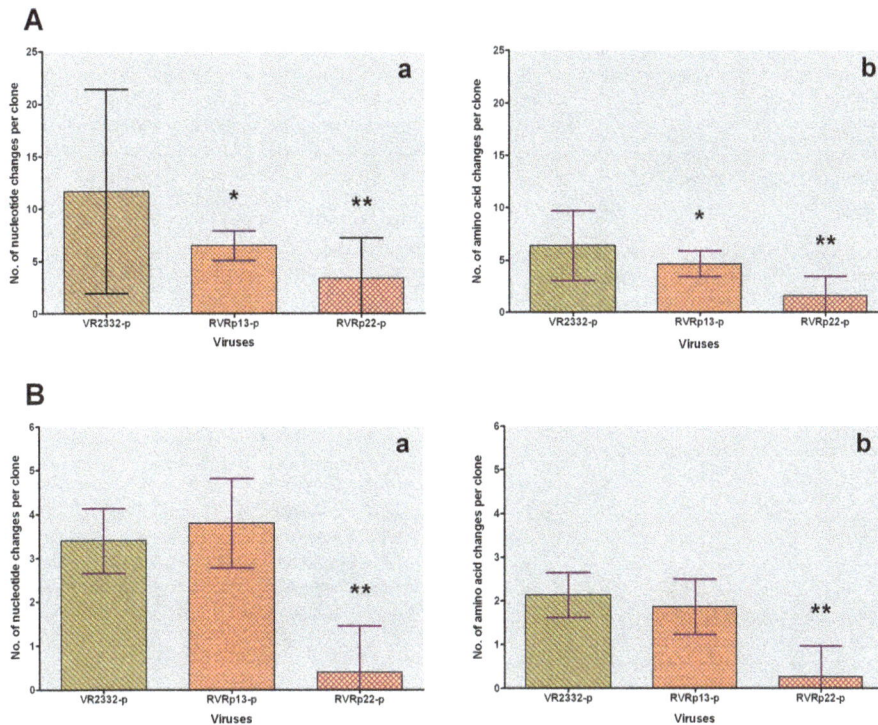

Figure 4 *In vitro* **assessment of the genetic stability of ribavirin-resistant PRRSV mutants during serial passages in cells.** The genetic stability of the plaque-purified, ribavirin-resistant mutants (RVRp13-P and RVRp22-P) was compared with that of plaque-purified VR2332 (VR2332-p) over 10 passages in MARC-145 cells. Fifteen viral clones obtained from cell culture fluids collected at the completion of 10 passages of each virus by plaque purification and nsp2 **(A)** and ORF5 **(B)** regions of each virus clone were sequenced and compared with their parental viruses (RVRp13-P, RVRp22-P, and VR2332-p) to determine nucleotide mutations **(a)** and amino acid **(b)** substitutions during the sequential passages. Asterisks represent significant differences in the mutation rate compared with VR2332 (*$p < 0.05$, **$p < 0.001$).

absence of ribavirin compared to VR2332. Therefore, the genetic stability of the ribavirin-resistant mutants was assessed by passaging the mutant viruses 10 times in MARC-145 cells without ribavirin in parallel with VR2332 to demonstrate that ribavirin-resistant mutants have increased genetic stability. The most variable genes (nsp2 and ORF5) in the PRRSV genome were sequenced to determine the mutation frequency of the viruses during sequential passages. RVRp13 and RVRp22 virus clones exhibited 1.8- and 3.4-fold lower numbers of nucleotide substitutions and 1.4- and 4-fold lower numbers of amino acid substitutions, respectively, in the nsp2 region compared with VR2332 virus clones {Table 2 and Figure 4 (A)}. In the ORF5 region, the RVRp13 virus clones exhibited mutation rates similar to those observed in VR2332 virus clones, while RVRp22 virus clones had approximately 8.5-fold lower numbers of nucleotide substitutions and 8-fold lower numbers of amino acid substitutions compared with VR2332 virus clones {Table 2 and Figure 4 (B)}. Based on these results, it was concluded that the ribavirin-resistant mutants, especially RVRp22, have significantly higher genetic stability compared with their parental virus, VR2332.

Conclusions

In conclusion, ribavirin was very effective in suppressing PRRSV replication in MARC-145 cells at concentrations higher than 0.2 mM, suggesting that ribavirin could be used as a therapeutic drug against PRRSV; however, its potential usefulness against PRRSV infection remains to be confirmed in animal studies. As described in the current study, the resistant viruses emerged in the presence of low concentrations (<0.2 mM) of ribavirin, and those resistant viruses had significantly higher genetic stability compared with VR2332. Because rapid reversion of attenuated PRRS vaccines to virulence is of great concern, RVRp22, which has a higher level of genetic stability, could be a good candidate for the development of a safer vaccine. Nonetheless, the mechanisms and genetic determinants responsible for the high genetic stability of ribavirin-resistant PRRSV should be elucidated in detail in the near future.

Abbreviations
PRRSV: Porcine reproductive and respiratory syndrome virus; MLV: Modified live virus; EAV: Equine arteritis virus; LDV: Lactate dehydrogenase-elevating virus of mice; SHFV: Simian hemorrhagic fever virus; ORF: Open reading frame; FMDV: Foot-and-mouth disease virus; HCV: Hepatitis C virus; CVB3: Coxsackievirus

B3; FBS: Fetal bovine serum; MOI: Multiplicity of infection; CPE: Cytopathic effect; TCID: Tissue culture infective dose; AAF: Alanyl-alanylphenylalanyl-aminoluciferin; RLU: Relative luminescence units; nsp2: Nonstructural protein 2, RSV, Respiratory syncytial virus; RVF: Rift valley fever virus; VSV: Vesicular stomatitis virus; HIV-1: Human immunodeficiency virus 1.

Competing interests
The authors declared that they have no competing interests.

Authors' contributions
AK performed the experiments, carried out the statistical analysis, and drafted the manuscript. NS contributed to the statistical analysis. KJY contributed to the study design and critically reviewed the manuscript. KIW conceived the study, coordinated the work described, and contributed to the manuscript preparation. All authors read and approved the final manuscript.

Acknowledgments
This research was supported by the Basic Science Research Program through the National Research Foundation of Korea (NRF), which is funded by the Ministry of Education, Science and Technology (2011–0009937) and Technology Development Program for Bio-industry (313005–3), Ministry for Food, Agriculture, Forestry and Fisheries, Republic of Korea.

Author details
[1]College of Veterinary Medicine, Chonbuk National University Jeonju, Korea, 664-14 Deokjin-Dong 1 Ga, Jeonju, Jeonbuk 561-756, Republic of Korea. [2]Department of Veterinary Diagnostic and Production Animal Medicine, College of Veterinary Medicine, Iowa State University, Ames, IA, USA.

References
1. Holtkamp DJ, Kliebenstein JB, Neumann EJ, Zimmerman JJ, Rotto HF, Yoder TK, et al. Assessment of the economic impact of porcine reproductive and respiratory syndrome virus on United States pork producers. J Swine Health Prod. 2013;21:72–84.
2. Cavanagh D. Nidovirales: A new order comprising Coronaviridae and Arteriviridae. Arch Virol. 1997;142:629–33.
3. Meulenberg JJM, Hulst MM, Demeijer EJ, Moonen PLJM, Denbesten A, Dekluyver EP, et al. Lelystad virus, the causative agent of porcine epidemic abortion and respiratory syndrome (PEARS), is related to LDV and EAV. Virology. 1993;192:62–72.
4. Conzelmann KK, Visser N, Vanwoensel P, Thiel HJ. Molecular characterization of porcine reproductive and respiratory syndrome virus, a member of the arterivirus group. Virology. 1993;193:329–39.
5. Firth AE, Zevenhoven-Dobbe JC, Wills NM, Go YY, Balasuriya UBR, Atkins JF, et al. Discovery of a small arterivirus gene that overlaps the GP5 coding sequence and is important for virus production. J Gen Virol. 2011;92:1097–106.
6. Johnson CR, Griggs TF, Gnanandarajah J, Murtaugh MP. Novel structural protein in porcine reproductive and respiratory syndrome virus encoded by an alternative ORF5 present in all arteriviruses. J Gen Virol. 2011;92:1107–16.
7. Meulenberg JJM, DenBesten AP, DKluyver E, VanNieuwstadt A, Wensvoort G. Molecular characterization of Lelystad virus. Vet Microbiol. 1997;55:197–202.
8. Music N, Gagnon CA. The role of porcine reproductive and respiratory syndrome (PRRS) virus structural and non-structural proteins in virus pathogenesis. Anim Health Res Rev. 2010;11:135–63.
9. Hanada K, Suzuki Y, Nakane T, Hirose O, Gojobori T. The origin and evolution of porcine reproductive and respiratory syndrome viruses. Mol Biol Evol. 2005;22:1024–31.
10. Shi M, Lam TT, Hon CC, Hui RK, Faaberg KS, Wennblom T, et al. Molecular epidemiology of PRRSV: a phylogenetic perspective. Virus Res. 2010;154:7–17.
11. Lunney JK, Benfield DA, Rowland RR. Porcine reproductive and respiratory syndrome virus: an update on an emerging and re-emerging viral disease of swine. Virus Res. 2010;154:1–6.
12. Meng XJ, Paul PS, Halbur PG, Morozov I. Sequence comparison of open reading frames 2 to 5 of low and high virulence United States isolates of porcine reproductive and respiratory syndrome virus. J Gen Virol. 1995;76(Pt 12):3181–8.
13. Nelsen CJ, Murtaugh MP, Faaberg KS. Porcine reproductive and respiratory syndrome virus comparison: divergent evolution on two continents. J Virol. 1999;73:270–80.
14. Suarez P, Zardoya R, Martin MJ, Prieto C, Dopazo J, Solana A, et al. Phylogenetic relationships of european strains of porcine reproductive and respiratory syndrome virus (PRRSV) inferred from DNA sequences of putative ORF-5 and ORF-7 genes. Virus Res. 1996;42:159–65.
15. Yin G, Gao L, Shu X, Yang G, Guo S, Li W. Genetic diversity of the ORF5 gene of porcine reproductive and respiratory syndrome virus isolates in southwest China from 2007 to 2009. PLoS One. 2012;7:e33756.
16. Charerntantanakul W. Porcine reproductive and respiratory syndrome virus vaccines: Immunogenicity, efficacy and safety aspects. World J Virol. 2012;1:23–30.
17. Kim WI, Kim JJ, Cha SH, Yoon KJ. Different biological characteristics of wild-type porcine reproductive and respiratory syndrome viruses and vaccine viruses and identification of the corresponding genetic determinants. J Clin Microbiol. 2008;46:1758–68.
18. Madsen KG, Hansen CM, Madsen ES, Strandbygaard B, Botner A, Sorensen KJ. Sequence analysis of porcine reproductive and respiratory syndrome virus of the American type collected from Danish swine herds. Arch Virol. 1998;143:1683–700.
19. Nielsen HS, Oleksiewicz MB, Forsberg R, Stadejek T, Botner A, Storgaard T. Reversion of a live porcine reproductive and respiratory syndrome virus vaccine investigated by parallel mutations. J Gen Virol. 2001;82:1263–72.
20. Opriessnig T, Halbur PG, Yoon KJ, Pogranichniy RM, Harmon KM, Evans R, et al. Comparison of molecular and biological characteristics of a modified live porcine reproductive and respiratory syndrome virus (PRRSV) vaccine (ingelvac PRRS MLV), the parent strain of the vaccine (ATCC VR2332), ATCC VR2385, and two recent field isolates of PRRSV. J Virol. 2002;76:11837–44.
21. Storgaard T, Oleksiewicz M, Botner A. Examination of the selective pressures on a live PRRS vaccine virus. Arch Virol. 1999;144:2389–401.
22. Harris S, Robins R. Ribavirin: structure and antiviral activity relationships. In: Smith RA, Kirkpatrick W, editors. Ribavirin: A Broad Spectrum Antiviral Agent. New York: Academic; 1980. p. 1–21.
23. Wu JZ, Walker H, Lau JY, Hong Z. Activation and deactivation of a broad-spectrum antiviral drug by a single enzyme: adenosine deaminase catalyzes two consecutive deamination reactions. Antimicrob Agents Chemother. 2003;47:426–31.
24. Boumah CE, Setterfield G, Kaplan JG. Purine and pyrimidine analogues irreversibly prevent passage of lymphocytes from the G1 to the S phase of the cell cycle. Can J Biochem Cell Biol. 1984;62:280–7.
25. Piskala A, Sorm F. Nucleic Acids Components + Their Analogues.51. Synthesis of 1-Glycosyl Derivatives of 5-Azauracil + 5-Azacytosine. Collect Czech Chem Communications. 1964;29:2060–76.
26. Agudo R, Arias A, Domingo E. 5-fluorouracil in lethal mutagenesis of foot-and-mouth disease virus. Future Med Chem. 2009;1:529–39.
27. Agudo R, Ferrer-Orta C, Arias A, de la Higuera I, Perales C, Perez-Luque R, et al. A multi-step process of viral adaptation to a mutagenic nucleoside analogue by modulation of transition types leads to extinction-escape. PLoS Pathog. 2010;6:e1001072.
28. Crotty S, Cameron C, Andino R. Ribavirin's antiviral mechanism of action: lethal mutagenesis? J Mol Med (Berl). 2002;80:86–95.
29. Crotty S, Cameron CE, Andino R. RNA virus error catastrophe: Direct molecular test by using ribavirin. Proc Natl Acad Sci U S A. 2001;98:6895–900.
30. Crotty S, Maag D, Arnold JJ, Zhong WD, Lau JYN, Hong Z, et al. The broad-spectrum antiviral ribonucleoside ribavirin is an RNA virus mutagen. Nat Med. 2000;6:1375–9.
31. Gordon MP, Staehelin M. Studies on the Incorporation of 5-Fluorouracil into a Virus Nucleic Acid. Biochim Biophys Acta. 1959;36:351–61.
32. Gu CJ, Zheng CY, Zhang Q, Shi LL, Li Y, Qu SF. An antiviral mechanism investigated with ribavirin as an RNA virus mutagen for foot-and-mouth disease virus. J Biochem Mol Biol. 2006;39:9–15.
33. Perales C, Agudo R, Tejero H, Manrubia SC, Domingo E. Potential benefits of sequential inhibitor-mutagen treatments of RNA virus infections. PLoS Pathog. 2009;5:e1000658.
34. Sanchez-Jimenez C, Olivares I, de Avila Lucas AI, Toledano V, Gutierrez-Rivas M, Lorenzo-Redondo R, et al. Mutagen-mediated enhancement of HIV-1 replication in persistently infected cells. Virology. 2012;424:147–53.
35. Vignuzzi M, Stone JK, Arnold JJ, Cameron CE, Andino R. Quasispecies diversity determines pathogenesis through cooperative interactions in a viral population. Nature. 2006;439:344–8.

36. Ewart GD, Mills K, Cox GB, Gage PW. Amiloride derivatives block ion channel activity and enhancement of virus-like particle budding caused by HIV-1 protein Vpu. Eur Biophys J. 2002;31:26–35.

37. Gazina EV, Harrison DN, Jefferies M, Tan H, Williams D, Anderson DA, et al. Ion transport blockers inhibit human rhinovirus 2 release. Antiviral Res. 2005;67:98–106.

38. Harrison DN, Gazina EV, Purcell DF, Anderson DA, Petrou S. Amiloride derivatives inhibit coxsackievirus B3 RNA replication. J Virol. 2008;82:1465–73.

39. Premkumar A, Wilson L, Ewart GD, Gage PW. Cation-selective ion channels formed by p7 of hepatitis C virus are blocked by hexamethylene amiloride. FEBS Lett. 2004;557:99–103.

40. Wilson L, Gage P, Ewart G. Hexamethylene amiloride blocks E protein ion channels and inhibits coronavirus replication. Virology. 2006;353:294–306.

41. Levi LI, Gnadig NF, Beaucourt S, McPherson MJ, Baron B, Arnold JJ, et al. Fidelity variants of RNA dependent RNA polymerases uncover an indirect, mutagenic activity of amiloride compounds. PLoS Pathog. 2010;6:e1001163.

42. Feigelstock DA, Mihalik KB, Feinstone SM. Selection of hepatitis C virus resistant to ribavirin. Virol J. 2011;8:402.

43. Pfeiffer JK, Kirkegaard K. A single mutation in poliovirus RNA-dependent RNA polymerase confers resistance to mutagenic nucleotide analogs via increased fidelity. Proc Natl Acad Sci U S A. 2003;100:7289–94.

44. Sierra M, Airaksinen A, Gonzalez-Lopez C, Agudo R, Arias A, Domingo E. Foot-and-mouth disease virus mutant with decreased sensitivity to ribavirin: implications for error catastrophe. J Virol. 2007;81:2012–24.

45. Bouchard J, Walker MC, Leclerc JM, Lapointe N, Beaulieu R, Thibodeau L. 5-azacytidine and 5-azadeoxycytidine inhibit human immunodeficiency virus type 1 replication in vitro. Antimicrob Agents Chemother. 1990;34:206–9.

46. Dapp MJ, Clouser CL, Patterson S, Mansky LM. 5-Azacytidine Can Induce Lethal Mutagenesis in Human Immunodeficiency Virus Type 1. J Virol. 2009;83:11950–8.

47. Greig A. The use of a microtitration technique for the routine assay of African swine fever virus. Brief Report Arch Virol. 1975;47:287–9.

48. Reed LJ, Muench H. A simple method of estimating fifty percent endpoints. American J Hygiene. 1938;27:493–7.

49. Niles AL, Moravec RA, Eric Hesselberth P, Scurria MA, Daily WJ, Riss TL. A homogeneous assay to measure live and dead cells in the same sample by detecting different protease markers. Anal Biochem. 2007;366:197–206.

50. Han J, Liu G, Wang Y, Faaberg KS. Identification of nonessential regions of the nsp2 replicase protein of porcine reproductive and respiratory syndrome virus strain VR-2332 for replication in cell culture. J Virol. 2007;81:9878–90.

51. Han J, Wang Y, Faaberg KS. Complete genome analysis of RFLP 184 isolates of porcine reproductive and respiratory syndrome virus. Virus Res. 2006;122:175–82.

52. Mardassi H, Mounir S, Dea S. Molecular analysis of the ORFs 3 to 7 of porcine reproductive and respiratory syndrome virus, Quebec reference strain. Arch Virol. 1995;140:1405–18.

53. Nam E, Park CK, Kim SH, Joo YS, Yeo SG, Lee C. Complete genomic characterization of a European type 1 porcine reproductive and respiratory syndrome virus isolate in Korea. Arch Virol. 2009;154:629–38.

54. Tian K, Yu X, Zhao T, Feng Y, Cao Z, Wang C, et al. Emergence of fatal PRRSV variants: unparalleled outbreaks of atypical PRRS in China and molecular dissection of the unique hallmark. PLoS One. 2007;2:e526.

55. Hruska JF, Bernstein JM, Douglas Jr RG, Hall CB. Effects of ribavirin on respiratory syncytial virus in vitro. Antimicrob Agents Chemother. 1980;17:770–5.

56. Oxford JS. Inhibition of the replication of influenza A and B viruses by a nucleoside analogue (ribavirin). J Gen Virol. 1975;28:409–14.

57. Sierra S, Davila M, Lowenstein PR, Domingo E. Response of foot-and-mouth disease virus to increased mutagenesis: influence of viral load and fitness in loss of infectivity. J Virol. 2000;74:8316–23.

58. Kim Y, Lee C. Ribavirin efficiently suppresses porcine nidovirus replication. Virus Res. 2013;171:44–53.

59. Caplen H, Peters CJ, Bishop DHL. Mutagen-directed attenuation of Rift-Valley fever virus as a method for vaccine development. J Gen Virol. 1985;66:2271–7.

60. Holland JJ, Domingo E, Delatorre JC, Steinhauer DA. Mutation frequencies at defined single codon sites in vesicular stomatitis-virus and poliovirus can be increased only slightly by chemical mutagenesis. J Virol. 1990;64:3960–2.

61. Lee CH, Gilbertson DL, Novella IS, Huerta R, Domingo E, Holland JJ. Negative effects of chemical mutagenesis on the adaptive behavior of vesicular stomatitis virus. J Virol. 1997;71:3636–40.

62. Perales C, Agudo R, Domingo E. Counteracting quasispecies adaptability: extinction of a ribavirin-resistant virus mutant by an alternative mutagenic treatment. PLoS One. 2009;4:e5554.

63. Pringle CR. Genetic characteristics of conditional lethal mutants of vesicular stomatitis virus induced by 5-fluorouracil, 5-azacytidine, and ethyl methane sulfonate. J Virol. 1970;5:559–67.

64. Sadeghipour S, Bek EJ, McMinn PC. Ribavirin-resistant mutants of human enterovirus 71 express a high replication fidelity phenotype during growth in cell culture. J Virol. 2013;87:1759–69.

65. Zeng J, Wang H, Xie X, Yang D, Zhou G, Yu L. An increased replication fidelity mutant of foot-and-mouth disease virus retains fitness in vitro and virulence in vivo. Antiviral Res. 2013;100:1–7.

66. Zeng J, Wang H, Xie X, Li C, Zhou G, Yang D, et al. Ribavirin-resistant variants of foot-and-mouth disease virus: the effect of restricted quasispecies diversity on viral virulence. J Virol. 2014;88:4008–20.

10

An inactivated vaccine made from a U.S. field isolate of porcine epidemic disease virus is immunogenic in pigs as demonstrated by a dose-titration

Emily A Collin[1,2,3], Srivishnupriya Anbalagan[1], Faten Okda[2,4], Ron Batman[1*], Eric Nelson[2] and Ben M Hause[1,3*]

Abstract

Background: Porcine epidemic diarrhea virus (PEDV), a highly pathogenic and transmissible virus in swine, was first detected in the U.S. in May, 2013, and has caused tremendous losses to the swine industry. Due to the difficulty in isolating and growing this virus in cell culture, few vaccine studies using cell culture propagated PEDV have been performed on U.S. strains in pigs. Therefore, the objective of this study was to evaluate the humoral immune response to the selected inactivated PEDV vaccine candidate in a dose-titration manner.

Results: PEDV was isolated from a pig with diarrhea and complete genome sequencing found >99% nucleotide identity to other U.S. PEDV. Inactivated adjuvanted monovalent vaccines were administered intramuscularly to five week old pigs in a dose titration experimental design, ranging from 6.0-8.0 $\log_{10}$ tissue culture infective dose ($TCID_{50}$/mL), to evaluate immunogenicity using a fluorescent foci neutralization assay (FFN), fluorescent microsphere immunoassay (FMIA), and enzyme-linked immunosorbent assay (ELISA) on sera. Pigs vaccinated with 8.0 $\log_{10}$ $TCID_{50}$/mL inactivated virus showed significantly higher FFN titers as well as FMIA and ELISA values than 6.0 $\log_{10}$ $TCID_{50}$/mL vaccinates and the negative controls.

Conclusions: These results demonstrate the immunogenicity of a PEDV inactivated viral vaccine with a U.S. strain via dose-titration. A future vaccination-challenge study would illustrate the efficacy of an inactivated vaccine and help evaluate protective FFN titers and ELISA and FMIA responses.

Keywords: Porcine, Epidemic, Diarrhea, Virus, PEDV, Inactivated, Vaccine, Immunogenicity

Background

Porcine epidemic diarrhea virus (PEDV) circulated throughout Europe and Asia during the past three decades before being detected in swine in the United States in May, 2013 [1-7]. Since its introduction to the U.S., PEDV has been identified in 33 states by the National Animal Health Laboratory Network, as of December, 2014 (www.aasv.org). It is characterized by watery diarrhea, vomiting, dehydration, and high mortality rates in suckling pigs [8-10]. The U.S. PEDV strains are phylogenetically subgroup IIa, which is similar to PEDV circulating in Asia in 2011 and 2012 [6,7].

Modified-live vaccines (MLVs) have long been used in Asia for the control of PEDV [11-13]. The strain 83P-5, attenuated by one-hundred cell culture passages, is a subgroup I isolate that has been licensed in Japan as an attenuated live PEDV vaccine [13]. During the attenuation process, this strain acquired fourteen amino acid changes in the immunodominant spike (S) protein, which is critical for virus binding to cell receptors and is the target of neutralizing antibodies [14-19]. The live attenuated DR13 vaccine strain of PEDV, whose parent strain was a subgroup II had thirteen of these fourteen mutations as well, and subsequently clustered with subgroup I [13]. Serial passage of 83P-5 in Vero cells resulted in attenuation of virulence *in vivo* and the strong

* Correspondence: rbatman@newportlabs.com; bhause@vet.k-state.edu
[1]Newport Laboratories Inc., Worthington, MN, USA
Full list of author information is available at the end of the article

selection for the viral spike (S) gene was associated with these phenotypic changes.

Classically attenuated cell culture passaged PEDV also shows mutations in open reading frame 3 (ORF) and changes to restriction fragment length polymorphism (RFLP) cut patterns, which have been used to distinguish MLV from field strains [10,20]. *In vivo*, high-passage (x > 100) MLVs were attenuated in sows and piglets while still capable of inducing a robust immune response [20]. While attenuated in their ability to cause disease, the safety of using MLV has been questioned, as MLV are shed in the environment. Virus was detected in feces of 3-day old piglets up to seven days after oral inoculation with DR13 passage 100 [12,21] . In 2010, PEDV was isolated from diarrheic pigs in China that had a close phylogenetic relationship to two MLV vaccines, suggesting it may have evolved from a MLV [22].

While modified live vaccines generally elicit a more robust and protective immune response than inactivated virus vaccines [13], long-term efficacy is often lacking due to viral mutations and accompanying antigenic changes [23]. In late 2010, China experienced a severe outbreak of PEDV in suckling pigs, causing drastic economic losses [24]. This outbreak was caused by a strain with a phylogenetically distinct S gene from other Chinese strains and from vaccine strain CV777 [24]. In 2012, the PEDV infection rates in vaccinated herds in China increased dramatically. Phylogenetic analysis of new variants from the outbreak showed insertions and deletions in antigenic regions of the S gene that may have influenced the efficacy of the CV777 MLV [25]. Investigation into whether an inactivated vaccine can elicit a protective immune response could lead to the development of vaccines more closely related to field strains and avoid potential antigenic changes due to excessive *in vitro* cultivation.

There are currently two conditionally licensed PEDV vaccines in the U.S, with label claims for use in sows; an inactivated virus vaccine and an alphavirus vectored subunit vaccine. With mortality rates as high as 100% in suckling piglets and total losses estimated over 5 million animals in the U.S. in less than one year, PEDV vaccines are critically needed (www.aasv.org). The U.S. Department of Agriculture (USDA) allows for the production of autogenous vaccines to address emerging diseases; however the difficulty in isolating PEDV in cell culture increases the difficulty in producing efficacious inactivated vaccines. Here, PEDV was isolated from pooled intestinal homogenate and passaged in cell culture. Inactivated cell culture derived viral vaccines were immunogenic when administered to naïve pigs. To our knowledge, this is the first demonstration of immunogenicity of an inactivated U.S. PEDV vaccine trial in pigs in the U.S.

Methods

Ethics statement

Swine studies were performed at Newport Laboratories and were approved by the Newport Laboratories' Institutional Animal Care and Use Committee.

Virus isolation

In May, 2013, intestines from pigs in Iowa experiencing PEDV-like symptoms were submitted to Newport Laboratories for diagnostic testing. Intestines were homogenized in phosphate buffered saline and debris was removed by centrifugation at 10,000 × g for 10 minutes followed by filtration through a 0.2 μm filter. Virus isolation was performed on Vero (ATCC® CCL-81™), Vero 76 (ATCC® CRL-1586™), and MARC-145 (M145) cells [26]. All cells were maintained in Dulbecco's modification of Eagles medium (DMEM) with five percent fetal bovine serum and one percent L-glutamine. Confluent monolayers were washed three times with DMEM without serum prior to inoculation. For the initial infection of cells in 12-well plates, 200 μL of inoculum was adsorbed at 37°C with + 5% CO_2 for 1–2 hours with small amount of viral growth media (DMEM with 0.75 μg/mL), L-1-Tosylamide-2-phenylethyl chloromethyl ketone (TPCK)-treated trypsin, and Normocin™ antibiotic (Invivogen)). The inoculum was rinsed from the plates with viral growth media and the cells were refed with viral growth media. Plates were incubated up to 5 days before being frozen, thawed, and passaged. Subsequent passages were performed by inoculating 200 μL of cell culture harvest onto confluent monolayers in 12-well plates. Viral replication was verified by Real time reverse transcription polymerase chain reaction (rt-RT-PCR) (below) and indirect immunofluorescence (IFA). Viral cultures were scaled up in M145 25 cm^2 flasks and 1700 cm^2 roller bottles, resulting in NPL PEDV 2013 P10.1PEDV.

Indirect immunofluorescence

IFA was performed on Vero or M145 96-well monolayers. Infected wells were fixed in cold ethyl alcohol and polyclonal rabbit anti-PEDV nucleoprotein (NP) antiserum (South Dakota State University Animal Disease Research and Diagnostic Laboratory (SDSU)) was added at 1:500. Cells were rinsed and then incubated with fluorescein isothiocyanate (FITC) labeled goat anti-rabbit IgG (Jackson Immunoresearch) at a dilution of 1:50, and then read using a fluorescent microscope. Tissue culture infective dose ($TCID_{50}$/mL) was calculated using the Spearman-Karber method.

Molecular analysis

Viral RNA from cell culture passages was extracted by using the MagMAX™-96 viral RNA isolation kit (Life Technologies) according to the manufacturer's instructions. rt-

RT-PCR was performed by using QIAGEN Quantitect® RT-PCR with the following PEDV primers and probe: PEDV forward: 5'-ACG TCC GTA ACA CCT TCA AG -3', PEDV reverse: 5'-GCT AGT GCC TGT ACC ATA GAT C-3', and PEDV Probe: 5'-/5HEX/ CGT GCC AGT AAT CAA CTC ACC CTT TGT /3IABkFQ/-3'. For analytical purposes, negative samples were assigned a Ct value of 37.1, which corresponds to the detection limit of the method (approximately -1.0 $TCID_{50}$/mL). Method specificity was assessed by using various porcine enteric viruses, including transmissible gastroenteritis virus, group A rotavirus and porcine enterovirus, and no cross-reaction was observed. A standard curve was generated by serial dilution of M145 cell harvests containing 5.7 $\log_{10}$ $TCID_{50}$/mL of PEDV, as determined by titration on M145 cells.

RNA isolation for next generation sequencing

M145 cells that showed 100% cytopathic effects (CPE) following virus infection at passage x + 9 were used for RNA extraction for sequencing. 20 mL of cell culture supernatant was filtered using the 0.2 μm bottle top filters (Thermo Scientific, Lenexa, Kansas). The filtrate was centrifuged at 50,000 × g for 2 hours. Supernatant was discarded and the pellet was suspended in 1000 μL of water. Samples were concentrated to a final 100 μL volume using Amicon® ultra centrifugal filters (0.5 mL; 50KDa) (Millipore, Tullagreen, Ireland). Cellular DNA and RNA were removed by incubation with DNase I (25 units) (New England Biolabs, NEB, Ipswich, MA) and RNase A (25units) (Qiagen, Valencia, CA) at 37°C for 1 hour. RNA was extracted using Trizol® LS Reagent (Life Technologies, Grand Island, NY) according to manufacturer's instructions. The pellet containing RNA was resuspended in 20 μL of sterile H₂O.

Sequencing and data analysis

10 μg of total RNA was depleted of ribosomal RNA using GeneRead™ rRNA depletion kit (Qiagen) and RNA sequencing libraries were generated using the Ion Total RNA-seq kit v2 (Ion Torrent™, Life Technologies) according to manufacturer's instructions. Sequencing was carried out using Ion Personal Genome Machine® (PGM) sequencing platform (Life Technologies, Grand Island, NY) as previously described [27]. Sequence reads were assembled into contigs using the SeqMan® NGen program (DNAstar, Madison, WI). Phylogenetic analysis on full genome sequences was performed using MEGA™ 6.0 software using Maximum Likelihood analysis with 1000 bootstrap replicates to verify tree topology. Sequence alignments were performed using the ClustalW algorithm in MegAlign (DNAstar, Madison WI). The complete genome of NPL PEDV 2013 P10.1 was compared to the sequence derived from the original clinical sample [Genbank:KJ778615] and various reference

strains. The reference strains included: CV777 [Genbank:EF353511] from Belgium; DR13 attenuated [Genbank:JQ023162], DR13 virulent [Genbank:JQ023161], and SM98 [Genbank:GU937797] from South Korea; LZC [Genbank:EF185992], JS2008 [Genbank:KC109141], and CHS [Genbank:JN547228] from China; CO13 [Genbank:KF272920], MN [Genbank:KF468752], and a variant strain OH851 [Genbank:KJ399978] from the United States. The genome sequence for NPL PEDV 2013 P10.1 was deposited in GenBank under the accession number KM052365 [Genbank:KM052365].

Assessment of immunogenicity in swine

Swine vaccination studies were approved by the Institutional Biosafety Committee, under Institutional Animal Care and Use Committee (IACUC) guidelines. The studies were performed at Newport Laboratories under biosafety level 1. Sixty pigs approximately 4 weeks of age were obtained from a commercial high-health herd. They were of mixed sexes of crossbred American Yorkshire-Landrace-Duroc. Prior to study commencement pigs were verified as serologically negative to PEDV by FFN and IFA. Pigs were also negative for PEDV shedding by rt-RT-PCR on fecal swabs. Pigs were divided into 8 vaccination groups of 5–9 pigs and a nonvaccinated control group of 5 pigs, co-mingled among two different rooms. Pigs were allowed 1 week to acclimate prior to study commencement.

Virus NPL PEDV 2013 P10.1 (6.6 $\log_{10}$ $TCID_{50}$/mL) was inactivated and concentrated 30X for use as vaccine. Inactivation was performed by the addition of 0.1 M binary ethyleneimine (BEI) to a final volume of 5% and incubating at 37°C for 24 hours. Excess BEI was neutralized with sodium thiosulfate. Virus inactivation was verified by passaging the inactivated fluids three times on permissive cells, resulting in no evidence of CPE or increase in rt-RT-PCR titer. Concentration was performed using a 10kD hollow fiber filter (Spectrum Labs). Due to the space constraints and the number of study groups, vaccination groups receiving 8.0 $\log_{10}$ $TCID_{50}$/mL antigen consisted of more pigs than groups receiving lower levels of antigen as they were anticipated to show the most robust immune response (Table 1). Groups 1–3 were vaccinated intramuscularly (IM) in the neck with 2 mL of 8.0, 7.0 or 6.0 $\log_{10}$ $TCID_{50}$/mL, respectively, of inactivated virus. Groups 5–7 were vaccinated IM in the neck with 2 mL of 8.0, 7.0 or 6.0 $\log_{10}$ $TCID_{50}$/mL, respectively, of inactivated virus treated with Triton® X-100 (added to 0.1% and incubated at room temperature 30 minutes) (Sigma). Groups 4 and 8 were vaccinated in the rear flank with 8.0 $\log_{10}$ $TCID_{50}$/mL of inactivated virus and inactivated virus treated with Triton® X-100, respectively. This was done to evaluate any potential changes in immune response due to a change in

Table 1 Vaccination groups and treatment

Group	Vaccine*	Pigs
0	Negative control	5
1	8.0 IM	8
2	7.0 IM	5
3	6.0 IM	5
4	8.0 RF	9
5	8.0 IM + Triton® X-100	9
6	7.0 IM + Triton® X-100	5
7	6.0 IM + Triton® X-100	5
8	8.0 RF + Triton® X-100	9

*PEDV titer in vaccine prior to inactivation (log_{10} $TCID_{50}$/mL) and route of administration (IM, intramuscular neck; RF, rear flank).

vaccination site. All vaccines were formulated to contain 67% TS6, a proprietary oil in water adjuvant. Pigs were vaccinated on days 0 and 21 and observed for adverse vaccine reactions for one hour. Animals were also observed daily for signs of disease. Serum was collected on days 0, 21 and 35, and the study was terminated at day 35. Fecal swabs were collected three days post vaccination and were tested by rt-RT-PCR to confirm absence of PEDV shedding.

Serology

The fluorescent foci neutralization assay (FFN) was performed at SDSU using a National Veterinary Services Laboratory (NVSL) reference isolate, USA/Colorado/2013 (CO/13). Briefly, test and control serum samples were heat inactivated at 56°C for 30 minutes, then serially diluted in serum-free Modified Eagles Medium (MEM) containing 1.0 μg/mL TPCK treated trypsin in 96-well plates with a final volume of 100 μL/well. Next, 100 μL of PEDV stock diluted to 100–200 fluorescent focus units (FFU)/100 μL was added to each well and plates were incubated at 37°C for 1 hour. Plates containing confluent 3 day old monolayers of Vero-76 cells were washed 3 times with serum-free MEM prior to transfer of the serum/virus mixtures to corresponding wells of these plates. After 1 hour incubation at 37°C, the serum/virus mixture was removed, monolayers washed once with serum-free MEM and 150 μL/well replacement media (MEM with 1.0 μg/mL TPCK treated trypsin) was added to each well. Plates were incubated 24 hours at 37°C, then monolayers fixed for 15 minutes with 80% acetone in water, dried and stained with fluorescein conjugated PEDV anti-nucleoprotein (NP) monoclonal antibody SD6-29. Titers were reported as the reciprocal of the greatest serum dilution resulting in a 90% or greater reduction in FFU relative to virus control well. A FFN titer <20 was considered negative.

Enzyme-linked immunosorbent assay (ELISA) was performed at the University of Minnesota (UMN) Veterinary

Diagnostic Laboratory. The assay utilizes a recombinant PEDV NP antigen and samples with a sample to positive ratio (S/P) value greater than 0.5 are considered positive. An experimental ELISA using a recombinant PEDV NP was also performed at SDSU to verify the UMN results. The SDSU cutoff for positive results was an S/P of 0.4, according to ROC analysis using Medcalc software (unpublished conference proceedings). Both ELISAs detected only swine IgG.

To further investigate the immune response to the inactivated PEDV vaccine, a fluorescent microsphere immunoassay (FMIA) was performed at SDSU using the same purified, full-length 51 kDa PEDV nucleoprotein antigen used in the ELISA. Briefly, the full length nucleocapsid open reading frame of PEDV was cloned into the pET-28a prokaryotic expression vector (Novagen). Recombinant proteins were expressed as His-tagged fusion proteins and purified using Ni-NTA agarose column chromatography prior to fluorescent microsphere coupling. The FMIA was performed as previously described [28,29]. Coupled microspheres were analyzed through a dual-laser Bio-Rad Bio-Plex 200 instrument. The mean fluorescence intensity (MFI) for 100 microspheres corresponding to each individual bead analyte was recorded for each well. All reported MFI measurements were normalized via $F - F_0$, where F_0 was the background signal determined from the fluorescence measurement of a test sample in uncoated beads and F was the MFI for a serological test sample in antigen-coated beads.

Statistical analysis

Statistical analysis was performed using SPSS 14 software. One-way ANOVA and Tukey HSD was performed on all groups, using harmonic mean sample size of 6.171 to account for unequal group sizes. Also, a comparison between the groups that had the same titer of the virus and different treatment was done by t-test.

Results
Virus isolation
The rt-RT-PCR Ct value of the PEDV positive intestinal homogenate was 21.4. After initial isolation attempts on Vero and Vero 76 cell lines, passaging of samples continued on Vero cells as viral replication was evident by rt-RT-PCR. CPE was evident after two passages and confirmed as PEDV by rt-RT-PCR and IFA. The Ct values for passages x + 1 through x + 5 ranged from 17.8-23.5. Cultures were scaled to a T25 Vero flask for x + 6 (17.97 Ct, 4.4 log_{10} $TCID_{50}$/mL). Cell cultures were adapted to M145 cells at x + 7 (18.55 Ct, 4.4 log_{10} $TCID_{50}$/mL) and x + 8 (23.31 Ct and 5.2 $TCID_{50}$/mL) due to their USDA-licensed status for autogenous vaccine production. After two passages in M145 25 cm^2 flasks, the culture was

scaled up to 1700 cm^2 roller bottles of M145 cells. This passage, X + 9, had a Ct = 21.2 and a titer of 6.6 log$_{10}$ TCID$_{50}$/mL as determined by IFA. The isolated PEDV was designated NPL PEDV 2013 P10.1.

Genetic analysis

Phylogenetic analysis of complete genome sequences showed >99% identity to U.S. PEDV virus CO/13 [Genbank:KF272920] and the original intestinal sample [Genbank:KJ778615]. The Minnesota isolate [Genbank:KF 468752] and an isolate from Ohio [Genbank:KJ408801] were also closely related to the NPL PEDV2013 strain (Figure 1). The ORF1ab, S, ORF3, envelope (E), membrane (M), and NP genes of eleven PED reference viruses were aligned and the percent nucleotide identity to NPL PEDV2013 P10.1 was determined (Table 2). ORF3 showed the greatest divergence, with 93.1-100% nucleotide identity. The S gene was the next most divergent, with 93.5-99.9% nucleotide identity. Amongst the US strains, ORF3, E, M, and NP were highly conserved with greater than 99.8% nucleotide identity. The S gene showed the greatest variability amongst U.S. strains, with OH851 having 96.9% identity to NPL PEDV 2013 P10.1 [30].

Pig vaccination and serology

All pigs in the study were confirmed seronegative for PEDV antibodies at day 0 by IFA and FFN (data not shown). Pig fecal swabs collected on day 3 post vaccination were negative for PEDV, further confirming that no infectious PEDV was present in the vaccine. No adverse reactions were noted following vaccination on days 0 and 21.

All vaccine groups had positive mean titers by the FFN (Table 3). Post Hoc analysis of the FFN results showed that all 8.0 log$_{10}$ TCID$_{50}$/mL groups [1,4,5,8], along with 7.0 log$_{10}$ TCID$_{50}$/mL Triton® X-100 treated

group (group 6), had statistically significant higher mean FFN titers than the control group 0 at p = 0.05 level and did not have a significant difference in means compared to each other per Tukey HSD. No groups were statistically similar to the control group by Tukey HSD analysis (using harmonic mean sample size of 6.171 due to unequal group sizes). The t-test was also performed on groups that had the same titer of virus and different treatment (Table 4). There was no statistical difference in FFN titers between vaccination groups of the same titer with and without Triton® X-100 treatment for the FFN assay.

Only one of the 9 animals in group 8, the 8.0 log$_{10}$ TCID$_{50}$/mL of inactivated Triton® X-100 treated virus to the rear flank, showed positive ELISA results at UMN (data not shown). To further clarify these results, an ELISA test was performed at SDSU and the results supported the UMN results in that no anti-nucleoprotein antibody from the Triton® X-100 treated groups was recognized. The ELISA results showed highly significant increases in S/P ratios in the 8.0 log$_{10}$ TCID$_{50}$/mL of inactivated virus to the IM neck and rear flank (groups 1 and 4, respectively) compared to control group 0 for both UMN and SDSU assays (Table 3). There was no significance between groups 1 and 4 by Tukey HSD, but both had significantly higher results compared to the remaining groups for the UMN ELISA. For the SDSU ELISA, group 2 (7.0 log$_{10}$ TCID$_{50}$/mL) also had significantly higher results than groups 3, 5, 6, and 8, per Tukey HSD. The t-test shows significant differences in ELISA results for the 8.0 log$_{10}$ TCID$_{50}$/mL groups 1 and 5 (IM, with and without Triton® X-100, respectively), as well as the 8.0 log$_{10}$ TCID$_{50}$/mL groups 4 and 8 (flank, with and without Triton® X-100, respectively). Also, the SDSU ELISA showed near significant difference between the 7.0 log$_{10}$ TCID$_{50}$/mL groups 2 and 6

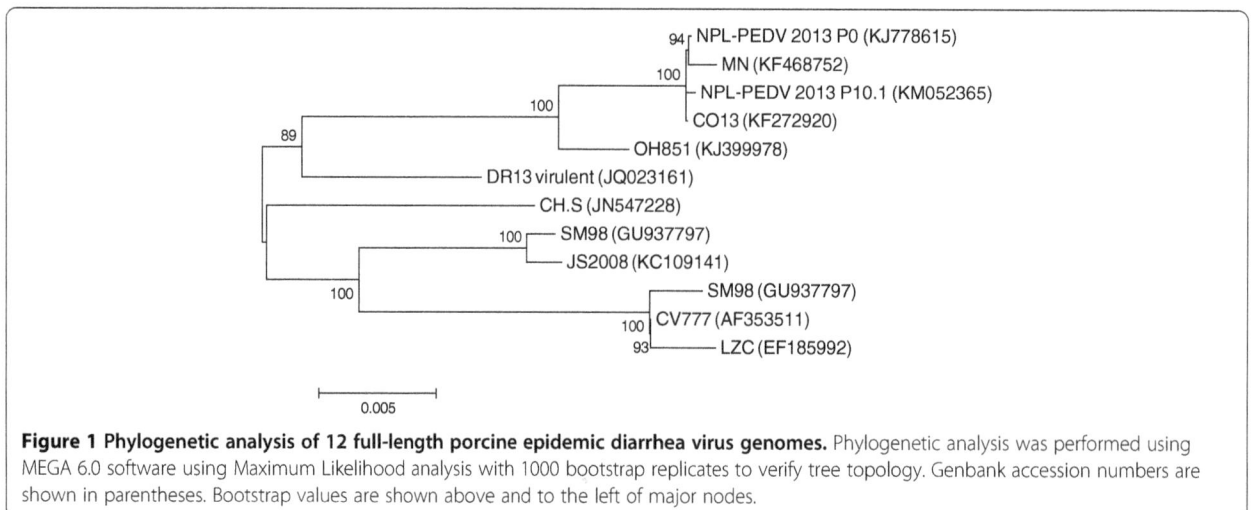

Figure 1 Phylogenetic analysis of 12 full-length porcine epidemic diarrhea virus genomes. Phylogenetic analysis was performed using MEGA 6.0 software using Maximum Likelihood analysis with 1000 bootstrap replicates to verify tree topology. Genbank accession numbers are shown in parentheses. Bootstrap values are shown above and to the left of major nodes.

Table 2 Genogroup and percent nucleotide identity of reference porcine epidemic diarrhea viruses to NPL PEDV 2013 P10.1

Virus (accession number)	Genogroup	ORF 1ab	S	ORF3	E	M	NP
CHS (JN47228)	G1	98.0	93.8	98.2	96.5	98.1	96.8
CO13 (KF272920)	G2	100.0	99.9	99.9	100.0	100.0	100.0
CV777 (AF353511)	G1	97.3	94.0	96.9	97.0	98.2	96.0
DR13 Attenuated (DQ462404)	G1	97.8	93.6	93.1	96.7	97.9	96.8
DR13 Virulent (JQ023161)	G2	98.2	95.0	98.5	98.3	98.4	97.4
JS2008 (KC109141)	G1	98.0	94.2	93.1	96.1	97.8	96.8
LZC (EF185992)	G1	97.2	93.5	95.6	96.1	97.2	95.8
MN (KJ468752)	G2	99.8	99.7	100.0	100.0	100.0	100.0
OH851 (KJ399978)	G2	99.5	96.9	100.0	100.0	99.9	99.8
SM98 (GU937797)	G1	97.2	93.7	96.8	96.1	98.1	95.9
NPL PEDV2013 p0 (KJ778615)	G2	100.0	99.8	100.0	100.0	100.0	100.0

(with and without Triton® X-100, respectively) with a p value of 0.057.

FMIA was performed and groups 1, 2, and 4 (8.0 $\log_{10}$ $TCID_{50}$/mL and 7.0 $\log_{10}$ $TCID_{50}$/mL IM and 8.0 $\log_{10}$ $TCID_{50}$/mL flank) and MFI values were significantly higher than the control by Tukey HSD analysis (Table 3). Again, the 8.0 $\log_{10}$ $TCID_{50}$/mL vaccine groups and the 7.0 $\log_{10}$ $TCID_{50}$/mL group without Triton® X-100 had statistically higher MFI than the Triton® X-100 treated groups by t-test (Table 4). Group 2, the 7.0 $\log_{10}$ $TCID_{50}$/mL group, had statistically lower MFI than groups 1 and 4, and significantly higher MFIs than all other groups. The 6.0 $\log_{10}$ $TCID_{50}$/mL groups [3,7] MFI showed no difference in Triton® X-100 treatment by t-test and were not significantly higher than controls via Tukey HSD. This is probably due to low antibody titers at the 6.0 $\log_{10}$ $TCID_{50}$/mL level. These results indicate that the Triton® X-100 treatment created significant differences in both ELISAs and the FMIA assay results, but did not affect FFN results.

Discussion

The severity of disease caused by an outbreak of PEDV makes it imperative that an efficacious vaccine be developed. Due to the difficulties of *in vitro* cultivation and high virus transmissibility leading to biosecurity concerns, limited research has been performed in pigs in the U.S. With a four percent success rate for virus isolation being reported, the development of diagnostic tests and research of U.S. field strains has been hampered [6]. After successfully isolating and passaging a U.S. PEDV isolate, growth was maintained on M145 cells between 5.0-6.6 $TCID_{50}$/mL.

The genetic characterization of NPL PEDV2013 P10.1 found that it is 99% identical to the strains circulating in Asia in the early 2010s. Its high genetic homology to the other circulating strains in the U.S. makes it a suitable candidate for investigation of U.S. PEDV inactivated vaccine immunogenicity in pigs. While there is data published regarding the efficacy of attenuated MLVs in Asia, there is limited published data on the immunogenicity of inactivated or subunit PEDV vaccines. This study demonstrates that inactivated PEDV vaccines are immunogenic is pigs.

Vaccine groups in this study were designed investigate at the effects of virus titer, site of administration and detergent treatment of antigen on immunogenicity in pigs. A dose response was observed by FFN for vaccines containing different virus titers, with 8.0 $\log_{10}$ $TCID_{50}$/mL groups all being significantly greater than 6.0 $\log_{10}$ $TCID_{50}$/mL groups. Vaccines were administered IM or in the rear flank to determine if the site of administration would affect overall immunogenic response. The flank vaccination site was only tested on the 8.0 $\log_{10}$ $TCID_{50}$/mL groups, as we expected them to have the highest immune response; however there was no significant difference between the two sites of administration. Likewise, there was no significant difference between vaccines formulated with Triton® X-100 treated antigen, by FFN. A challenge model is needed to correlate FFN and/or ELISA titers to protection.

Surprisingly, with the exception of one pig, negative ELISA results were obtained from pigs vaccinated with Triton® X-100 treated virus formulated at 8.0 $\log_{10}$ $TCID_{50}$/mL despite high FFN mean titers. The t-test shows Triton® X-100 treated groups were significantly different from non- Triton® X-100 treated groups at the same titer for ELISA and FMIA. Triton® X-100 detergent is used to create split-virion vaccines of influenza virus that are immunogenic and non-reactogenic [31]. Our data suggests that Triton® X-100 treatment of the PEDV antigen altered the antigenicity or immunogenicity of the NP, leading to negative ELISA results, while other immunogens capable of inducing a neutralizing antibody

Table 3 One way Anova and Tukey HSD

Group		FFN[†]	UM ELISA[#]	SDSU ELISA[#§]	FMIA[£]
0 (control)	Mean	1.93 [D]	0.00[B]	0.05[C]	0.04[C]
N = 5	Std.Deviation	2.66	0.00	0.05	0.04
	Std. Error	1.19	0.00	0.02	0.02
1 - 8.0 $\log_{10}$ TCID$_{50}$/mL	Mean	7.32[*A,B]	1.06[*A]	1.79[*A]	1.14[*A]
N = 8	Std.Deviation	1.2	0.17	0.79	0.04
	Std. Error	0.42	0.06	0.28	0.01
2 - 7.0 $\log_{10}$ TCID$_{50}$/mL	Mean	5.06[B,C]	0.29[B]	0.57[B]	0.51[*B]
N = 5	Std.Deviation	3.24	0.39	0.54	0.42
	Std. Error	1.45	0.17	0.24	0.19
3 - 6.0 $\log_{10}$ TCID$_{50}$/mL	Mean	4.66[C]	0.01[B]	0.07[C]	0.08[C]
N = 5	Std.Deviation	2.74	0.02	0.04	0.07
	Std. Error	1.23	0.01	0.02	0.03
4 - 8.0 $\log_{10}$ TCID$_{50}$/mL (Flank)	Mean	7.99[*A]	1.04[*A]	2.11[*A]	1.16[*A]
N = 9	Std.Deviation	1.32	0.40	0.26	0.03
	Std. Error	0.44	0.13	0.09	0.01
5 - 8.0 $\log_{10}$ TCID$_{50}$/mL (Triton® X-100)	Mean	6.99[*A,B]	0.00[B]	0.04[C]	0.06[C]
N = 9	Std.Deviation	1.80	0.01	0.03	0.07
	Std. Error	0.60	0.00	0.01	0.02
6 - 7.0 $\log_{10}$ TCID$_{50}$/mL (Triton® X-100)	Mean	6.52[*A,B,C]	0.11[B]	0.03[C]	0.04[C]
N = 5	Std.Deviation	0.84	0.03	0.04	0.05
	Std. Error	0.37	0.011	0.02	0.23
7 - 6.0 $\log_{10}$ TCID$_{50}$/mL (Triton® X-100)	Mean	5.12[B,C]	0.01[B]	0.36[C,B]	0.14[C]
N = 5	Std.Deviation	0.84	0.02	0.59	0.13
	Std. Error	0.37	0.01	0.27	0.06
8 - 8.0 $\log_{10}$ TCID$_{50}$/mL (Triton® X-100, Flank)	Mean	7.54[*A]	0.14[B]	0.06[C]	0.02[C]
N = 9	Std.Deviation	1.20	0.41	0.45	0.03
	Std. Error	0.40	0.14	0.02	0.11

[A,B,C,D] Tukey HSD lists different letters between groups whose means that are statistically significant. Those with same letters means no significant difference among their means. Tukey HSD used harmonic mean sample size = 6.171 to account for differences in group sizes.
[†]The FFN results were log2 transformed before analysis.
[#]The ELISA results are sample to positive (S/P) ratios. The UMN ELISA cutoff is 0.5. [#§]The SDSU cutoff for ELISA is S/P of 0.4.
[£]The FMIA MFI cutoff is 0.1.
*The mean difference is significant at the 0.05 level compared to the control group.

Table 4 T-test comparison between groups with same titer and different treatment (with and without Triton® X-100 treatment), results considered significant at p <0.05 level

Group	FFN	UM ELISA	SDSU ELISA	FMIA
2,6	.356	.143	.057	.038
3,7	.727	.986	.305	.438
1,5	.657	.000	.000	.000
4,8	.466	.000	.000	.000

response detected by the FFN assay remained intact. The two ELISA tests and the FMIA all utilize NP antigen. Triton® X-100 treatment of the vaccine may have altered the conformation of the virion NP such that antibody induced by this antigen was not able to recognize the recombinant NP used in the ELISA or FMIA. An assay, such as the FFN, that detects functional neutralizing antibody associated with epitopes on the S protein may be better at quantifying antibody response to Triton® X-100 treated viruses. Few ELISAs targeting the S protein are readily available and they may also be subject to variations in protein conformation associated with Triton® X-100 treatment.

Though the vaccine in this trial was able to generate an antibody response, as indicated by FFN, FMIA, and

ELISA assays, a protective titer is unknown. Previous work with attenuated virus used to vaccinate sows showed an immune response by ELISA in serum and colostrum, but could not draw a specific correlation to the level of mucosal immunity needed to confer protection [32]. Another study showed antibody was detected in serum from piglets and colostrum from pregnant sows after being inoculated with attenuated PEDV, though finding a specific protective antibody titer of the colostrum was complicated due to varying factors including litter size, colostrum uptake per piglet, antibody concentration, and quality of colostrum [20]. Due to biosecurity concerns, a post-vaccination challenge was not performed for this study. This should be done in the future to determine immune correlates of protection.

With reports that farms can be re-infected after a primary outbreak, disease will continue to be an ongoing problem due to lack of complete immunity after infection. In one case, piglets born from re-infected sows were reported to suffer around 30% mortality instead of near 100% during the first outbreak [33]. Further research is necessary to determine if secondary outbreaks in sows could be prevented via vaccination and or boosters. While this study focused on the humoral immune response in sera from vaccinated pigs, the post-vaccination immune response in sows and antibody titers in colostrum should be studied as the optimal vaccination regimen would utilize maternal antibodies to protect pigs when they are most susceptible to PEDV. Additionally, inactivated vaccines may prove efficacious when used as a booster in conjunction with live exposure or following MLV. If there is risk of re-infection among previously exposed herds, an inactivated vaccine booster to pregnant sows could reduce the occurrence of re-infection and limit secondary outbreaks. PEDV continues to be a source of economic loss and will continue to have a profound impact on the swine market in the U.S.

Conclusions

These results demonstrate the immunogenicity of the PEDV inactivated viral vaccines with a U.S. strain. Information from this immunogenicity study shows the potential for inactivated vaccine development for U.S. PEDV strains. Further work is needed to evaluate protective FFN titers and ELISA and FMIA responses in a vaccination-challenge study.

Abbreviations
PEDV: Porcine epidemic diarrhea virus; TCID50: Tissue culture infective dose; FFN: Fluorescent foci neutralization assay; FMIA: Fluorescent microsphere immunoassay; ELISA: Enzyme-linked immunosorbent assay; MLV: Modified live vaccine; S: Spike; ORF: Open reading frame; RFLP: Restriction fragment length polymorphism; USDA: United States Department of Agriculture; M145: MARC-145 cells; DMEM: Dulbecco's modification of Eagles Medium; TPCK: L-1-Tosylamide-2-phenylethyl chloromethyl ketone; rt-RT-PCR: Real time reverse transcription polymerase chain reaction; IFA: Indirect immunofluorescent assay; SDSU: South Dakota State University; FITC: Fluorescein isothiocyanate; CPE: Cytopathic effect; IACUC: Institutional Animal Care and Use Committee; BEI: Binary ethyleneimine; IM: Intramuscularly; NVSL: National Veterinary Services Laboratory; MEM: Modified Eagles Medium; FFU: Fluorescent focus units; NP: Nucleoprotein; UMN: University of Minnesota; S/P: Sample to positive ratio; MFI: Mean fluorescence intensity; E: Envelope; M: Membrane.

Competing interests
The authors have the following interest. EAC, RB, SA and BMH were employed by Newport Laboratories Inc. at the time of this study. Newport Laboratories Inc., a for-profit organization that offers diagnostic testing and produces vaccines for the livestock industries, is the funder for this study. This does not alter the authors' adherence to all the policies on sharing data and materials, as detailed online in the guide for authors.

Authors' contributions
EAC performed virus isolation, performed molecular analysis, co-wrote paper. SA performed next generation sequencing and contributed to materials and methods for that section. FO assisted with serological assays and statistical analysis. RB prepared vaccine and assisted in design of pig study. EN performed serological assays and contributed to serological materials and methods section, provided critical review. BMH supervised overall project and contributed to critical review of manuscript, co-wrote paper. All authors read and approved the final manuscript.

Acknowledgements
We would like to express our thanks to the Molecular and Viral departments at Newport Laboratories (Danielle McKeown, Jessica Peterson, Brent Wassman, Karen Schwartz, Josh Elston, Tina Spaans, and Pat Klumper) for their assistance in the growth and characterization of this U.S. PEDV strain. We also would like to thank the technicians who assisted with the animal studies at our research farm facility.

Disclaimer
This document is provided for scientific purposes only. Any reference to a brand or trademark herein is for information purposes only and is not intended for a commercial purpose or to dilute the rights of the respective owners(s) or the brand(s) or trademark(s).

Author details
[1]Newport Laboratories Inc., Worthington, MN, USA. [2]Department of Veterinary and Biomedical Sciences, South Dakota State University, Brookings, SD, USA. [3]Present Address: Veterinary Diagnostic Laboratory, Kansas State University, Manhattan, KS, USA. [4]National Research Center, Giza, Egypt.

References
1. Pensaert MB, de Bouck P. A new coronavirus-like particle associated with diarrhea in swine. Arch Virol. 1978;58:243–7. doi:10.1007/BF01317606.
2. Horvath I, Mocsari E. Ultrastructural changes in the small intestinal epithelium of suckling pigs affected with a transmissible gastroenteritis (TGE)-like disease. Arch Virol. 1981;68:103–13.
3. Kweon CH, Kwon BJ, Jung TS, Kee YJ, Hur DH, Hwang ED, et al. Isolation of porcine epidemic diarrhea virus (PEDV) in Korea. Korean J Vet Res. 1993;33:249–54.
4. Sueyoshi M, Tsuda T, Yamazaki K, Yoshida K, Nakazawa M, Sato K, et al. An immunohistochemical investigation of porcine epidemic diarrhoea. J Comp Path. 1995;113:59–67.
5. Arriba ML, Carvajal A, Pozo J, Rubio P. Mucosal and systemic isotype-specific antibody responses and protection in conventional pigs exposed to virulent or attenuated porcine epidemic diarrhoea virus. Vet Immunol Immunopathol. 2002;85(2002):85–97.
6. Chen Q, Li G, Stasko J, Thomas JT, Stensland WR, Pillatzki AE, et al. Isolation and characterization of porcine epidemic diarrhea viruses associated with the 2013 disease outbreak among swine in the United States. J Clin Microbiol. 2014;52:234–43.
7. Huang YW, Dickerman AW, Pineyro P, Li L, Fang L, Kiehne R, et al. Origin, evolution, and genotyping of emergent porcine epidemic diarrhea virus

strains in the united states. mBio. 2013;4(5):e00737–13. doi:10.1128/mBio.00737-13 15 Oct 2013.

8. Shibata I, Tsuda T, Mori M, Ono M, Sueyoshi M, Uruno K. Isolation of porcine epidemic diarrhea virus in porcine cell cultures and experimental infection of pigs of different ages. Vet Microbiol. 2000;72(2000):173–82.

9. Park JE, Cruz DJM, Shin HJ. Receptor-bound porcine epidemic diarrhea virus spike protein cleaved by trypsin induces membrane fusion. Arch Virol. 2011;156:1749–56.

10. Yang X, Huo JY, Chen L, Zheng FM, Chang HT, Zhao J, et al. Genetic variation analysis of reemerging porcine epidemic diarrhea virus prevailing in central China from 2010 to 2011. Virus Genes. 2012;46:337–44.

11. Li C, Li Z, Zou Y, Wicht O, van Kuppeveld FJM, Rottier PJM, et al. Manipulation of the porcine epidemic diarrhea virus genome using targeted RNA recombination. PLoS One. 2013;8(8):e69997.

12. Song DS, Oh JS, Kang BK, Yang JS, Moon HJ, Yoo HS, et al. Oral efficacy of Vero cell attenuated porcine epidemic diarrhea virus DR13 strain. Res Vet Sci. 2007;82:134–40.

13. Sato T, Takeyama N, Katsumata A, Tuchiya K, Kodama T, Kusanagi K. Mutations in the spike gene of porcine epidemic diarrhea virus associated with growth adaptation in vitro and attenuation of virulence in vivo. Virus Genes. 2011;43:72–8.

14. Bosch BJ, van der Zee R, de Haan CA, Rottier PJ. The coronavirus spike protein is a class I virus fusion protein: structural and functional characterization of the fusion core complex. J Virol. 2003;77:8801–11.

15. Sun D, Feng L, Shi H, Chen J, Cui X, Chen H, et al. Identification of two novel B cell epitopes on porcine epidemic diarrhea virus spike protein. Vet Microbiol. 2008;131:73–81.

16. Cruz DJM, Kim CH, Shin HJ. The GPRLQPY motif located at the carboxy-terminal of the spike protein induces antibodies that neutralize porcine epidemic diarrhea virus. Virus Res. 2008;132:192–6.

17. Song D, Park B. Porcine epidemic diarrhoea virus: a comprehensive review of molecular epidemiology, diagnosis, and vaccines. Virus Genes. 2012;44:167–75.

18. Meng F, Ren Y, Suo S, Sun X, Li X, Li P, et al. Evaluation on the efficacy of immunogenicity of recombinant DNA plasmids expressing spike genes from porcine transmissible gastroenteritis virus and porcine epidemic diarrhea virus. PLoS ONE. 2013;8(3):e57468.

19. Shirato K, Matsuyama S, Ujike M, Taguchi F. Role of proteases in the release of porcine epidemic diarrhea virus from infected cells. J Virol. 2011;85(15):7872–80.

20. Song DS, Yang JS, Oh JS, Han JH, Park BK. Differentiation of a Vero cell adapted porcine epidemic diarrhea virus from Korean field strains by restriction fragment length polymorphism analysis of ORF3. Vaccine. 2003;21:1833–42.

21. Song DS, Oh JS, Kang BK, Yang JS, Song JY, Moon H, et al. Fecal shedding of a highly cell-culture-adapted porcine epidemic diarrhea virus after oral inoculation in pigs. J Swine Health Prod. 2005;13(5):269–72.

22. Chen J, Wang C, Shi H, Qiu H, Liu S, Chen X, et al. Molecular epidemiology of porcine epidemic diarrhea virus in China. Arch Virol. 2010;155:1471–6.

23. Chen JF, Sun DB, Wang CB, Shi HY, Cui XC, Liu SW, et al. Molecular characterization and phylogenetic analysis of membrane protein genes of porcine epidemic diarrhea virus isolates in China. Virus Genes. 2008;36:355–64.

24. Sun RQ, Cai RJ, Chen YQ, Liang PS, Chen DK, Song CX. Outbreak of porcine epidemic diarrhea in suckling piglets, china. Emerg Infect Dis. 2012;18(1):161–3.

25. Tian Y, Yu Z, Cheng K, Liu Y, Huang J, Xin Y, et al. Molecular characterization and phylogenetic analysis of new variants of the porcine epidemic diarrhea virus in Gansu, China in 2012. Viruses. 2013;2013(5):1991–2004.

26. Kim HS, Kwang J, Yoon IJ, Joo HS, Frey ML. Enhanced replication of porcine reproductive and respiratory syndrome (PRRS) virus in a homogenous subpopulation of MA-104 cell line. Arch Virol. 1993;133(2–4):477–83.

27. Anbalagan S, Cooper E, Klumper P, Simonson R, Hause B. Whole genome analysis of epizootic haemorrhagic disease virus identified limited genome constellations and preferential reassortment. J Gen Virol. 2014;95:434–41.

28. Lawson S, Lunney J, Zuckermann F, Osorio F, Nelson E, Welbon C, et al. Development of an 8-plex Luminex assay to detect swine cytokines for vaccine development: Assessment of immunity after porcine reproductive and respiratory syndrome virus (PRRSV) vaccination. Vaccine. 2010;28:5383–91.

29. Langenhorst R, Lawson S, Kittawornrat A, Zimmerman J, Sun Z, Li Y, et al. Development of a fluorescent microsphere immunoassay for detection of antibodies against PRRSV using oral fluid samples as an alternative to serum-based assays. Clin Vaccine Immunol. 2012;19:180–9.

30. Wang L, Byrum B, Zhang Y. New variant of porcine epidemic diarrhea virus, United States, [letter]. Emerg Infect Dis. 2014, doi:10.3201/eid2005.140195.

31. Gross PA, Ennis FA, Gaerlan PF, Denning CR, Setia U, Davis WJ, et al. Comparison of new triton X-100- and tween-ether-treated split-product vaccines in children. J Clin Microbiol. 1981;14:534–8.

32. Kweon CH, Kwon BJ, Lee JG, Kwon GO, Kang YB. Derivation of attenuated porcine epidemic diarrhea virus (PEDV) as vaccine candidate. Vaccine. 1999;17:2546–53.

33. Polansek T. "Exclusive: Deadly pig virus re-infects U.S. farm, fuels supply fears." Reuters. Thomson Rueters. 28 May, 2014. Web. 26 June 2014.

11

Feeding a high-grain diet reduces the percentage of LPS clearance and enhances immune gene expression in goat liver

Guangjun Chang[1], Kai Zhang[1], Tianle Xu[1], Di Jin[1], Hans-Martin Seyfert[3], Xiangzhen Shen[1*] and Su Zhuang[2*]

Abstract

Background: The effects of feeding a high-grain (HG) diet on lipopolysaccharide (LPS) clearance and innate immune defence responses in the liver remain unclear. Therefore, we conducted the present study in which twelve female goats were randomly assigned to either a treatment group fed a HG diet (60% grain, n = 6) or a control group fed a low grain diet (LG; 40% grain, n = 6) for 6 weeks. Catheters were installed in the mesenteric, portal and hepatic veins, as well as one femoral artery of the goats, for determining blood flow and net clearance rate of LPS in the liver. Plasma and tissue samples were collected in the week 6 for analyzing pro-inflammatory cytokines, acute phase protein and biochemical parameters, as well as expression of genes involved in immune response.

Result: HG diet feeding increased blood flow and LPS concentration in the portal vein, hepatic vein and artery. Hepatic net LPS clearance showed that HG diet feeding elevated the rate of hepatic LPS clearance, but decreased the percentage of removed LPS accounting for the total entry of LPS into the liver. Our results demonstrated that the feeding of HG diet increased plasma concentrations of pro-inflammatory cytokines and acute phase proteins and triggered a systemic inflammatory response. In addition, peripheral blood plasma concentrations of alanine aminotransferase, alkaline phosphatase and total bilirubin were increased in the HG group compared to the LG group. This indicated that the impairment of hepatocytes occurred after 6 weeks of HG diet feeding. The expression of genes involved in immune response and Toll-like receptor (TLR)4 protein in the liver was up-regulated in the HG group compared to the LG group, indicating that increased entry of LPS enhanced hepatic immune defence responses and contributed to hepatic inflammatory responses.

Conclusion: These results provide insight into the capacity of the liver to clear LPS. The increased entry of LPS into liver enhanced hepatic immune defence responses, thereby elevated the rate of LPS clearance. However, the reduction of the percentage of hepatic LPS clearance could be due to the formation of hepatocyte lesion during HG diet feeding.

Keywords: High grain diet, Lipopolysaccharide, Immune gene expression, Liver

Background

Ruminants are fed a high grain diet to support high milk yields or induce rapid weight gain in modern animal husbandry. However, the long-term consumption of high grain diet is harmful to the health of ruminants. It has been reported that the feeding of high grain diet resulted in reduced pH values and increased lipopolysaccharide (LPS) concentrations in the digestive tract [1-3]. These changes cause local inflammatory responses of digestive tract and injury to the gastrointestinal barrier [4-6], which facilitates the translocation of LPS from the digestive tract into the bloodstream [7,8].

Many studies have demonstrated that increased circulating LPS cause a systemic inflammatory response [8-10]. Acute phase proteins (APPs), such as serum amyloid A (SAA), haptoglobin (Hp) and LPS-binding protein (LBP), are biomarkers for the diagnosis of inflammation and infection [11]. An increase of SAA and

---

* Correspondence: xzshen@njau.edu.cn; zhuangsu@njau.edu.cn
[1]College of Veterinary Medicine, Nanjing Agricultural University, Nanjing 210095, PR, China
[2]College of Animal Science and Technology, Nanjing Agricultural University, Nanjing 210095, PR, China
Full list of author information is available at the end of the article

Hp concentrations in the peripheral blood of cows fed a high proportion of grain diet showed that a systemic inflammatory response was activated [8]. The concentration of LBP in peripheral blood is an important indicator for systemic inflammation caused by circulating LPS. An increase of plasma LBP concentration in a grain-induced subacute ruminal acidosis (SARA) experimental model indicated that LPS translocated from the digestive tract into the bloodstream to elicit a systemic inflammatory response [1]. In addition, the increased levels of circulating LPS also can elevated the concentration of blood pro-inflammatory cytokines (interleukin (IL)-1, IL-6 and tumour necrosis factor (TNF)-α). A recent study showed that the concentration of pro-inflammatory cytokines was significantly increased in an LPS intra-mammary infusion experiment [12]. The feeding of a high concentrate corn straw diet also resulted in increased pro-inflammatory cytokines in mammary arteries caused by the translocation of LPS from the digestive tract into the bloodstream [13].

Experimentally-induced endotoxic shock demonstrated that the liver is a major contributor of inflammatory cytokines in the bloodstream [14]. Circulating LPS entering the liver is recognized by Toll-like receptor (TLR) 4, which is expressed on the surface of Kupffer cells (liver macrophages) and other immune cells, to orchestrate the synthesis and secretion of cytokines and chemokines [15-17]. Subsequently, those cytokines can activate intracellular signalling pathways between immune cells and hepatocytes to regulate hepatic APP synthesis [18]. The synthesis of SAA and Hp was enhanced in primary bovine hepatocytes in response to stimulation with recombinant human pro-inflammatory cytokines [19]. Intravenous or intra-mammary infusion of LPS is frequently used in an *Escherichia coli*-induced mastitis model [12,20,21], where expression of cytokines and APPs was significantly increased in the liver of experimental animals. However, the production of excessive cytokines in the liver can cause functionally- impaired hepatocytes [22,23].

It is well known that the liver is the main site for clearance of circulating LPS [24,25], and these hepatic removing mechanisms have been well documented [26,27]. The significant increase in LPS concentrations in the bloodstream during feeding with high grain diet has received increasing attentions [1,28]. However, few investigations have reported on the rate of hepatic LPS clearance and the percentage of removed LPS accounting for the total entry of LPS into liver. Furthermore, little information is available regarding hepatic immune responses induced by the increased entry of LPS into the liver during the feeding of high grain diet. Therefore, we hypothesized that feeding a high grain diet to goats resulted in the increased entry of LPS into liver, thereby enhanced hepatic immune defence response heightening the rate of hepatic LPS clearance.

Methods

The experimental design and sampling procedures were approved by the Nanjing Agricultural University Institutional Animal Care and Use Committee before the beginning of this experiment.

Animals, diets and experimental design

Goats were housed in individual metabolic cage in the Centre of Experimental Animal at Nanjing Agricultural University (Nanjing, China). Twelve non-lactating and non-pregnant GuanZhong dairy goats (body weight 40.56 ± 1.34 kg, mean ± SEM) aged 2–3 years were used in experiments. All goats received a low grain diet (LG; forage: concentrate = 6:4) for weeks before the start of the formal experiment as an adaption period to obtain a similar metabolic status in all individuals. The goats were randomly assigned to two groups: goats were fed an LG diet ($n = 6$) as the control group or fed a high grain diet (HG; forage: concentrate = 4:6; $n = 6$) as the treatment group (Table 1). During the experimental period of six weeks, goats were fed two times daily at 8.30 and 16.30, had free access to fresh water, and the feed amount met or exceeded the animal's nutritional requirements.

Table 1 Chemical composition and nutrient levels of diets

Ingredient	Percentage (%) of ingredients (dry matter)	
	LG diet	HG diet
Chinese wildrye hay	48.00	32.00
Alfalfa hay	12.00	8.00
Corn	28.78	43.17
Soybean meal	8.45	12.68
limestone	0.77	1.25
Calcium phosphate dibasic	1.10	1.65
Salt	0.40	0.50
Premix [a]	0.50	0.75
Forage: Concentrate	6:4	4:6
Nutrient levels, % of dry matter		
Dry mater, %	88.90	88.60
Net energy, MJ/kg	5.40	5.89
CP, %	12.24	13.45
NDF, %	36.55	27.69
ADF, %	24.04	17.54

[a]Premix provided: 3000, 1250, and 40 IU kg^{-1} of diet of vitamin A, D and E, and 6.25, 62.5, 62.5, 50, 0.25, 0.125, 0.125 mg kg^{-1} of diet of Cu, Fe, Zn, Mn, I, Se, Co, respectively. CP: crude protein; NDF: neutral detergent fibre; ADF: acid detergent fibre.

In the first week of the adaption period, Catheters were administered in the mesenteric, portal and hepatic veins, as well as one femoral artery of the goats, for determining blood flow and net clearance rate of LPS in the liver. According to previous study [29], concentration of arterial content is homogeneous, so we used the femoral artery to substitute for hepatic artery. Animals were looked after for 3 weeks after surgery. Sterilized heparin saline (500 IU/mL, 0.3 mL/time) was used to prevent catheter blocking at 8-hour intervals per day until the end of the experiment.

Sample collection

On the first 3 days of the 6th week, blood samples were collected from the portal vein, hepatic vein, and femoral artery at 0 h (15 min before feeding), and at 2, 4, 6, and 8 h after feeding and injected into a blank 5 mL heparinised evacuated glass tube. Blood samples from the jugular vein were taken at 0 h (15 min before feeding), and at 4 and 8 h after feeding. Samples were kept on ice until transported to the laboratory. Plasma was harvested by centrifuging heparinised evacuated glass tubes at $1900 \times g$ for 15 min. Plasma from the portal vein, hepatic vein and femoral artery were transferred into pyrogen-free glass tubes and stored at $-20°C$ for LPS analysis. Plasma from the jugular vein was preserved in sterilized Eppendorf plastic tubes and stored at $-20°C$ for analysis of APPs, cytokines, and biochemical parameters.

After 2 days of blood sampling, goats were measured the body weight and then administered a continuous infusion of a sterilized aqueous solution (pH 7.4) of *para*-aminohippuric acid (pAH, 1% (wt/vol), CAS 94-16-6, from Alfa Aesar China Co., Ltd) into the mesenteric vein. The initial rate of infusion was 4 mL/min for 10 min, and then the infusion rate was kept constant (0.8 mL/min) until the end of sampling. Blood samples were collected from the portal vein, hepatic vein, and femoral artery at 0 h (15 min before feeding), and at 2, 4, 6, and 8 h after feeding and injected into a blank 5 mL heparinised evacuated glass tube. Plasma was harvested by centrifuging heparinised evacuated glass tubes at $1900 \times g$ for 15 min and transferred into Eppendorf plastic tubes and stored at $-20°C$ for measurement of pAH.

On the last day of the 6th week, liver samples were excised immediately after euthanasia. Small frozen tubes (2 mL) were snap-frozen and stored in liquid nitrogen.

Measurements of plasma parameters

The concentration of pAH in the portal vein, hepatic vein and artery were determined as described previously [30]. In brief, plasma was deproteinised by addition of 0.5 mL/L trichloroacetic acid and then spun down at $1000 \times g$ for 15 min. A portion (2 g) of supernatant was mixed with 0.5 g of 1.2 mol/L HCL, heated at 95°C for 65 min without charring, and left to cool at room temperature for 15 min. Then, 0.25 mL of 1% sodium nitrite, 0.25 mL of 0.5% ammonium sulphamate and 0.25 mL of 0.1% N-1-napthyl-ethylene-diamino-dihydrochloride were added in time sequence. After 60 min at room temperature, the absorbance of samples and standards was read at 540 nm in a spectrophotometer (V-5600, METASH, Shanghai, China). The concentration of pAH was calculated according to the standard curve.

The concentration of LPS in the plasma of the portal vein, hepatic vein and femoral artery was determined by a chromogenic endpoint assay (CE80545, Chinese Horseshoe Crab Reagent Manufactory Co., Ltd., Xiamen, China) with a minimum detection limit of 0.01 EU/mL. The procedures were performed in accordance with the manufacturer's instruction, as described by Dong *et al.* [31].

Radioimmunoassay was applied to determine the concentrations of master cytokines, including IL-1β, IL-6 and TNF-α in circulating blood. The concentrations of IL-1β, IL-6 and TNF-α were determined with commercially available human radioimmunoassay kits purchased from Beijing North Institute of Biological Technology. The detected range of radioimmunoassay kits for IL-1β (cat. C09DJB), IL-6 (cat. C12DJB) and TNF-α (cat. C06PJB) were 0.1–8.1 ng/mL, 50–4000 pg/ml and 9–590 fmol/mL, respectively.

APPs such as LBP (cat. BP-E93101, Shanghai Lengton), Hp (cat. ab108856, Shanghai Abcam), and SAA (cat. ab100635, Shanghai Abcam) were detected by enzyme-linked immunosorbent assay (ELISA) kits according to the manufacturer's instructions. ELISA kits for SAA and Hp were already validated by Dong *et al.* [31]. The assay range of the LBP ELISA kit was 62.5–2000 ng/mL. Plasma samples were diluted until the LBP concentration was in the range of this kit.

The plasma concentrations of alanine aminotransferase (ALT), aspartate aminotransferase (AST), total proteins (T-PRO), albumin (ALB), total bilirubin (T-BIL) and alkaline phosphatase (ALP) were determined using enzymatic colorimetric assay kits on an automatic biochemical analyser (Mindray BS-300, Mindray Medical International Limited, Shenzhen, China).

RNA extraction and real-time quantitative PCR (RT-qPCR)

RT-qPCR was performed using an ABI 7300 instrument to determine the relative copy numbers of the different mRNA. Liver samples were powdered in a mortar under liquid nitrogen and total RNA was extracted with TRIZOL (Takara) according to the manufacturer's protocol. For cDNA synthesis, 1.5 µg of total RNA was prepared in reverse transcriptional reaction with oligo(dT) for all mRNAs. After reverse transcription (cat. RR036A, Takara) and cDNA purification (cat. D0033, Beyotime), RT-qPCR was run with gene-specific primer pairs to amplify the target segment of cDNA using the SYBR Premix EX Taq™ kit (DRR420A, Takara). Relative copy numbers of the individual mRNA were calculated from a dilution series of 10^6 to 10^2 copies of the respective cDNA subclones. All samples were checked twice from two independent cDNA preparations. All primers used for amplification are listed in Table 2.

Western blotting

Liver tissue was crushed in a mortar under liquid nitrogen and total protein was extracted with RIPA Lysis Buffer (cat. SN338, Sunshine Biotechnology (Nanjing) Co., Ltd). Protein concentration was determined using the BCA assay (Pierce, Rockford, IL, USA). Fifty μg of protein extracted from each sample was applied to electrophoresis on a 7.5% sodium dodecyl sulphate-polyacrylamide gel electrophoresis (SDS-PAGE) gel, and the separated proteins were transferred onto nitrocellulose membranes (Bio Trace, Pall Co., USA). Western blotting analysis for TLR4 (sc-293072, Santa Cruz Biotechnology Inc., 1:200) was performed with the primary antibody and corresponding HRP-conjugated secondary antibody. β-actin (KC-5A08, Kang Chen Bio-Tech, China, 1:5000) was used as a reference protein for normalization in western blotting analyses. Then the blot was washed and detected by enhanced chemiluminescence (ECL) using the Lumi-Glo substrate (Super Signal West Pico Trial Kit, Pierce, USA). ECL signals were recorded by an imaging system (Bio-Rad, USA) and analyzed with Quantity One software (Bio-Rad, USA). Gray values of TLR4 protein were presented as fold change relative to the mean value of the control group.

Calculation and statistical analysis

The calculation of blood flow was previously described by Huntington et al. [32] and Wieghart et al. [33] as follows:

$$F_P(L/h) = C_0 I / (C_P - C_A); F_H(L/h) = C_0 I / (C_H - C_A);$$

$$F_A = F_H - F_P;$$

where I (L/h) is the rate of initial infusion, C_0 represents the initial content of pAH (mg/L); C_P, C_H, C_A are pAH concentration (mg/L) in plasma of portal vein, hepatic vein and artery, respectively. F_P, F_H and F_A represent the mean blood flow in the portal vein, hepatic vein and artery. Net clearance rate and ratio in liver were calculated in accordance with the following equations, modified by Lobley [29] and Galindo [34]:

$$Net\ clearance\ rate(EU/h) = F_P \times P_{LPS} + F_A \\ \times A_{LPS} - F_H \times H_{LPS};$$

$$Net\ clearance\ ratio = (F_P \times P_{LPS} + F_A \times A_{LPS} - F_H \times H_{LPS}) / \\ (F_P \times P_{LPS} + F_A \times A_{LPS}) \times 100\%$$

where P_{LPS}, H_{LPS} and A_{LPS} are the concentrations of LPS in plasma of portal vein, hepatic vein and artery.

Data of blood flow, LPS concentration, LPS clearance, and plasma parameters (cytokines, biochemical parameter, and APPs) were analysed with repeated measures using the MIXED procedure of SAS (SAS version 9.2, SAS Institute Inc.). The effects of diet and time were considered fixed. The effects of goats, diet × goats and diet × time × goats were considered random. Time within diet and goat was considered a repeated measure, and compound symmetry (CS) was used as the type of covariance. Data analysis of the expression of mRNAs encoding selected genes involved in immune response and

Table 2 The list of primers for amplification of RT-qPCR

Gene	Forward primer	Reverse primer	Length
TLR4	CTGAGAACCGAGAGCTGGGAC	GCCTTGAAATGTGTTGTCTTCA	207 bp
TLR2	GCTCAGGTGGAAGCTTTCCAG	GGTGATCTCGTTGTTGGACAG	241 bp
IL-1A	GATGATGACCTGGAAGCCATTG	GCTGAGAATCCTCTTCTGATAC	259 bp
IL-1B	CCGTGATGATGACCTGAGGAG	CAAGACAGGTATAGATTCTTGTC	303 bp
IL-6	CGAAGCTCTCATTAAGCACATC	CCAGGTATATCTGATACTCCAG	241 bp
TNF-α	CAACAGGCCTCTGGTTCAGAC	GGACCTGCGAGTAGATGAGG	209 bp
IL-8	CTGAGAGTTATTGAGAGTGGGC	CAGTACTCAAGGCACTGAAGTAG	259 bp
IL-10	GTGATGCCACAGGCTGAGAAC	GAAGATGTCAAACTCACTCATGG	213 bp
CCL5	CTACACCAGCAGCAAGTGCT	CAAGCTGCTTAGGACAAGAGG	190 bp
CCL20	GAAGCAGCAAGCAGCTTTGAC	GTTCCATTCCAGGGAGCATC	244 bp
SAA3	GACATTCCTCAGGGAAGCTG	CTTCGAATCCTTCCGTACCTG	247 bp
Hp	GGAGTACTCGGTTCGCTATCA	CCATCGTTCATTGATGAGTGTG	280 bp
LBP	GAGCTGTCCACCACCAAGATG	CACACTCAGATCAAATGTACCG	243 bp

TLR4 protein was performed using the t-test of paired values. A correlation between TLR4 mRNA and protein was analyzed by the Pearson model. Effects were considered significant when $P < 0.05$.

Results

Blood flow of hepatic vein, portal vein and artery

The mean blood flows in the hepatic vein ($P = 0.005$), portal vein ($P < 0.001$) and artery ($P = 0.024$) in the HG group were higher than those in the LG group. The highest blood flow in hepatic vein, portal vein and artery was observed at 4 h after feeding in both groups. Results also showed that blood flow was fastest in the hepatic vein, and slowest in arteries (Table 3). In addition, Body weights of both groups did not change during the experiment and averaged 41.23 ± 0.97 kg (not shown in table).

LPS concentration in the hepatic vein, portal vein and artery and LPS clearance in liver

Plasma LPS concentrations in the hepatic vein ($P = 0.001$), portal vein ($P < 0.001$) and artery ($P < 0.001$) in the HG group were increased in comparison to those in the LG group. The concentration of LPS in the portal vein was higher than that in the hepatic vein and artery in both groups. The effect of diet × time ($P < 0.01$) on plasma LPS concentrations in the portal vein showed a significant

difference between the LG group and HG group. The effect of sampling time on plasma LPS concentrations in the hepatic vein or artery was not significant (Table 4).

According to the calculation of net LPS clearance, the mean rate of hepatic LPS clearance in the HG group was faster than that in the LG group (5.46 EU/sec *vs* 2.83 EU/sec; HG group *vs* LG group, $P = 0.022$, Figure 1a). However, feeding the HG diet to goats declined the percentage of hepatic LPS clearance accounting for the total entry of LPS into liver in the HG group compared to the LG group (10.57% *vs* 18.27%; HG group *vs* LG group, Figure 1b). Yet, the data of the individual percentage of LPS clearance were highly variable and the difference did not obtain statistical significance.

Pro-inflammatory cytokines and APPs in peripheral blood

After 6 weeks feeding, the plasma concentrations of pro-inflammatory cytokines TNF-α and IL-1β were significantly increased in the HG group compared to the LG group ($P < 0.001$ for both). Although the plasma concentration of IL-6 was increased, there was no significant difference between HG and LG groups ($P = 0.09$, Table 5). Time os sampling did not affect the plasma concentrations of these cytokines.

Compared with feeding of the LG diet, HG diet feeding increased the concentration of LBP ($P < 0.01$), Hp ($P = 0.021$) and SAA ($P = 0.024$) in peripheral blood. The effects of time

Table 3 The average blood flows in hepatic vein, portal vein and artery of goats

Blood flow (L/h)	Diet		SED[a]	Effect, P-value		
	LG	HG		Diet	Time	Diet × Time
Hepatic vein						
0 h	120.04	144.87	10.35	0.005	0.419	0.951
2 h	124.35	151.73				
4 h	128.42	167.84				
6 h	128.64	157.67				
8 h	118.01	148.29				
Portal vein						
0 h	100.96	122.26	7.72	<0.001	0.210	0.879
2 h	105.56	129.75				
4 h	111.57	142.71				
6 h	118.99	133.73				
8 h	103.52	127.88				
Artery						
0 h	19.08	22.61	4.76	0.024	0.726	0.627
2 h	18.79	21.98				
4 h	16.85	25.14				
6 h	9.64	23.94				
8 h	14.49	20.42				

[a]SED: standard error of difference between treatment and control.

Table 4 The average concentrations of LPS in plasma of hepatic vein, portal vein and artery of goats

LPS conc. (EU/mL)	Diet		SED[a]	Effect, P-value		
	LG	HG		Diet	Time	Diet × Time
Hepatic vein						
0 h	0.41	1.11	0.07	0.001	0.066	0.419
2 h	0.28	1.09				
4 h	0.48	1.23				
6 h	0.39	1.13				
8 h	0.42	1.01				
Portal vein						
0 h	0.47	1.32	0.05	<0.001	0.672	0.011
2 h	0.45	1.28				
4 h	0.52	1.32				
6 h	0.48	1.35				
8 h	0.59	1.13				
Artery						
0 h	0.36	1.08	0.06	<0.001	0.415	0.451
2 h	0.34	1.09				
4 h	0.43	1.15				
6 h	0.39	1.08				
8 h	0.41	0.97				

[a]SED: standard error of difference between treatment and control.

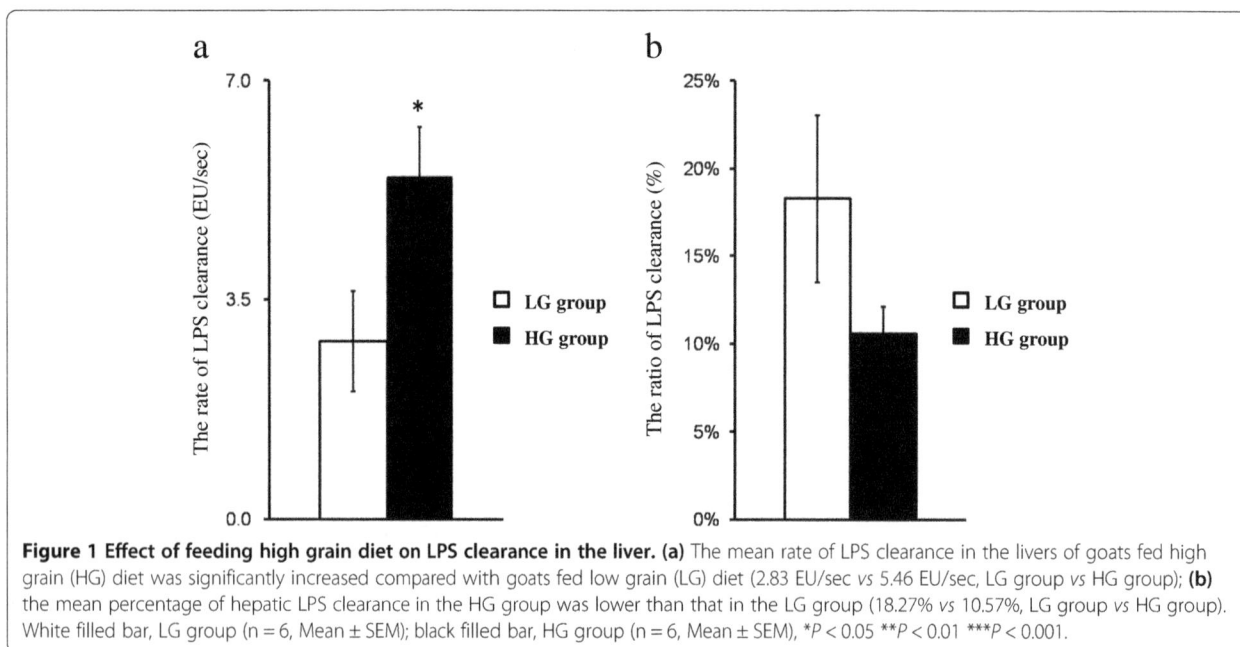

Figure 1 Effect of feeding high grain diet on LPS clearance in the liver. (a) The mean rate of LPS clearance in the livers of goats fed high grain (HG) diet was significantly increased compared with goats fed low grain (LG) diet (2.83 EU/sec *vs* 5.46 EU/sec, LG group *vs* HG group); **(b)** the mean percentage of hepatic LPS clearance in the HG group was lower than that in the LG group (18.27% *vs* 10.57%, LG group *vs* HG group). White filled bar, LG group (n = 6, Mean ± SEM); black filled bar, HG group (n = 6, Mean ± SEM), *P < 0.05 **P < 0.01 ***P < 0.001.

or interactions with diet on APPs were not significant (Table 5).

Biochemical parameters of liver function in peripheral blood

The measurement of biochemical parameters refer to ALT, AST, ALP, T-PRO, T-BIL and ALB in peripheral blood was used to determine liver functions. The concentrations of ALT (P < 0.001), ALP (P = 0.002) and T-BIL (P = 0.005) in peripheral blood were higher in the goats fed HG diet compared to the goats fed LG diet. However, feeding a HG diet to goats did not affect plasma concentration of AST (P = 0.231), T-PRO (P = 0.343) and ALB (P = 0.438) in the HG group in comparison to the LG group (Table 6). The effect of interactions of diet with time on plasma concentrations of ALT was significant; however, the effects of time or its interactions with diet on plasma concentrations of the other were not significant.

Expression of mRNAs encoding genes involved in immune response in the liver

Hepatic mRNA expression of 13 different genes involved in immune response, encoding pro- and anti-inflammatory cytokines, chemokines, APPs, TLR4 and TLR2 were assessed. The expression levels of most these genes were up-regulated in the liver of goats fed the HG diet (Figure 2). Expression of TLR4, but not TLR2, was increased (P = 0.006) in the liver of goats in the HG group compared to the LG group. A similar fold change in pro-inflammatory cytokine-encoding gene expression in the liver was observed between HG group and LG group (Figure 2). The differences in IL-1β (P < 0.001) and TNF-α (P = 0.014) gene

expression differed between groups, but not for IL-1α (P = 0.058) and IL-6 (P = 0.074). Expression of IL-10, an anti-inflammatory cytokine produced by dendritic cells, monocytes and particularly macrophages, was 2.04-fold increased, but no significance was observed (P = 0.059) in the livers of goats fed different diets. Moreover, feeding with the HG diet significantly enhanced the expression of mRNAs encoding APPs SAA3 (P = 0.02), Hp (P = 0.023) and LBP (P = 0.007), as well as up-regulated the expression of mRNAs encoding key chemokines IL-8 (P = 0.042), CCL5 (P = 0.02) and CCL20 (P = 0.037) in the liver of goats in the HG group compared to the LG group.

Expression of TLR4 protein in the liver

Western blotting analyses showed that TLR4 protein expression was enhanced in the liver of goats fed HG diet compared with that in the liver of goats fed LG diet (P = 0.043, Figure 3a). In addition, plotting individual relative TLR4 protein expression with the mRNA relative copy numbers revealed a strong correlation (r 0.83; P < 0.001, Figure 3b).

Discussion

In recent years, intensive production systems for ruminants have encouraged the use of the HG diet or easily fermentable carbohydrate diet to support high milk yields or rapid weight gain. Although this feeding practice can enhance economic efficiency in the short-term, the feeding of HG diet leads to the translocation of LPS from the digestive system into the circulating blood. In an experiment conducted by replacing 21% of dry matter from a total

Table 5 The average concentrations of pro-inflammatory cytokines and acute phase proteins in plasma of peripheral blood of goats

Item	Diet		SED[a]	Effect, P-value		
	LG	HG		Diet	Time	Diet × Time
TNFα (fmol/mL)						
0 h	15.54	52.36	6.98	<0.001	0.681	0.774
4 h	11.51	71.67				
8 h	19.24	53.92				
IL-1B (ng/mL)						
0 h	0.05	0.11	0.02	<0.001	0.089	0.127
4 h	0.06	0.14				
8 h	0.06	0.09				
IL-6 (pg/mL)						
0 h	93.99	107.02	23.81	0.097	0.372	0.717
4 h	120.56	150.95				
8 h	116.58	161.07				
LBP (µg/mL)						
0 h	13.58	42.22	4.23	<0.001	0.612	0.734
4 h	14.50	42.34				
8 h	16.25	37.91				
Hp (µg/mL)						
0 h	79.55	365.58	50.42	0.021	0.477	0.636
4 h	183.39	307.53				
8 h	112.66	350.52				
SAA (µg/mL)						
0 h	57.31	348.56	37.49	0.024	0.726	0.627
4 h	78.18	386.66				
8 h	63.06	324.88				

[a]SED: standard error of difference between treatment and control.

Table 6 The average concentrations of biochemical parameters in plasma of peripheral blood of goats

Item	Diet		SED[a]	Effect, P-value		
	LG	HG		Diet	Time	Diet × Time
ALT (IU/L)						
0 h	16.96	26.54	3.16	<0.001	0.529	0.031
4 h	16.20	21.20				
8 h	10.66	33.18				
AST (IU/L)						
0 h	46.92	47.20	5.76	0.231	0.881	0.394
4 h	47.88	50.76				
8 h	45.27	43.25				
ALP (IU/L)						
0 h	55.40	74.20	6.75	0.002	0.787	0.131
4 h	54.20	82.60				
8 h	45.68	67.23				
T-PRO (g/L)						
0 h	64.36	63.88	10.87	0.343	0.682	0.530
4 h	72.18	79.14				
8 h	58.37	57.76				
ALB (g/L)						
0 h	19.58	21.37	50.42	0.438	0.504	0.477
4 h	25.13	29.14				
8 h	29.67	27.48				
T-BIL (µmol/L)						
0 h	2.56	3.38	0.86	0.005	0.845	0.278
4 h	2.64	4.79				
8 h	1.68	3.97				

[a]SED: standard error of difference between treatment and control. IU: international unit.

mixed ration control diet with pellets containing 50% wheat and 50% barley, LPS concentration in the peripheral blood were significantly increased [1]. Other studies showed that feeding a diet containing 60% concentrate to lactating goats or feeding cattle with 70 g grain/kg body weight elevated blood LPS concentrations [28,31]. Moreover, an *in vitro* study by Emmanuel *et al.*, showed five fold increased of the permeability of the rumen wall when this tissue was bathed in pH 5.5 solution, which promoted the translocation of LPS across the rumen wall [10], and Chin *et al.* found that LPS induced cell apoptosis of intestinal epithelial cell lines, disrupted tight junction proteins and enhanced epithelial permeability [35]. *In vivo* studies in which high grain diets were fed to goats caused ruminal and caecal mucosal injury as well as colonic epithelial barrier disruption [4-6]. Taken together, these breaches contribute to the translocation of harmful compounds, such as LPS and histamine, released in the digestive tract into the

portal vein occurs during HG diet feeding. In the present study, the feeding of HG diet increased LPS concentrations in circulating blood, especially in the portal vein. In addition, LBP was directly involved in the clearance of LPS in the blood [26,36]. Therefore, an increase of LBP in the peripheral blood of goats fed HG diet support the translocation of LPS from the digestive tract into the bloodstream [1,7]. Alterations of blood flow in response to dietary changes have been reported in previous studies. In a study by Reynolds *et al.*, an increase of dry matter intake significantly increased blood flow in the portal vein and liver of heifers fed 75% alfalfa diet or 75% concentrate diet [37], although the significant difference of blood flow between both diets was not obtained. In present study, the increase of blood flow in the portal vein, hepatic vein and artery indicated that the feeding of HG diet resulted in accelerated blood flow. In addition, it is known that blood flow is affected by body weight, our study observed that

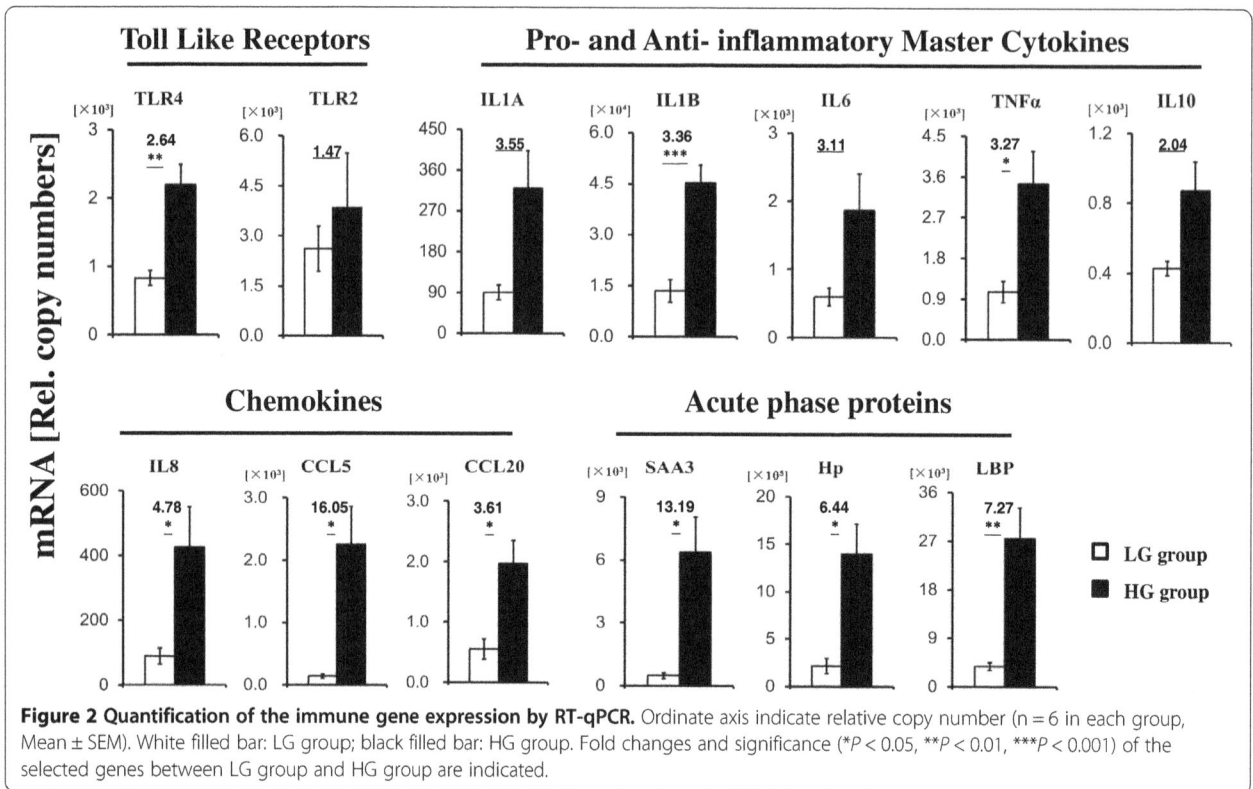

Figure 2 Quantification of the immune gene expression by RT-qPCR. Ordinate axis indicate relative copy number (n = 6 in each group, Mean ± SEM). White filled bar: LG group; black filled bar: HG group. Fold changes and significance (*P < 0.05, **P < 0.01, ***P < 0.001) of the selected genes between LG group and HG group are indicated.

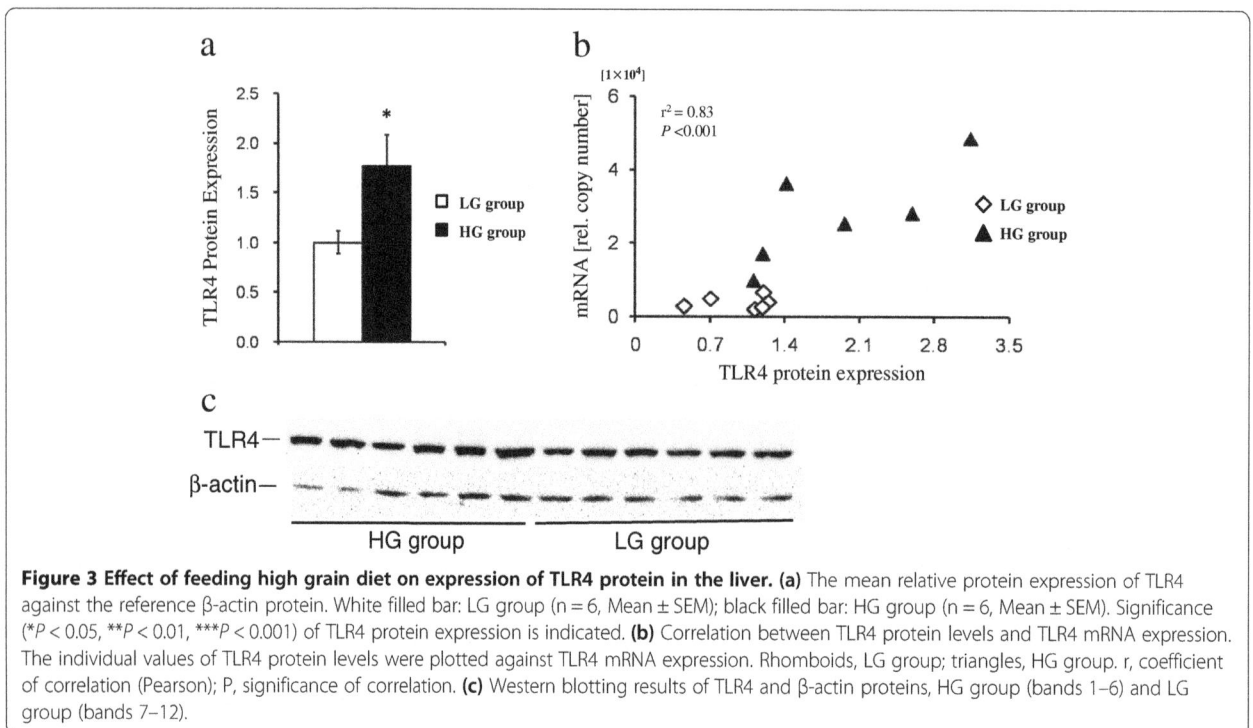

Figure 3 Effect of feeding high grain diet on expression of TLR4 protein in the liver. (a) The mean relative protein expression of TLR4 against the reference β-actin protein. White filled bar: LG group (n = 6, Mean ± SEM); black filled bar: HG group (n = 6, Mean ± SEM). Significance (*P < 0.05, **P < 0.01, ***P < 0.001) of TLR4 protein expression is indicated. **(b)** Correlation between TLR4 protein levels and TLR4 mRNA expression. The individual values of TLR4 protein levels were plotted against TLR4 mRNA expression. Rhomboids, LG group; triangles, HG group. r, coefficient of correlation (Pearson); P, significance of correlation. **(c)** Western blotting results of TLR4 and β-actin proteins, HG group (bands 1–6) and LG group (bands 7–12).

the average value of body weight did not change through this experiment. These findings suggest that the feeding of HG diet can promote blood flow entering or exiting the liver, and the increased entry of LPS into the liver through the portal vein. In addition, these findings also demonstrate that the rate of hepatic LPS clearance was significantly increased, but that the percentage of hepatic removed LPS was decreased during HG diet feeding.

There has been increasing attentions on inflammatory responses triggered by HG diet feeding in recent years. Acute phase response (APR) is the early stage of a systemic inflammatory response and was shown in a number of studies investigating the effects of the alterations of the grain proportion in the diet on the health of ruminants. During APR, the concentration of APPs in circulating blood is increased remarkably, and thus, SAA and Hp are often used as inflammatory markers in cattle. Determination of the serum SAA and Hp concentrations demonstrated that Hp but not SAA was notably increased when a diet administered to steers was switched from 0% concentrate diet to 61% concentrate diet [38]. And when this proportion of concentrate was further increased to induce SARA, a rumen metabolic disorder, the serum concentration of SAA was also elevated. These studies confirm another study that also showed that serum concentrations of SAA and Hp were increased when cows received a HG diet [8]. Similar results for serum SAA and Hp levels were observed in a study by Khafipour et al., where LBP plasma concentrations were also increased in this experimental model by increasing the grain percentage of the diet to induce SARA [1]. In the present study, concentrations of SAA, Hp and LBP in peripheral blood were markedly increased, suggesting that feeding the HG diet to goats causes an systemic inflammatory responses.

In addition, we also observed that HG diet feeding elevated plasma concentrations of the pro-inflammatory cytokines TNF-α and IL-1β, but did not affect plasma IL-6 concentrations. The increase in blood pro-inflammatory cytokines also provides evidence for the translocation of LPS and activation of inflammatory responses. The liver is an important immune organ where foreign antigens from the digestive tract encounter the immune system, and immune cells (mononuclear phagocytes) are activated to synthesize or secrete cytokines [39-42]. Thus, during the feeding of HG diet, an increased entry of LPS into the liver via the portal vein probably stimulates Kupffer cells (liver macrophages), the major cytokine-producing liver cells, to release cytokines that subsequently enhance the secretion of APPs from hepatocytes.

Excessive production of cytokines in the liver can damage hepatocytes [22,43]. The biochemical parameters ALT, AST, ALP, T-PRO, ALB and T-BIL in peripheral blood are common indicators used to assess the status of liver function [44]. In particular, ALT is a specific parameter that reflects hepatocyte damage [45]. In the present study, increased plasma concentrations of ALT, ALP and T-BIL suggested that feeding the HG diet resulted in the breach of hepatocytes releasing those parameters into circulation. In previous studies conducted by Scott et al., hepatocytes were shown to be critical for clearance of circulating LPS in the liver [46,47]. Thus, the impairment of hepatocytes during HG diet feeding could contribute to the decreased percentage of LPS clearance in the liver.

There are few studies reporting changes of immune gene expression in the liver in response to variation in diet. The current study showed that HG diet feeding enhanced the expression of many genes involved in immune response, including TLR4, pro- and anti-inflammatory cytokines, chemokines and APPs. Although other hazardous substances in blood and in digesta that can be translocted into circulating blood, LPS is thought to be the major contributor to the induction of synthesis of APPs and cytokines in the liver. An early study demonstrated that expression of cytokines and APPs in the liver was up-regulated during LPS intra-mammary gland infusion [12]. The liver is continually exposed to small amounts of LPS translocated from the digestive tract through the mesentery vein directly into the liver via the portal vein [48]. However, the increased concentration of LPS in the portal vein during HG diet feeding in the present study might explain why the enhanced immune gene expression and subsequent inflammatory response in the liver.

Recognition of inflammatory stimuli by the innate immune system is orchestrated by pattern recognition receptors that recognize external stimuli such as pathogen associated molecular patterns (PAMPs) and internal stimuli (damaged associated molecular patterns) [49]. LPS, a well known PAMP, binds to LBP and activates the TLR4-signaling pathway resulting in the production of IL-1β, IL-6 and TNF-α. These pro-inflammatory cytokines play an important role in orchestrating the synthesis of APPs as well as the secretion of other cytokines and chemokines. In our study, the increase of TLR4 and LBP expression in the liver confirmed that the TLR4 signalling pathway was activated by LPS translocated from the digestive tract into the circulating blood. Moreover, the feeding of HG diet elevated the level of mRNAs encoding for the chemokines IL-8, CCL5 and CCL20 in the liver. All these chemokines trigger diapedesis of polymorph nuclear granulocytes, mononuclear cells, macrophages and T-cells through the endothelia of blood vessels into the hepatic inflamed site. Furthermore, expressions of SAA and Hp were also up-regulated in HG group in the present study. Both SAA and Hp have major roles in the innate immune system by opsonising pathogens and removing the potential toxic substances [50].

The general understanding is that a severe local inflammation in peripheral tissues can lead to the release of pro-inflammatory cytokines (IL-1β, IL-6, TNF-α) and anti-inflammatory cytokine IL-10 [51] as well as APPs [52] in the liver. In accordance with previous studies, feeding HG diet to goats resulted in injury to the gastrointestinal barrier and local inflammation [4-6], which might be the cause of the up-regulation of immune genes in the liver. In addition, the reduction of the percentage of hepatic LPS clearance during the feeding of HG diet indicated the accumulation of LPS in systemic circulation. This condition contribute to further explain the conclusion of recent study [53] in which feeding high-starch diets to cows have successful induced subacute ruminal acidosis, which caused the endotoxin tolerance in the mammary gland of cows and suppressed the response of mammary gland to LPS challenge.

Conclusions

Results obtained in the present study suggest that the feeding of HG diet results in increased blood flow and LPS concentration in the hepatic vein, portal vein and artery, thereby increasing the rate of hepatic LPS clearance, but decreased the percentage of removed LPS accounting for the total entry of LPS into liver. The increase in the rate of hepatic LPS clearance could be due to enhancement of hepatic immune defence response to synthesize and secret cytokines and APPs, and the reduction in the percentage of hepatic LPS clearance might be caused by impaired hepatocytes elicited by the increased entry of LPS into the liver via the portal vein. Overall, our findings provide a fundamental understanding of the effect of the feeding of HG diet on hepatic LPS clearance and immune responses. Future work should focus on the regulation mechanisms of immune relevant gene expression, such as epigenetic modulations, to further elaborate etiology of liver inflammation elicited by the feeding of HG diet.

Abbreviations
LPS: Lipopolysaccharide; TLR: Toll-like receptor; SARA: Subacute ruminal acidosis; pAH: para-aminohippuric acid; IL-1α: −1β, −6, Interleukin-1α, 1β, −6; TNF-α: Tumor necrosis factor-α; APR: Acute phase response; APPs: Acute phase proteins; SAA: Serum amyloid A; Hp: Haptoglobin; LBP: Lipopolysaccharide; ALT: Alanine aminotransferase; AST: Aspartate aminotransferase; T-PRO: Total proteins; ALB: Albumin; T-BIL: Total bilirubin; ALP: Alkaline phosphatase; RT-qPCR: Real-time quantitative PCR.

Competing interests
None of the authors has any financial or personal competing interests that would have influenced the content of the paper or interfered with their objective assessment of the manuscript.

Authors' contributions
GC carried out the most of measurements of parameters in this study and drafted the manuscript, KZ prepared the blood and the liver samples, TX and DJ contributed to the statistical analyses, XS and SZ together conceived the idea, and designed the experiment. HMS and XS finalized the manuscript. All authors contributed to interpret and discuss the manuscript. All authors read and approved the final manuscript.

Acknowledgements
This work was supported by grants from the National Basic Research Program of China (project No. 2011 CB100802), the National Nature Science Foundation of China (project No.31172371) and the Priority Academic Program Development of Jiangsu Higher Education Institutions (PAPD).

Author details
[1]College of Veterinary Medicine, Nanjing Agricultural University, Nanjing 210095, PR, China. [2]College of Animal Science and Technology, Nanjing Agricultural University, Nanjing 210095, PR, China. [3]Leibniz Institute for Farm Animal Biology, Wilhelm-Stahl-Allee 2, 18196 Dummerstorf, Germany.

References
1. Khafipour E, Krause DO, Plaizier JC. A grain-based subacute ruminal acidosis challenge causes translocation of lipopolysaccharide and triggers inflammation. J Dairy Sci. 2009;92:1060–70.
2. Li S, Khafipour E, Krause DO, Kroeker A, Rodriguez JC, Gozho GN, et al. Effects of subacute ruminal acidosis challenges on fermentation and endotoxins in the rumen and hindgut of dairy cows. J Dairy Sci. 2012;95:294–303.
3. Li S, Kroeker A, Khafipour E, Rodriguez JC, Krause DO, Plaizier JC. Effects of subacute ruminal acidosis challenges on lipopolysaccharide endotoxin (LPS) in the rumen, cecum, and feces of dairy cows. J Dairy Sci. 2010;93:433–4.
4. Liu JH, Xu TT, Zhu WY, Mao SY. High-grain feeding alters caecal bacterial microbiota composition and fermentation and results in caecal mucosal injury in goats. Brit J Nutr. 2014;112:416–27.
5. Liu JH, Xu TT, Zhu WY, Mao SY. A high-grain diet alters the omasal epithelial structure and expression of tight junction proteins in a goat model. Vet J. 2014;201:95–100.
6. Tao S, Duanmu Y, Dong H, Tian J, Ni Y, Zhao R. A high-concentrate diet induced colonic epithelial barrier disruption is associated with the activating of cell apoptosis in lactating goats. BMC Vet Res. 2014;10:235.
7. Emmanuel DGV, Dunn SM, Ametaj BN. Feeding high proportions of barley grain stimulates an inflammatory response in dairy cows. J Dairy Sci. 2008;91:606–14.
8. Gozho GN, Krause DO, Plaizier JC. Ruminal lipopolysaccharide concentration and inflammatory response during grain-induced subacute ruminal acidosis in dairy cows. J Dairy Sci. 2007;90:856–66.
9. Plaizier JC, Khafipour E, Li S, Gozho GN, Krause DO. Subacute ruminal acidosis (SARA), endotoxins and health consequences. Anim Feed Sci Tech. 2012;172:9–21.
10. Emmanuel DGV, Madsen KL, Churchill TA, Dunn SM, Ametaj BN. Acidosis and lipopolysaccharide from Escherichia coli B : 055 cause hyperpermeability of rumen and colon tissues. J Dairy Sci. 2007;90:5552–7.
11. Eckersall PD, Bell R. Acute phase proteins: Biomarkers of infection and inflammation in veterinary medicine. Vet J. 2010;185:23–7.
12. Vels L, Rontved CM, Bjerring M, Ingvartsen KL. Cytokine and acute phase protein gene expression in repeated liver biopsies of dairy cows with a lipopolysaccharide-induced mastitis. J Dairy Sci. 2009;92:922–34.
13. Zhou J, Dong GZ, Ao CJ, Zhang S, Qiu M, Wang X, et al. Feeding a high-concentrate corn straw diet increased the release of endotoxin in the rumen and pro-inflammatory cytokines in the mammary gland of dairy cows. BMC Vet Res. 2014;10:172.
14. Ji XH, Sun KY, Feng YH, Yin GQ. Changes of inflammation-associated cytokine expressions during early phase of experimental endotoxic shock in macaques. World J Gastroentero. 2004;10:3026–33.
15. Peri F, Piazza M. Therapeutic targeting of innate immunity with Toll-like receptor 4 (TLR4) antagonists. Biotechnol Adv. 2012;30:251–60.
16. Takeda K, Akira S. Toll-like receptors in innate immunity. Int Immunol. 2005;17:1–14.
17. Yoshioka M, Ito T, Miyazaki S, Nakajima Y. The release of tumor necrosis factor-alpha, interleukin-1, interleukin-6 and prostaglandin E-2 in bovine Kupffer cells stimulated with bacterial lipopolysaccharide. Vet Immunol Immunop. 1998;66:301–7.
18. Gabay C, Kushner I. Acute-phase proteins and other systemic responses to inflammation. New Engl J Med. 1999;340:448–54.
19. Yoshioka M, Watanabe A, Shimada N, Murata H, Yokomizo Y, Nakajima Y. Regulation of haptoglobin secretion by recombinant bovine cytokines in

primary cultured bovine hepatocytes. Domest Anim Endocrin. 2002;23:425–33.

20. Zheng J, Watson AD, Kerr DE. Genome-wide expression analysis of lipopolysaccharide-induced mastitis in a mouse model. Infect Immun. 2006;74:1907–15.

21. Kabaroff LC, Rodriguez A, Quinton M, Boermans H, Karrow NA. Assessment of the ovine acute phase response and hepatic gene expression in response to escherichia coli endotoxin. Vet Immunol Immunop. 2006;113:113–24.

22. Schattenberg JM, Schuchmann M, Galle PR. Cell death and hepatocarcinogenesis: dysregulation of apoptosis signaling pathways. J Gastroen Hepatol. 2011;26:213–9.

23. Brenner C, Galluzzi L, Kepp O, Kroemer G. Decoding cell death signals in liver inflammation. J Hepatol. 2013;59:583–94.

24. Petzl W, Zerbe H, Günther J, Yang W, Seyfert HM, Nürnberg G, et al. Escherichia coli, but not Staphylococcus aureus triggers an early increased expression of factors contributing to the innate immune defense in the udder of the cow. Vet Res. 2008;39:18.

25. Gozho GN, Plaizier JC, Krause DO, Kennedy AD, Wittenberg KM. Subacute ruminal acidosis induces ruminal lipopolysaccharide endotoxin release and triggers an inflammatory response. J Dairy Sci. 2005;88:1399–403.

26. Munford RS. Detoxifying endotoxin: time, place and person. J Endotoxin Res. 2005;11:69–84.

27. Satoh M, Ando S, Shinoda T, Yamazaki M. Clearance of bacterial lipopolysaccharides and lipid A by the liver and the role of argininosuccinate synthase. Innate Immun. 2008;14:51–60.

28. Andersen PH, Hesselholt M, Jarløv N. Endotoxin and arachidonic acid metabolites in portal, hepatic and arterial blood of cattle with acute ruminal acidosis. Acta Vet Scand. 1994;35:223–34.

29. Lobley GE, Connell A, Lomax MA, Brown DS, Milne E, Calder AG, et al. Hepatic detoxification of ammonia in the ovine liver: possible consequences for amino acid catabolism. Brit J Nutr. 1995;73:667–85.

30. Katz ML, Bergman EN. Simultaneous measurements of hepatic and portal venous blood flow in the sheep and dog. Am J Physiol. 1969;216:946–52.

31. Dong HB, Wang SQ, Jia YY, Ni YD, Zhang YS, Zhuang S, et al. Long-term effects of subacute ruminal acidosis (SARA) on milk quality and hepatic gene expression in lactating goats fed a high-concentrate diet. PLoS One. 2013;8:e82850.

32. Huntington GB, Reynolds CK, Stroud BH. Techniques for measuring blood flow in splanchnic tissues of cattle. J Dairy Sci. 1989;72:1583–95.

33. Wieghart M, Slepetis R, Elliot JM, Smith DF. Glucose absorption and hepatic gluconeogenesis in dairy cows fed diets varying in forage content. J Nutr. 1986;116:839–50.

34. Galindo CE, Ouellett DR, Pellerin D, Lemosquet S, Ortigues MI, Lapierre H. Effect of amino acid or casein supply on whole-body, splanchnic, and mammary glucose kinetics in lactating dairy cows. J Dairy Sci. 2011;94:5558–68.

35. Chin AC, Flynn AN, Fedwick JP, Buret AG. The role of caspase-3 in lipopolysaccharide-mediated disruption of intestinal epithelial tight junctions. Can J Physiol Pharm. 2006;84:1043–50.

36. Vesy CJ, Kitchens RL, Wolfbauer G, Albers JJ, Munford RS. Lipopolysaccharide-binding protein and phospholipid transfer protein release lipopolysaccharides from gram-negative bacterial membranes. Infect Immun. 2000;68(5):2410–7.

37. Reynolds CK, Tyrrell HF, Reynolds PJ. Effects of diet forage to concentrate ratios and intake on energy metabolism in growing beef heifers: whole body energy and nitrogen balance and visceral heat production. J Nutr. 1991;121:994–1003.

38. Gozho GN, Krause DO, Plaizier JC. Rumen lipopolysaccharide and inflammation during grain adaptation and subacute ruminal acidosis in steers. J Dairy Sci. 2006;89:4404–13.

39. Czaja AJ, Manns MP. Advances in the diagnosis, pathogenesis, and management of autoimmune hepatitis. Gastroenterology. 2010;139:58–101.

40. Hewett JA, Roth RA. Hepatic and extrahepatic pathobiology of bacterial lipopolysaccharides. Pharmacol Rev. 1993;45:381–411.

41. Gegner JA, Ulevitch RJ, Tobias PS. Lipopolysaccharide (LPS) signal transduction and clearance: dual roles for LPS binding protein and membrane CD14. J Biol Chem. 1995;270:5320–5.

42. Kitchens RL, Munford RS. CD14-dependent internalization of bacterial lipopolysaccharide (LPS) is strongly influenced by LPS aggregation but not by cellular responses to LPS. J Immunol. 1998;160:1920–8.

43. Fabregat I. Dysregulation of apoptosis in hepatocellular carcinoma cells. World J Gastroentero. 2009;15:513–20.

44. Sevinc M, Basoglu A, Birdane FM, Boydak M. Liver function in dairy cows with fatty liver. Rev Med Vet-toulouse. 2001;152(4):297–300.

45. William M. Alanine aminotransferase (serum, plasma). [http://www.acb.org.uk/Nat%20Lab%20Med%20Hbk/ALT.pdf]

46. Scott MJ, Billiar TR. β2-integrin-induced p38 MAPK activation is a key mediator in the CD14/TLR4/MD2-dependent uptake of lipopolysaccharide by hepatocytes. J Biol Chem. 2008;283:29433–46.

47. Scott MJ, Liu SB, Shapiro RA, Vodovotz Y, Billiar TR. Endotoxin uptake in mouse liver is blocked by endotoxin pretreatment through a suppressor of cytokine signaling-1-dependent mechanism. Hepatology. 2009;49:1695–708.

48. Mimura Y, Sakisaka S, Harada M, Sata M, Tankawa K. Role of hepatocytes in direct clearance of lipopolysaccharide in rats. Gastroenterology. 1995;109:1969–76.

49. Bieghs V, Trautwein C. The innate immune response during liver inflammation and metabolic disease. Trends Immunol. 2013;34:446–52.

50. Gruys E, Toussaint MJM, Niewold TA, Koopmans SJ. Acute phase reaction and acute phase proteins. J Zhejiang Univ Sci B. 2005;6:1045–56.

51. Zhong J, Deaciuc JV, Burikhanov R, de Villiers WJS. Lipopolysaccharide-induced liver apoptosis is increased in interleukin-10 knockout mice. Bba-mol Basis Dis. 2006;1762:468–77.

52. Murata H, Shimada N, Yoshioka M. Current research on acute phase proteins in veterinary diagnosis: an overview. Vet J. 2004;168:28–40.

53. Gott PN, Hogan JS, Weiss WP. Effects of various starch feeding regimens on responses of dairy cows to intramammary lipopolysaccharide infusion. J Dairy Sci. 2015;in press.

12

Molecular characterization and phylogenetic analysis of transmissible gastroenteritis virus HX strain isolated from China

Xiaoliang Hu Jr[1,2], Nannan Li Jr[1], Zhige Tian Jr[3], Xin Yin Jr[2], Liandong Qu[4*] and Juanjuan Qu[1*]

Abstract

Background: Porcine transmissible gastroenteritis virus (TGEV) is the major etiological agent of viral enteritis and severe diarrhea in suckling piglets. In China, TGEV has caused great economic losses, but its role in epidemic diarrhea is unclear. This study aims to reveal the etiological role of TGEV in piglet diarrhea via molecular characterization and phylogenetic analysis.

Results: A TGEV-HX strain was isolated from China, and its complete genome was amplified, cloned, and sequenced. Sequence analysis indicated that it was conserved in the 5' and 3'-non-translated regions, and there were no insertions or deletions in nonstructural genes, such as ORF1a, ORF1b, ORF3a, ORF3b, and ORF7, as well as in genes encoding structural proteins, such as the envelope (E), membrane (M), and nucleoprotein (N) proteins. Furthermore, the phylogenetic analysis indicated that the TGEV-HX strain was more similar to the TGEV Purdue cluster than to the Miller cluster.

Conclusions: The present study described the isolation and genetic characterization of a TGEV-HX strain. The detailed analysis of the genetic variation of TGEVs in China provides essential information for further understanding the evolution of TGEVs.

Keywords: Porcine transmissible gastroenteritis virus, Sequence alignment, Phylogenetic analysis

Background

Transmissible gastroenteritis virus (TGEV) is the etiological agent of transmissible gastroenteritis (TGE), and it can cause viral enteritis and severe diarrhea with high morbidity in pigs of all ages, as well as high mortality in suckling piglets [1]. It occurs at swine-raising farms and results in significant economic losses [2,3].

TGEV is an enveloped virus belonging to the *Coronaviridae* (CoV) family and the *Nidovirales* order. It possesses a large 28.5-kb single-stranded, positive-sense RNA genome. About two-thirds of the entire RNA comprises open reading frames (ORFs) 1a and 1b, encoding RNA replicase. The 3' one-third of the genome comprises genes encoding structural and non-structural proteins [4,5]. The genes of TGEV are arranged in the order of 5'-rep-S-3a-3b-E-M-N-ORF7-3'.

The spike (S) gene of TGEV encodes an approximately 1,450-amino acid protein, with a molecular weight ranging from 128–160 kDa without glycosylation and 150–200 kDa after glycosylation. Functionally, the S glycoprotein is the major target of neutralizing antibodies, and it is also related to host cell tropism [6], interaction with its cellular receptor, pathogenicity, fusion, and hemagglutination activity [7-9]. ORF7 encodes a small hydrophobic protein (HP) during viral replication. The intracellular localization of the HP suggests that it may play an important role in the process of membrane integrity during viral replication and/or virion assembly [10,11].

In this report, we isolated a TGEV-HX strain of TGEV from the feces of piglets in Heilongjiang province in China. To better understand the molecular characteristics of this isolate, its complete genome sequence was

* Correspondence: qld@hvri.ac.cn; juanjuanqu@126.com
[4]National Key Laboratory of Veterinary Biotechnology, Harbin Veterinary Research Institute, Chinese Academy of Agricultural Sciences, Harbin 150001, People's Republic of China
[1]College of Resources and Environment, Northeast Agricultural University, Harbin 150030, People's Republic of China
Full list of author information is available at the end of the article

obtained, and a phylogenetic tree was constructed based on the complete ORF sequence of the S gene. The results provide molecular and phylogenetic information for a Chinese isolate of TGEV, which may assist in elucidating the genetic evolution of TGEV in China.

Methods

Ethics statement

Pigs used in this study were approved by the Institutional Animal Care and Use Committee (IACUC) of the Harbin Veterinary Research Institute (HVRI), the Chinese Academy of Agricultural Sciences. No animals were sacrificed specifically for this study. Feces samples were collected at the farm.

Viral isolation and identification

Five fecal samples were collected from piglets with diarrhea in a suburb of Harbin, the capital of Heilongjiang province, P. R. China. As both TGEV and PEDV can cause diarrhea, two pairs of specific primers (TGEV-NF; TGEV-NR; PEDV-NF, PEDV-NR) were employed to identify the kinds of viruses in the above samples (Table 1). PCRs were conducted as below, and the cycling parameters for the PCR included 94°C for 5 min, followed by 30 cycles of 94°C for 0.5 min, 55°C for 0.5 min, and 72°C for 1 min, and a final extension at 72°C for 10 min. Then, PCR-positive viral samples were inoculated into PK-15 cells, which were grown as a monolayer in Dulbecco's modified Eagle medium (DMEM) (GIBCO, Grand Island, NY, USA) containing 10% fetal calf serum (GIBCO, Grand Island, NY, USA) and 5% CO_2 in air. Viruses were passaged three times and were harvested by three cycles of freezing and thawing. Cellular debris was removed by low speed centrifugation at $3,000 \times g$ (Eppendorf, Hamburg, Germany) for 10 min, and the supernatant was aliquoted and stored at –80°C. Viral titers were determined using the Reed-Muench method [12].

Extraction of viral RNA, reverse transcribed-polymerase chain reaction (RT-PCR) and complete genome sequencing

Viral RNA was extracted from PK-15 cells infected with TGEV-HX using the TRIzol reagent (Invitrogen, Carlsbad, CA, USA). cDNA was generated by adding 4 μl of RNA to the following components: 4 μl of 5× reverse transcription buffer, 4 μl of dNTPs mixture (2.5 mM), 0.5 μl of RNase inhibitor, 5 μl of random primer (50 μM), 0.5 μl (10 U) of AMV reverse transcriptase, and 2 μl of sterile water. The components were gently mixed in an Eppendorf tube and incubated at room temperature for 10 min, then transferred to a water incubator at 42°C for 1 h prior to storage at –20°C . The resulting cDNA was amplified by PCR using LA Taq DNA polymerase (TaKaRa, Tokyo, Japan). Ten pairs of primers were

Table 1 Primers used for identifying and completely sequencing the TGEV-HX strain

Primer	Sequence 5'-3'	Position
TGEV-NF	TCATGCAGATGCCAAATTTAAAGA	27,213-27,236
TGEV-NR	TCATCCTTCTTGTTATTGAATTGT	27,456-27,479
PEDV-NF	TTTCTAAGGTACTTGCAAATAATG	26,382-26,405
PEDV-NR	TTGGAGATCTGGACCTGTTGTTGC	26,757-26,780
P1	ATGAGTTCCAAACAATTCAAGA	315-336
P2	ATCAAA ACATCCAAAGCACCCT	4,318-4,339
P3	AATTCA AAGTCCTAA AAACGAT	4,250-4,271
P4	GCGTAGATGATCATA AAGAACG	8,470-8,491
P5	CATTGTCACCCTTGTTGTGAAC	8,420-8,441
P6	GTAGATGTCAAA AGCTCTACTA	12,400-12,421
P7	TCTATGCAGAGTTTTACTGTTG	12,300-12,321
P8	TAATGAATTTATGCTTTGTTCC	15,200-15,221
P9	AGGCATGTGTGTAGTATGTGGT	15,100-15,121
P10	AAGCTTAGCAAA AGCTCTT	18,169-18,187
P11	CGCACTCGCTCTAAATTGTCTT	18,080-18,101
P12	ACTACGTTTAACCGTTGTCTGT	20,660-20,681
P13	ATGAAA AAACTATTTGTGG	20,365-20,383
P14	TTA ATGGACGTGCACTTTT	24,690-24,708
P15	GCTGTGGATGCATAGGTTGTTT	24,608-24,629
P16	TTGGAGGGTTATGGGGTTGAAG	27,021-27,042
P17	CTTCTAAATGGCCAACCAGGGAC	26,910-26,932
P18	CGAGCATCTCGTTTAGTTCGTT	28,056-28,077
P19	AGA AAGGTCAGAGCAAGATGTG	27,963-27,984
P20	GTATCACTATCA AAAGGA AAAT	28,559-28,580
P-F	CAAACTGAATGGAAATAATCAA	139-160
P-R	ATTTGGCAATGCTAGATTTAGTAA	28,441-28,464

designed based on conserved regions of TGEV strain H165 (Table 1). PCRs were conducted in a total of volume of 50 μl containing 5 μl of 10× buffer, 3 μl of dNTPs mixture (2.5 mM), 8 μl of cDNA, 1 μl of forward primer (10 μM), 1 μl of reverse primer (10 μM), 5 U of LA Taq polymerase (TaKaRa, Tokyo, Japan), and 31 μl of sterile water. The cycling parameters for the PCR included 94°C for 1 min, followed by 30 cycles of 94°C for 1 min, 50°C for 1 min and 72°C for 1 min, and a final extension at 72°C for 10 min. Two primers (P-F, P-R) were employed to confirm the 5′ and 3′ ends of the viral genome by rapid amplification of cDNA ends (RACE) using the RACE cDNA Amplification Kit (Invitrogen, Carlsbad, CA, USA). The PCR products were run on agarose gels, and correctly sized amplicons were observed. Then, the PCR products were purified using the Axygen Gel Extraction Kit (Axygen, USA) and cloned into pMD18-T (TaKaRa, Tokyo, Japan). Three to five independent clones of each TGEV amplicon were sequenced. The DNA was

Table 2 Source of transmissible gastroenteritis virus (TGEV) sequences used in the experiment

Isolate	Accession no.	Origin	Collection date
96-1933	AF104420	UK	2001
H16	FJ755618.2	CHN	2010
H165	EU074218	CHN	2010
TGEV-HX	KC962433	CHN	2013
ISU-1	DQ811787	USA	2009
Miller 6	DQ811785	USA	2009
Miller 60	DQ811786.2	USA	2011
Purdue	DQ811789	USA	2011
Purdue 115	DQ811788.1	USA	2009
SC-Y	DQ443743	CHN	2006
TS	DQ201447	CHN	2006
WH-1	HQ462571.1	CHN	2011

sequenced using an ABI 3730XL Sanger-based Genetic Analyzer (Applied Biosystems, Waltham, MA, USDA).

Electron microscopy

PK-15 cells infected with TGEV were harvested by freezing and thawing three times. One mL of cell culture was centrifuged for 5 min at $800 \times g$. The supernatant was transferred into a new microfuge tube and centrifuged for 10 min at $13,400 \times g$. Then, the pellet was negatively stained with 2% phosphotungstic acid and analyzed on a transmission electron microscope (H-7650, Hitachi, Tokyo, Japan) [13].

Sequence alignment and phylogenetic analysis

Sequence data were assembled and analyzed using Clustal X software (1.83) and DNASTAR. To determine the relationship between the TGEV representative isolates and the HX strain, phylogenetic trees based on the S gene were constructed using molecular evolutionary genetics analysis (MEGA) software (version 4.0) using the neighbor-joining (NJ) method. Bootstrap values were estimated for 1,000 replicates. The sequences of the TGEV reference strains were obtained from GenBank, and the details are summarized in Table 2. The sequences obtained in this study were assembled and submitted to GenBank under the accession number KC962433.

Results

Virus culture and electron microscopy analysis

The PCR results confirmed that one of five samples was TGEV-positive, designated TGEV-HX; the other four samples were TGEV-negative and all five samples were PEDV-negative (Figure 1A). After three passages, cytopathic effects (CPE) were found in the PK-15 cells, as evidenced by the cells rounding up and enlarging, the formation of syncytia, and the detachment of cells into

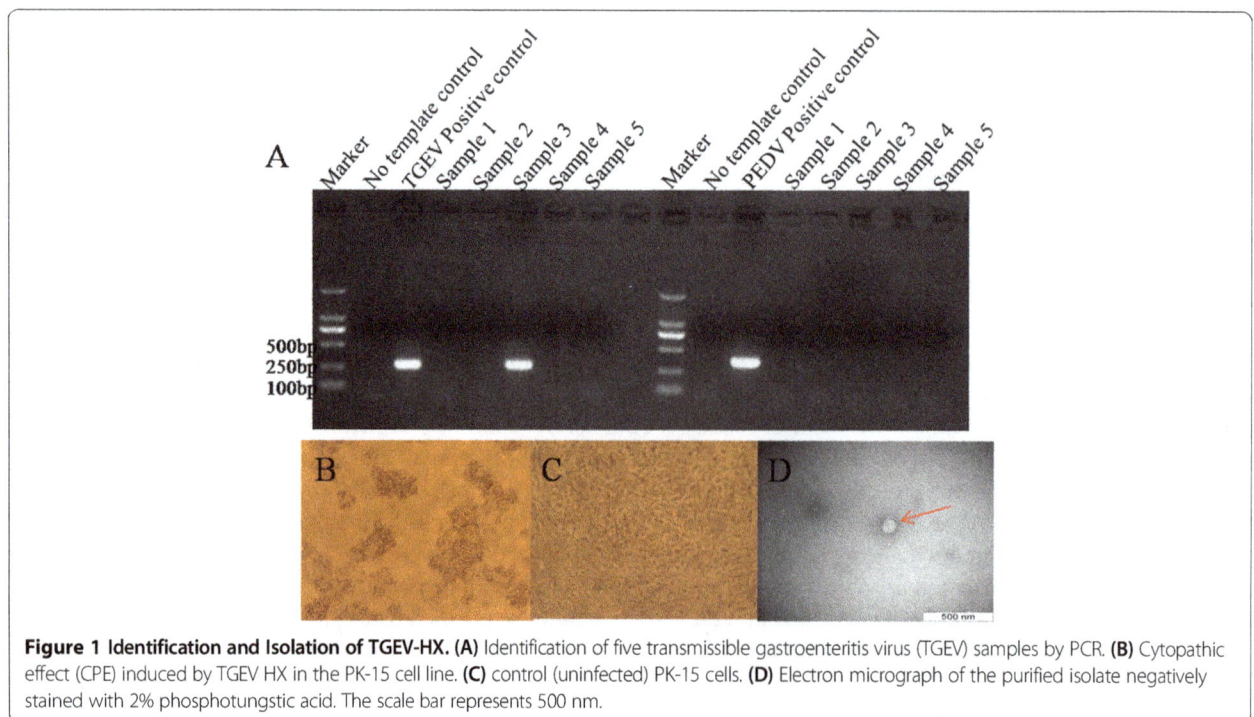

Figure 1 Identification and Isolation of TGEV-HX. (A) Identification of five transmissible gastroenteritis virus (TGEV) samples by PCR. **(B)** Cytopathic effect (CPE) induced by TGEV HX in the PK-15 cell line. **(C)** control (uninfected) PK-15 cells. **(D)** Electron micrograph of the purified isolate negatively stained with 2% phosphotungstic acid. The scale bar represents 500 nm.

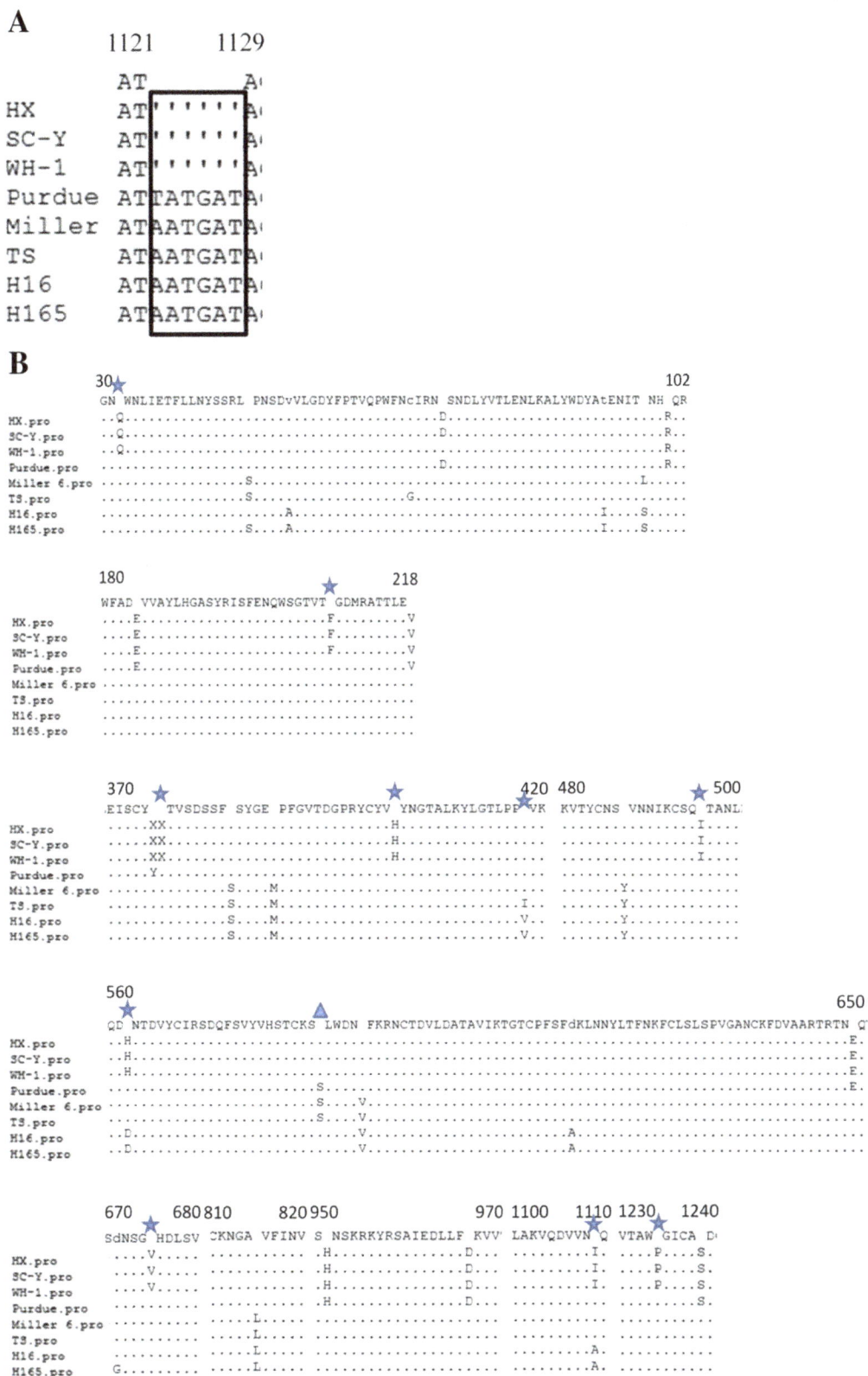

Figure 2 Multiple sequence alignment of S among TGEV strains. (A) A 6-nt deletion in the S gene at nt position 1123–1128 of the HX, SC-Y, and WH-1 strains. **(B)** Amino acid alignments of deduced S sequences compared with strain HX. (▲) indicates amino acid 585, (★) indicates amino acids of the HX, SC-Y, and WH-1 strains that are different from those of other transmissible gastroenteritis viruses.

the medium (Figure 1B and C). The median tissue culture infective dose (TCID$_{50}$) of TGEV-HX ($10^{7.25}$/0.1 ml) was measured using the Reed-Muench method. When observed by electron microscopy, the virus displayed a circular shape, and the surface projections were petal-shaped, with a diameter ranging from 100 to 150 nm, which is similar in size to known TGEVs (Figure 1D).

Complete genome sequence of the TGEV-HX strain

The full-length genome sequence of the TGEV-HX strain was deduced by combining the sequences of 10 overlapping cDNA fragments. The genome sequence of the TGEV-HX strain was 28,580 nucleotides (nt) long, including the poly A tail. The 5′ portion of the genome contained a 314-nt non-translated region (NTR), and ORF1a (315–12,368) and ORF1b (12,326–20,368), encoding the viral RNA-dependent RNA replicase. The structural proteins S, E, M, and N were found to be encoded by ORFs S (nt 20,365–24,708), E (nt 25,857–26,105), M (nt 26,116–26,904), and N (nt 26,917–28,065), respectively. The three non-structural protein-coding genes were ORF3a (nt 24,827–25,042), ORF3b (nt 25,136–25,870), and ORF7 (nt 28,071–28,307). The 5′ NTR included a potential short AUG-initiated ORF (nt 114–121), beginning within a Kozak sequences (5′-UCUAUGAA-3′). The 3′ end of the genome contained a 273-nt untranslated sequence and a poly (A) tail. Upstream from the poly (A) tail, there was a 5′-GGAA GAGC-3′ octameric sequence .

The non-structural genes

The replicase genes were composed of ORF1a and ORF1b, which contained a 43-nt common region (nt 12,326–12,368) and a "slippery site" (5′-UUUAAAC-3′, nt 12,333–12,339). The ORF1a gene of TGEV-HX was predicted to encode a protein of 4,017 amino acids (aa), while ORF1b was predicted to encode a 2,680-aa protein. Nucleotide sequence analysis indicated that there were no deletions or insertions in the ORF1ab region of the Miller 6 and Purdue TGEV strains.

ORF3a and ORF3b of TGEV-HX were predicted to encode 72-aa and 244-aa proteins, respectively. No deletions or insertions were found in the ORF3a or ORF3b genes of TGEV-HX. The ORF7 gene of TGEV-HX was predicted to encode a 78-aa protein, which contained the common PP1c-binding motif 5′-RVIFLVI-3′ [14]. No deletions or insertions were found in ORF7 of TGEV-HX.

The structural genes

The nucleotide sequence of the S gene of TGEV-HX was 4,344 nt in length, encoding a predicted protein of 1,447 aa. A 6-nt deletion was found in the S gene at nt 1,123–1,128 of the TGEV-HX, SC-Y, and WH-1 strains,

which caused the S protein to be two amino acids shorter than those of the Purdue, Miller 6, TS, H16 and H165 strains (Figure 2A). Amino acid 585 of the Purdue, Miller 6, and TS strains was S, while in the TGEV-HX, SC-Y, WH-1, H16, and H165 strains, it was A (Figure 2B). Amino acids 32, 208, 376, 403, 418, 496, 562, 675, 1,109, and 1,234 of TGEV-HX were identical to those of strains SC-Y and WH-1, but different from those of strains TS, H16, and H165.

Sequence analysis revealed no deletions or insertions in the E and N genes of any of the TGEVs. The predicted E, M, and N proteins were 82-, 264-, and 382-aa long, respectively (Table 3).

Homology comparison

To investigate the homology of TGEV-HX to other TGEVs, the nucleotide and predicted amino acid sequences of the nonstructural and structural protein coding genes were compared (Table 4). The results suggested that TGEV-HX showed higher identity to strains SC-Y, WH-1, and Purdue, and less identity to TS, Miller 6, and H165.

Phylogenetic analysis

Phylogenetic analysis of the complete S gene showed that TGEV strains could be divided into two groups (Figure 3). The TGEV-HX strain had a close relationship with the Purdue strain and is more distant evolutionarily from the Miller strains group and strain ISU-1.

Discussion

As an enteropathogenic coronavirus, TGEV is the major cause of viral enteritis and diarrhea in neonatal pigs, resulting in significant economic losses. Currently, TGEV occurs sporadically in parts of Europe, North America, and Asia. The fact that wild and domestic carnivores (foxes, dogs, cats, and possibly minks) seroconvert to

Table 3 Length, in nucleotide acids and amino acids, of the predicted structural and nonstructural proteins of the transmissible gastroenteritis virus (TGEV)-HX strain

HX	Position	nt	aa
Replicase 1a	315-12368	12054	4017
Replicase 1b	12326-20368	8043	2680
S	20365-24708	4344	1447
ORF3a	24827-25042	216	72
ORF3b	25136-25870	735	244
E	25857-26105	249	82
M	26116-26904	789	264
N	26917-28065	1149	382
ORF7	28071-28307	237	78

Table 4 Nucleotide and amino acid sequence identities (%) of various transmissible gastroenteritis virus (TGEV) strains

	SC-Y	WH-1	Purdue	Purdue 115	H16	H165	M6	M60	TS
ORF1A	99.4/99.1	99.9/99.9	99.8/99.6	99.8/99.8	98.9/98.8	98.9/98.8	99.0/99.0	98.9/98.9	98.8/98.6
ORF1B	99.8/99.8	100.0/100.0	99.9/100.0	99.9/100.0	99.0/99.6	99.0/99.6	99.0/99.6	99.0/99.6	98.9/99.6
S	99.7/99.4	100.0/99.9	99.5/99.0	99.9/99.8	98.1/97.7	98.0/97.6	98.3/98.0	98.2/97.8	98.3/98.0
ORF3A	100.0/100.0	100.0/100.0	99.5/98.6	100.0/100.0	93.1/88.9	92.6/87.5	93.1/88.9	92.6/87.5	92.1/86.1
ORF3B	99.9/99.6	99.9/99.6	99.7/99.2	99.9/99.6	98.9/97.6	98.8/97.1	98.9/97.6	57.4/44.1	98.5/96.3
E	100.0/100.0	100.0/100.0	99.6/98.8	100.0/100.0	98.0/95.2	97.2/92.8	98.4/95.2	98.4/95.2	98.8/96.4
M	99.7/99.2	99.9/99.6	99.7/99.2	99.9/99.6	98.1/97.3	98.1/97.3	98.2/97.7	98.2/97.7	98.0/97.0
N	99.9/99.7	100.0/100.0	99.7/99.7	99.9/99.7	98.2/98.4	98.1/98.4	98.2/98.4	98.0/98.2	98.1/98.2
ORF7	100.0/100.0	100.0/100.0	100.0/100.0	100.0/100.0	96.2/93.7	96.2/93.7	95.8/93.7	95.8/92.4	96.2/93.7

TGEV indicates that they are potential subclinical carriers of TGEV. [15]. In summation, TGEV has become a new challenge for the pig farming industry. As few TGEV genome sequences have been published, little is known about TGEV evolution. The results of this study will provide necessary information for further understanding the evolution of TGEV.

A complete sequence analysis indicated that no deletions or insertions were found in the 5′- and 3′- NTR regions of TGEV-HX, suggesting that its replication and transcription mechanism was not changed. A 6-nt (nt 1,123–1,128) deletion in the S gene was found in the TGEV-HX, SC-Y, and WH-1 strains, but not in the Purdue, Miller 6, TS, H16, and H165 strains. It was showed that this deletion was observed in the attenuated Purdue strains PUR46-C8 and PUR46-MAD, and it was considered to play a role in viral attenuation [16]. Competition studies using monoclonal antibodies led to the prediction of at least four main antigenic sites, designated A, B, C, and D [17,18]. The A and B sites (aa 506–706) have

been mapped, and they serve as the major antigenic sites, including the binding site for the viruses host receptor, aminopeptidase N (APN). Single amino acid changes in the S protein can greatly impact its antigenicity [19]. The serine to alanine mutation at amino acid 585 may have a significant influence in receptor binding or neutralizing antibody interactions [18]. Five Chinese strains, TGEV-HX, SC-Y, WH-1, H16, and H165, ha and alanine residue at this position, while the Purdue, Miller 6, and TS strains had a serine residue, which suggested that the antigenicity of the S protein of the five Chinese strains may be changed. Furthermore, amino acids 32, 208, 376, 403, 418, 496, 562, 675, 1,109, and 1,234 of TGEV-HX were identical to those of strains SC-Y and WH-1, but different from those of strains TS, H16, and H165.

The nucleotide and amino acid sequence homology analysis of the structural proteins and non-structural proteins indicated that TGEV-HX was highly similar to the WH-1, SC-Y, and Purdue strains, and had a lower sequence similarity to the Miller 6, TS, H16, and H165 strains. The phylogenetic analysis showed that TGEV-HX was closely related to the SC-Y, WH-1, and Purdue strains, which belonged to the Purdue cluster, while the Miller 6, TS, H16, and H165 strains belonged to the Miller cluster, which was consistent with the results of the homology comparison. The data obtained in this study indicated that HX had different ancestors than the early Chinese strain H16, and it might be derived from the same ancestor as the SC-Y, WH-1, and Purdue strains.

Conclusions

The present study provides the complete genome sequence of a TGEV-HX strain from China. By comparing the S gene and protein with those of other TGEV strains, we have gained a further understanding of the genetic structure, diversity, and evolution of the TGEV-HX strain. Our next work is to evaluate the characteristics of mutations in the S gene using a reverse genetic approach in animal experiments.

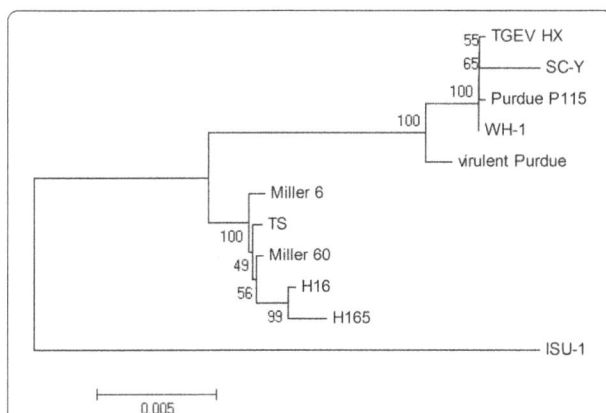

Figure 3 Phylogenetic tree based on the complete S nucleotide sequence. The tree was constructed based on the neighbor-joining (NJ) method using MEGA 4.0 software. Bootstrap values were calculated with 1,000 replicates of the alignment.

Abbreviations

TGEV: Transmissible gastroenteritis virus; CoV: Coronaviridae; ORF: Open reading frames; S: Spike; HP: Hydrophobic protein.

Competing interests

The authors declare that they have no competing interests.

Authors' contributions

HXL participated in the study design and collection of samples, conducted all laboratory and statistical analyses, participated in the interpretation of analyses, and drafted the manuscript. LNN, YX, and TZG participated in the study, provided oversight of the laboratory analysis, participated in interpretation of analyses, and helped to draft and critically revise the manuscript. QJJ and QLD participated in the study design and in the interpretation of analyses, and helped to draft and critically revise the manuscript. All authors have read and approved the final manuscript.

Acknowledgment

This work was supported by the National Ministry of Science and Technology of China (no. 2012BAD46B01).

Author details

[1]College of Resources and Environment, Northeast Agricultural University, Harbin 150030, People's Republic of China. [2]College of Life Sciences, Northeast Agricultural University, Harbin, Harbin 150030, People's Republic of China. [3]College of Wildlife Resources, Northeast Forestry University, Harbin 150040, People's Republic of China. [4]National Key Laboratory of Veterinary Biotechnology, Harbin Veterinary Research Institute, Chinese Academy of Agricultural Sciences, Harbin 150001, People's Republic of China.

References

1.   Enjuanes L, Smerdou C, Castilla J, Anton IM, Torres JM, Sola I, et al., editors. Development of Protection Against Coronavirus Induced Diseases. New York: Spinger; 1995. p. 197–211.

2.   Enjuanes L, Smerdou C, Castilla J, Anton IM, Torres JM, Sola I, et al. Development of protection against coronavirus induced diseases. Adv Exp Med Biol. 1995;380:197–211.

3.   Wesley R, Woods R, Cheung A. Genetic analysis of porcine respiratory coronavirus, an attenuated variant of transmissible gastroenteritis virus. J Virol. 1991;65(6):3369–73.

4.   Enjuanes L, Brian D, Cavanagh D, Holmes K, Lai MMC, Laude H, et al. In: van Regenmortel MHV, Fauquet SG, Bishop CM, Carsten DHLEB, Lemon MK, McGeoch SM, Maniloff DJ, Mayo MA, Pringle CR, Wicker RB, editors. Virus Taxonomy: Classification and Nomenclature of Viruses. New York: Academic; 2000. p. 835–49.

5.   Vaughn EM, Halbur PG, Paul PS. Sequence comparison of porcine respiratory coronavirus isolates reveals heterogeneity in the S, 3, and 3–1 genes. J Virol. 1995;69(5):3176–84.

6.   Krempl C, Schultze B, Laude H, Herrler G. Point mutations in the S protein connect the sialic acid binding activity with the enteropathogenicity of transmissible gastroenteritis coronavirus. J Virol. 1997;71:3285–7.

7.   Ballesteros M, Sanchez C, Enjuanes L. Two amino acid changes at the N-Terminus of transmissible gastroenteritis coronavirus spike protein result in the loss of enteric tropism. Virology. 1997;227(2):378–88.

8.   Delmas B, Rasschaert D, Godet M, Gelfi J, Laude H. Four major antigenic sites of the coronavirus transmissible gastroenteritis virus are located on the amino-terminal half of spike glycoprotein S. J Gen Virol. 1990;71(6):1313–23.

9.   Sánchez C, Izeta A, Sánchez M, Alonso S, Sola I, Balasch M, et al. Targeted recombination demonstrates that the spike gene of transmissible gastroenteritis coronavirus is a determinant of its enteric tropism and virulence. J Virol. 1999;73(9):7607–18.

10. Ortego J, Sola I, Almazan F, Ceriani JE, Riquelme C, Balasch M, et al. Transmissible gastroenteritis coronavirus gene 7 is not essential but influences in vivo virus replication and virulence. Virology. 2003;308:13–22.

11. Tung FY, Abraham S, Sethna M, Hung S, Sethna P, Hogue B, et al. The 9-kDa hydrophobic protein encoded at the 3′ end of the porcine transmissible gastroenteritis coronavirus genome is membrane-associated. Virology. 1992;186(2):676–83.

12. Reed LJ, Muench H. A simple method of estimating fifty percent Endpoints. Am J Hygiene. 1937;27(3):493–7.

13. Hoshino K, Isawa H, Tsuda Y, Yano K, Sasaki T, Yuda M, et al. Genetic characterization of a new insect flavivirus isolated from Culex pipiens mosquito in Japan. Virology. 2007;359:405–14.

14. Cruz JLG, Sola I, Becares M, Alberca B, Plana J, Enjuanes L, et al. Coronavirus gene 7 counteracts host defenses and modulates virus virulence. PLoS Pathog. 2011;7(6):e1002090. doi:10.1371/journal.ppat.1002090.

15. Saif LJ, Sestak K. Transmissible gastroenteritis virus and porcine respiratory coronavirus. In: Straw BE, Zimmerman JJ, D'Allaire S, Taylor DJ, editors. Diseases of Swine. 9th ed. New York: Wiley; 2006. p. 489–516.

16. Penzes Z, Gonzalez JM, Calvo E, Izeta A, Smerdou C, Mendez A, et al. Complete genome sequence of transmissible gastroenteritis coronavirus PUR46-MAD clone and evolution of the purdue virus cluster. Virus Genes. 2001;23(1):105–18.

17. Godet M, Grosclaude J, Delmas B, Laude H. Major receptor-binding and neutralization determinants are located within the same domain of the transmissible gastroenteritis virus (coronavirus) spike protein. J Virol. 1994;68(12):8008–16.

18. Delmas B, Gelfi J, Laude H. Antigenic structure of transmissible gastroenteritis virus. I. Properties of monoclonal antibodies directed against virion proteins. J Gen Virol. 1986;67(1):119–30.

19. Zhang XS, Hasoksuz M, Spiro D, Halpin R, Wang S, Stollar S, et al. Complete genomic sequences, a key residue in the spike protein and deletions in nonstructural protein 3b of US strains of the virulent and attenuated coronaviruses, transmissible gastroenteritis virus and porcine respiratory coronavirus. Virology. 2007;358(2):424–35.

13

Protective immunity against influenza H5N1 virus challenge in chickens by oral administration of recombinant *Lactococcus lactis* expressing neuraminidase

Han Lei[1,2,3*], Xiaojue Peng[3], Jiexiu Ouyang[3], Daxian Zhao[3], Huifeng Jiao[3], Handing Shu[3] and Xinqi Ge[3]

Abstract

Background: Highly pathogenic H5N1 avian influenza viruses pose a debilitating pandemic threat in poultry. Current influenza vaccines predominantly focus on hemagglutinin (HA) which anti-HA antibodies are often neutralizing, and are used routinely to assess vaccine immunogenicity. However, Neuraminidase (NA), the other major glycoprotein on the surface of the influenza virus, has historically served as the target for antiviral drug therapy and is much less studied in the context of humoral immunity. The aim of this study was to evaluate the protective immunity of NA based on *Lactococcus lactis* (*L.lactis*) expression system against homologous H5N1 virus challenge in a chicken model.

Results: *L.lactis*/pNZ2103-NA which NA is derived from A/Vietnam/1203/2004 (H5N1) (VN/1203/04) was constructed based on *L.lactis* constitutive expression system in this study. Chickens vaccinated orally with 10^{12} colony-forming unit (CFU) of *L.lactis*/pNZ2103-NA could elicit significant NA-specific serum IgG and mucosa IgA antibodies, as well as neuraminidase inhibition (NI) titer compared with chickens administered orally with saline or *L.lactis*/pNZ2103 control. Most importantly, the results revealed that chickens administered orally with *L.lactis*/pNZ2103-NA were completely protected from a lethal H5N1 virus challenge.

Conclusions: The data obtained in the present study indicate that recombinant *L.lactis*/pNZ2103-NA in the absence of adjuvant can be considered an effective mucosal vaccine against H5N1 infection in chickens via oral administration. Further, these findings support that recombinant *L.lactis*/pNZ2103-NA can be used to perform mass vaccination in poultry during A/H5N1 pandemic.

Keywords: *L.lactis*/pNZ2103-NA, H5N1 virus, Protective immunity

Background

Rapid worldwide dissemination of highly pathogenic avian influenza (HAPI) H5N1 viruses among poultry and ongoing viral evolution through genetic drift and reassortment raise concerns of a potential influenza pandemic [1]. HAPI H5N1 virus has emerged in Southeast Asian and resulted in the destruction of millions of birds [2]. Concerns about the potential for the generation of a pandemic H5 strain and its concomitant morbidity and mortality are spurring the search for an effective vaccine. Vaccination is the most safe and effective way to prevent and control H5N1 infection in poultry. Currently, two commercial inactivated H5N1vaccines (Re-1 and Re-5) have been widely applied in domestic duck in many Asian countries [3]. However, these approved vaccines against H5N1 viruses produced in fertilized eggs have serious limitations, particularly the limited capability of producing conventional inactivated influenza H5N1 vaccines could severely hinder the ability to control the pandemic spread of avian influenza through vaccination [1,4]. In addition, conventional vaccines utilizing the hemagglutinin (HA) of H5N1 viruses have been poor immunogenicity and have safety issues [4]. Although novel approaches, such as

* Correspondence: hlei@binghamton.edu
[1]School of Medicine, Southwest Jiaotong University, Chengdu, 6111756, China
[2]Department of Biomedical Engineering, State University of New York, Binghamton 13902, USA
Full list of author information is available at the end of the article

recombinant DNA vaccines and virus-like particles (VLPs), show some promising signs against H5N1 infection in mice or poultry [5-8], the risk of generating a reassortant prohibit the use of this vaccine in most instances. Therefore, there is a clear need for a new vaccine strategy in poultry that provides increasing immunogenicity and safety.

For mucosal immunization, lactic acid bacterium (LAB) is more attractive vaccine delivery system than other live vaccine vehicles, such as *Shigella*, *Salmonella*, and *Listeria* [9-11]. *Lactococcus lactis* (*L.lactis*), a typical model of lactic acid bacteria, is an ideal vaccine delivery vector and has been engineered to express many viral antigens [12,13]. It was shown previously that *L.lactis*, expressing hemaglutinin (HA) from A/chicken/Henan/12/2004(H5N1) and then coated by enteric capsule, is a safe and effective vaccine against avian influenza H5N1 virus infection in mice [14]. Similarly, it was described that HA1 from A/chicken/ Henan/12/2004(H5N1) virus was displayed on the surface of *L.lactis*, and showed it to be protective against homologous H5N1 virus by oral co-administration with CTB in mice [15]. Recently, it also shown that intranasal immunization of *L.lactis*-HA combined with mucosal adjuvant LTB could provide protection against homologous H5N1 in chickens [16]. However, most of these vaccines focus on raising a humoral response against hemagglutintin (HA) of H5N1 viruses. Neuraminidase (NA) is another major glycoprotein on the surface of the virus and has historically served as the target for antiviral drug therapy and is much less studied in the context of humoral immunity [17]. It remains largely unknown regarding the immunogenicity of recombinant *L.lactis* expressing neuraminidase (NA) in poultry via oral administration.

In the present study, we develop a constitutive expression system by constructing recombinant *L.lactis* expressing NA gene from A/Vietnam/1203/2004 (H5N1) (VN/1203/04) and then evaluating its immunogenicity via oral administration without the use of adjuvant in a chicken model. This study reported here suggests that this system can be used as a platform technology to develop a mucosal NA vaccine for preventing and controlling H5N1 infection in poultry.

Methods
Construction of plasmid expressing NA and expression on *L.lactis*
The NA gene (1459 bp) of A/Vietnam/1203/2004 (H5N1) was PCR-amplified from pCDNA3.1-HA (kindly provided by St. Jude Children's Research Hospital, Memphis, TN, USA) using the following primers: NA-F: CTA*GCTAGC* GGTACCGCCGCCACCATGAA (*Nhe* I); NA-R: CCG*A AGCTT*ACAGGAAGTATTCAATC (*Hind* III) and cloned into *L.lactis* based constitutive expression plasmid pNZ2103 (purchased from MoBiTec, Goettingen,

Germany), the resulting plasmid was transformed into competent *L.lactis* NZ3000, the positive clone was named as *L.lactis*/pNZ2103-NA.

Western blot analysis was described previously [14] and *L.lactis*/pNZ2103 was used as a negative control.

Animal experiments and sample collection
For oral administration of chickens, 7-day-old specific-pathogen-free (SPF) single comb white leghorn chickens from an in-house flock (Institute of Jiangxi Agriculture, China) were used in this study. The concentration of recombinant *L.lactis*/pNZ2103-NA was adjusted to 10^{12} colony forming unit (CFU)/ml with sterile saline.

Three groups of 16 chickens each were immunized with oral administration of 1 ml of sterile saline, 10^{12} CFU of *L. lactis*/pNZ2103 or 10^{12} CFU of *L.lactis*/pNZ2103-NA, respectively. Prime immunization was performed at day 0, 1, 2, 3 and boosted at day 17, 18, 19, 20.

At day 15 and day 34 after the first immunization, blood samples were collected from the retro-orbital plexus. Sera were separated by centrifugation of blood at $2,000 \times g$ for 10 min and stored at -20°C until use. Intestine and upper respiratory were isolated from the vaccinated chickens and washed with 500 μL sterile saline, respectively.

At two weeks after the last immunization, chickens were lightly anesthetized with CO_2 and inoculated intranasally with 25 μl of 10^4 EID_{50} of VN/1203/04 virus through the choanal slit to determine protection efficacy. Chickens were observed for illness, weight loss, and death for 14 days after H5N1 virus infection. H5N1 virus challenge experiments must be strictly performed under the enhanced bio-safety level-3 laboratory (BSL-3).

The chickens were managed with pelleted feed and sterile water, maintained in a SPF environment and all efforts were made to minimize suffering following approval from the Institute Animal Care and Use Committee of the Nanchang University (Approval No. 726-14).

Enzyme-linked immunosorbent assay (ELISA)
Immune sera from the vaccinated chickens were collected by bleeding from the wing vein and treated with receptor-destroying enzyme from *Vibrio cholerae* (Denka-Seiken, San Francisco, CA) before being tested for the presence of H5-specific antibodies as described previously [16].

NA-specific immunoglobulin G (IgG) and secretory immunoglobulin A (IgA) antibodies were detected by enzyme-linked immunosorbent assay (ELISA) using recombinant NA protein as a coating antigen as described previously [14]. ELISA end point titers were expressed as the highest dilution that yielded an optical density greater than twice the mean plus one standard deviation of that of similarly diluted negative control samples.

Neuraminidase inhibition (NI) assay

The anti-NA immune response was evaluated by Bioluminescence-based neuraminidase inhibition kit. To perform this, 50 μl of chickens sera from each group was taken at 1/2 dilutions which were half diluted further till 1/1024 in a 96-well micro-titer plate. 50 μl of purified rNA (0.25 mg/ml) was added to each well and incubated at 37°C for 2 h. The neuraminidase inhibition titer was represented as the highest dilution until there was no neuraminidase activity observed.

Data analysis

Data are presented as the means ± standard deviations (S.D.) and are representative of at least three independent experiments. All analysis for statistically significant differences was performed by the Student t test and one-way ANOVA. A p value less than 0.05 was considered to be significant.

Results

Expression of NA protein on *L.lactis*

In this study, we generated a constitutive plasmid pNZ2103-NA containing NA gene from A/Vietnam/1203/2004 (H5N1) (Figure 1A). Expression of NA protein on *L. lactis* NZ3000 was confirmed by western blotting using anti-HA monoclonal antibody (Figure 1B). As we expected, there is no band shown in the *L.lactis*/pNZ2103 cells, while a specific band was observed at expected size for NA protein (approximately 54 kDa) (Figure 1B, Lane 3) in the *L.lactis*/pNZ2103-NA cells.

Immune responses elicited d by oral administration of *L.lactis*/pNZ2103-NA

At day 15 and day 34 after the prime immunization, sera samples were obtained from all chickens to screen for antibody responses as a marker of immunogenicity. There was no significant serum IgG detected between *L. lactis*/pNZ2103-NA and saline or *L.lactis*/pNZ2103 group at day 15 after the prime immunization. However,

at day 34 after the prime immunization, chickens administered orally with *L.lactis*/pNZ2103-NA could elicit a higher significant NA-specific IgG titer than other groups (saline or *L.lactis*/pNZ2103) (Figure 2A).

To assess the mucosal immune responses, the secretory mucosal IgA levels were determined by ELISA. Intestinal and upper respiratory washes were also collected at day 15 and day 34 after the prime immunization. As shown in Figure 2B and C, *L.lactis*/pNZ2103-NA induced significantly increased levels of NA-specific mucosal IgA compared to saline or *L.lactis*/pNZ2103 group at day 34 after the prime immunization in the intestinal and upper respiratory washes. These results are consistent with the detection of serum IgG antibody.

These data demonstrate that chickens vaccinated orally with *L.lactis*/pNZ2103-NA after prime-boost immunization can result in significant IgG and IgA levels which may contribute to protection against virus infection.

Neuraminidase inhibition (NI) titers induced by *L.lactis*/pNZ2103-NA

Similarly, oral vaccination with *L.lactis*/pNZ2103-NA induced a higher NI titer compared to other groups (saline or *L.lactis*/pNZ2103) (Figure 2D). These results support that recombinant *L.lactis*/pNZ2103-NA is immunogenic without the use of adjuvant in a chicken model.

Protection efficacy against H5N1 challenge

At two weeks after the last immunization, all chickens were challenged by intranasal inoculation with 25 μl of 10^4 EID_{50} of VN/1203/04 (H5N1). All chickens immunized orally with saline or *L.lactis*/pNZ2103 experienced substantial weight loss beginning at day 2 post challenge and death by 6 to 8 days post infection. In contrast, chickens immunized orally with *L.lactis*/pNZ2103-NA showed only mild and transient loss of body weight and survived the lethal challenge (Figure 3).

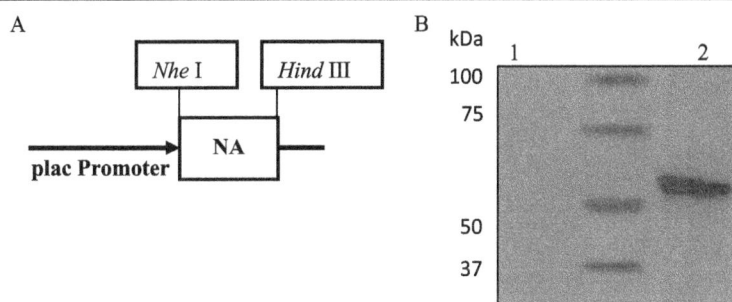

Figure 1 Construction of pNZ2103-NA and expression of NA protein on *L.lactis*. (A) A schematic diagram of constitutive plasmid pNZ2103-NA. **(B)** Western blot analysis of recombinant *L.lactis*/pNZ2103-NA expression. Lane 1: negative control *L.lactis*/pNZ2103; Lane 2: MagicMark™ XP Western Protein Standard; Lane 3: *L.lactis*/pNZ2103-NA. A specific protein band of around 54 kDa corresponding to NA was detected using anti-NA monoclonal antibody.

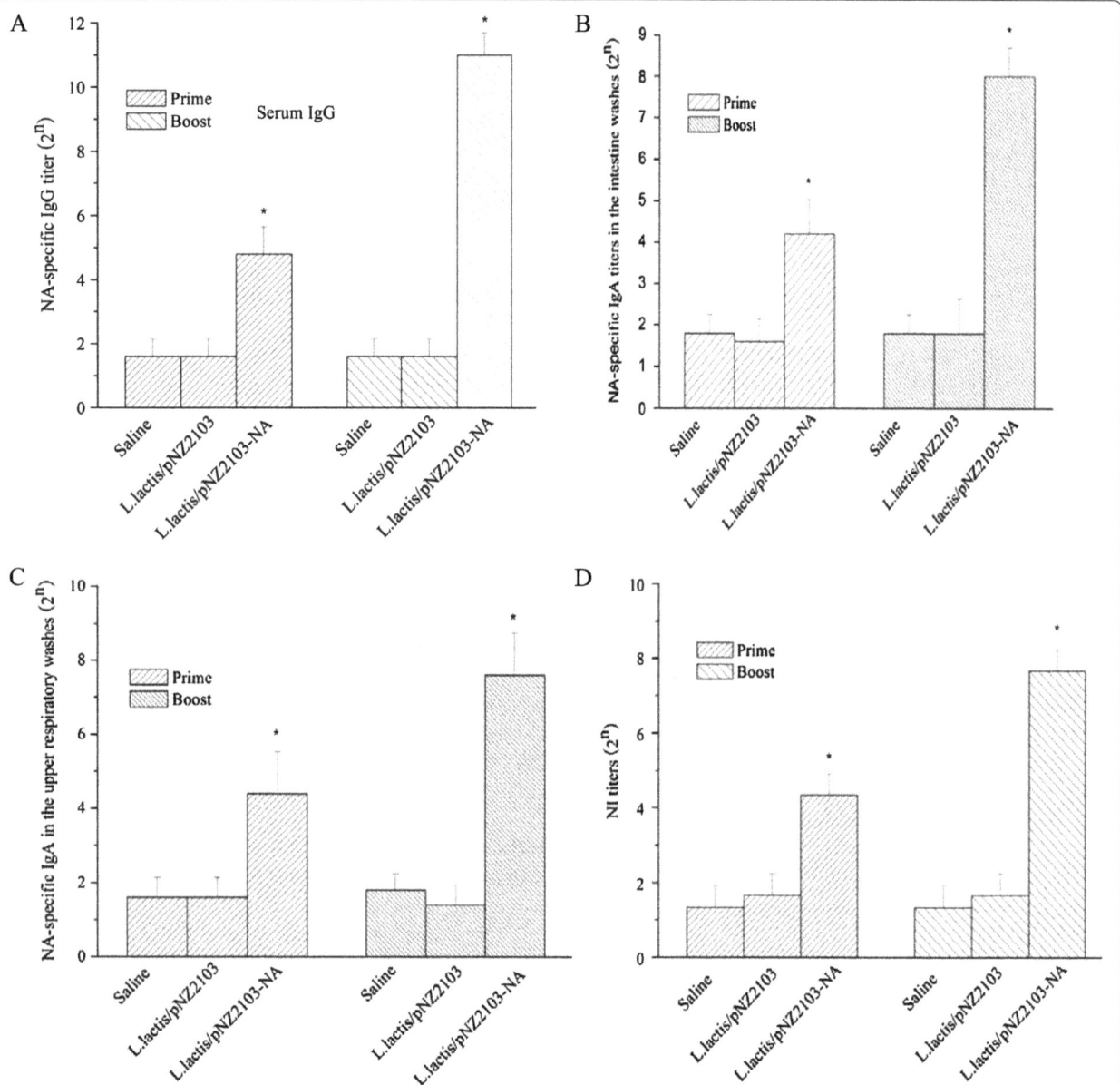

Figure 2 Oral administration of recombinant *L.lactis*/pNZ2103-NA induces NA-specific immune responses in chickens. Chickens were immunized orally with saline, *L.lactis*/pNZ2103 or *L.lactis*/pNZ2103-NA at day 0, 1, 2, 3 and day 17, 18, 19, 20. Sera (n = 16/group), intestine (n = 3/group) and upper respiratory (n = 3/group) washes were collected at day 15 and day 34 after the prime immunization. **(A)** NA-specific IgG antibody was measured by ELISA in the sera. **(B)** NA-specific IgA antibody was assessed in the intestinal washes. **(C)** NA-specific IgA antibody was assessed in the upper respiratory washes. **(D)** NI titers were determined using rNA protein. Data are presented as the means ± standard deviations (S.D.). The asterisk indicates a significant difference between *L.lactis*/pNZ2103-NA and other groups (saline or *L.lactis*/pNZ2103) (* $p < 0.05$).

Discussion

Vaccination is an integral component of strategies aiming to prevent and control pandemic influenza in poultry. Unfortunately, current commercial inactivated influenza H5N1 vaccines for poultry are generated from the whole viruses that have serious safety issues and poor immunogenic [8,18]. Therefore, it is crucial to develop a safe and effective influenza H5N1 vaccine that can be applied broadly and rapidly in poultry during

H5N1 pandemic. Our previous study has shown that intranasal immunization of *L.lactis*-HA combined with LTB can provide protective immunity in chicken [16]. However, most of influenza H5N1 vaccines focus on HA, it remains unclear that whether NA express on *L. lactis* has immunogenicity and poses potential for H5N1 vaccine development in poultry via oral administration. Further, it is well recognized in the NA field that a vaccine that purely raises antibodies to neuraminidase is

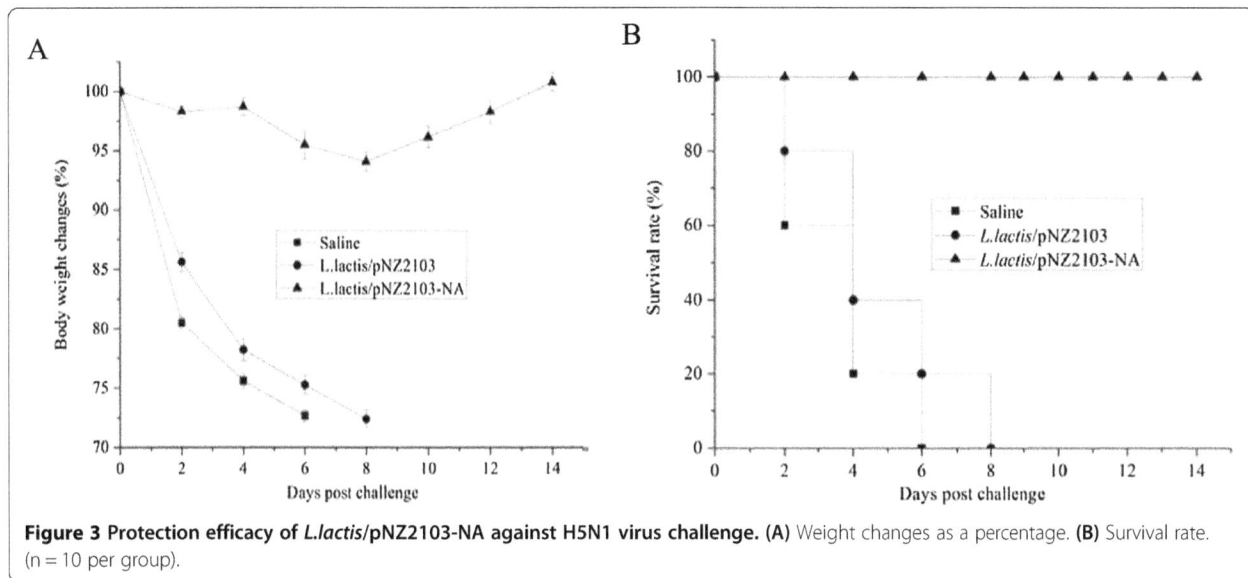

Figure 3 Protection efficacy of *L.lactis*/pNZ2103-NA against H5N1 virus challenge. **(A)** Weight changes as a percentage. **(B)** Survival rate. (n = 10 per group).

not desirable and would not be as effective as one which includes some combination of the NA and HA antigen [19]. Here, we hypothesize that recombinant *L.lactis* expressing NA can confer protective immunity against H5N1 challenge. To address this hypothesis, oral administration of *L.lactis*/pNZ2103-NA in the absence of adjuvant could induce protective immunity against H5N1 infection in a chicken model. This provides an evidence that *L.lactis*/pNZ2103-NA can serve as an effective mucosal vaccine to prevent and control H5N1 infection in poultry without the use of adjuvant.

The mucosal immune system is the first immunological barrier against the pathogens that invade the body via the mucosal surface. Thus, the induction of mucosal immunity via mucosal administration (oral or intranasal) is necessary to ensure protection against multiple subtypes of influenza A virus. Secretion of IgA is a representative antibody of mucosal immune response, and confers efficient protection against acquired mucosal infection [20]. It is an effective way to construct the incorporation of viral antigen to recombinant *L.lactis* that is considered essential to boost the interaction of the vaccine with the mucosal immune system [21]. This study revealed that chickens vaccinated orally with optional dosage as 10^{12} CFU of *L.lactis*/pNZ2103-NA was able to induce a significantly higher level mucosal IgA antibody in intestinal and upper respiratory washes (Figure 2B and C). Similarly, chickens administered orally with *L.lactis*/pNZ2103-NA also elicited a higher HA-specific IgG titer and NI titer which played an important role in providing protection against H5N1 lethal infection (Figure 2A and D). Collectively, these results support that *L.lactis*/pNZ2103-NA has a strong immunogenicity via oral immunization route without the use of adjuvant. In this regard, *L.lactis*/pNZ2103-NA can be considered an effective influenza H5N1 vaccine candidate for poultry.

The final protective immunity is most important for vaccine development [22]. Monitoring after post infection of H5N1 virus indicated that there was no significant decrease in the body weight of chickens vaccinated orally with *L.lactis*/pNZ2103-NA. In addition, the survival rate revealed that *L.lactis*/pNZ2103-NA could provide complete protection efficacy against highly pathogenic avian influenza H5N1 virus (Figure 3B). These findings suggest that *L.lactis*/pNZ2103-NA can be considered an effective influenza H5N1 vaccine candidate for mass vaccination in poultry. In addition, influenza vaccines based on *L.lactis* expression system have no safety issues, which make this technology has the potential of becoming one of the most promising platforms for avian influenza H5N1 vaccine development in poultry via oral vaccination. Our long-term goal is to translate these animal studies to preclinical studies, and determine the immunogenicity of recombinant *L.lactis* based vaccines in human, and to augment this technology to develop influenza universal vaccines against different influenza virus subtypes.

Conclusion

In conclusion, our findings strongly support oral administration of chickens with *L.lactis*/pNZ2103-NA in the absence of adjuvant can induce significant humoral and mucosal immune responses, as well as NI titers in chickens. Given the induction of protective immunity in the vaccinated chickens, widespread immunization of *L.lactis*/pNZ2103-NA in susceptible poultry would likely provide a significant barrier to the spread of H5N1 virus and also be economically advantageous. Thus, *L.lactis*/pNZ2103-NA may be a promising avian influenza H5N1 vaccine candidate for poultry in the event of the pandemic spread of H5N1 virus.

Competing interests

The authors declare that they have no competing interests.

Authors' contributions

All authors approved the manuscript. HL, XP, JO, DZ, HJ, HS and XG contributed to study design and data interpretation. HL was the principal investigator. All contributed to data analysis and results interpretation. HL wrote the manuscript and produced all figures. All authors read and approved the final manuscript.

Acknowledgements

This work was supported by grants from National Natural Science Foundation of China (No. 31360225) and Natural Science Foundation of Jiangxi Province (No. 20114BAB214014) to H. Lei.

Author details

[1]School of Medicine, Southwest Jiaotong University, Chengdu, 6111756, China. [2]Department of Biomedical Engineering, State University of New York, Binghamton 13902, USA. [3]Department of Biotechnology, College of Life Science, Nanchang University, Jiangxi 330031, China.

References

1. Subbarao K, Joseph T. Scientific barriers to developing vaccines against avian influenza viruses. Nat Rev Immunol. 2007;7:267–78.
2. Pantin-Jackwood MJ, Suarez DL. Vaccination of domestic ducks against H5N1 HPAI: a review. Virus Res. 2013;178:21–34.
3. Cha RM, Smith D, Shepherd E, Davis CT, Donis R, Nguyen T. Suboptimal protection against H5N1 highly pathogenic avian influenza viruses from Vietnam in ducks vaccinated with commercial poultry vaccines. Vaccine. 2013;31:4953–60.
4. Stephenson I, Nicholson KG, Wood JM, Zambon MC, Katz JM. Confronting the avian influenza threat: vaccine development for a potential pandemic. Lancet Infect Dis. 2004;4:499–509.
5. Singh N, Pandey A, Mittal SK. Avian influenza pandemic preparedness: developing prepandemic and pandemic vaccines against a moving target. Expert Rev Mol Med. 2010;12:e14.
6. Horimoto T, Kawaoka Y. Designing vaccines for pandemic influenza. Curr Top Microbiol Immunol. 2009;333:165–76.
7. Easterbrook JD, Schwartzman LM, Gao J, Kash JC, Morens DM, Couzens L, et al. Protection against a lethal H5N1 influenza challenge by intranasal immunization with virus-like particles containing 2009 pandemic H1N1 neuraminidase in mice. Virology. 2012;432:39–44.
8. Gao W, Soloff AC, Lu X, Montecalvo A, Nguyen DC, Matsuoka Y, et al. Protection of mice and poultry from lethal H5N1 avian influenza virus through adenovirus-based immunization. J Virol. 2006;80:1959–64.
9. Wells JM, Mercenier A. Mucosal delivery of therapeutic and prophylactic molecules using lactic acid bacteria. Nat Rev Microbiol. 2008;6:349–62.
10. Lee JS, Shin KS, Pan JG, Kim CJ. Surface displayed viral antigens on salmonella carrier vaccine. Nat Biotechnol. 2000;18:645–8.
11. Shata MT, Hone DM. Vaccination with a *Shigella* DNA vaccine vector induces antigen-specific CD8$^+$ T cells and antiviral protective immunity. J Virol. 2001;75:9665–70.
12. Van Huynegem K, Loos M, Steidler L. Immunomodulation by genetically engineered lactic acid bacteria. Front Biosci (Landmark Ed). 2009;14:4825–35.
13. Pontes DS, de Azevedo MS, Chatel JM, Langella P, Azevedo V, Miyoshi A. Lactococcus lactis as a live vector: heterologous protein production and DNA delivery systems. Protein Exp Purif. 2011;79:165–75.
14. Lei H, Xu Y, Chen J, Wei X, Lam DM. Immunoprotection against influenza H5N1 virus by oral administration of eneteric coated recombinant Lactococcus lactis mini-capsules. Virology. 2010;407:319–24.
15. Lei H, Sheng Z, Ding Q, Chen J, Wei X, Lam DM, et al. Evaluation of oral immunization with recombinant avian influenza virus HA1 displayed on the Lactococcus lactis surface and combined with the mucosal adjuvant cholera toxin subunit B. Clin Vaccine Immunol. 2011;18:1046–51.
16. Lei H, Peng X, Shu H, Zhao D. Intranasal immunization with live recombinant Lactococcus lactis combined with heat-labile toxin B subunit protects chickens from highly pathogenic avian influenza H5N1 virus. J Med Virol. 2014. doi: 10.1002/jmv.23983.
17. Wohlbold TJ, Krammer F. In the shadow of hemagglutinin: a growing interest in influenza viral neuraminidase and its role as a vaccine antigen. Viruses. 2014;6:2465–94.
18. Rappuoli R, Dormitzer PR. Influenza: options to improve pandemic preparation. Science. 2012;336:1531–3.
19. Doyle TM, Hashem AM, Li C, Van Domselaar G, Larocque L, Wang J, et al. Universal anti-neuraminidase antibody inhibiting all influenza A subtypes. Antiviral Res. 2013;100:567–74.
20. Yuki Y, Kiyono H. New generation of mucosal adjuvant for the induction of protective immunity. Rev Med Virol. 2003;13:293–310.
21. Bermúdez-Humarán LG. Lactococcus lactis as a live vector for mucosal delivery of therapeutic proteins. Hum Vaccin. 2009;5:264–7.
22. Nicholson KG, Wod JM, Zamvon M. Influenza. Lancet. 2003;362:1733–45.

14

Sero-epidemiology of Peste des petits ruminants virus infection in Turkana County, Kenya

Simon M Kihu[1,2*], John M Gachohi[3,4], Eunice K Ndungu[5], George C Gitao[1], Lily C Bebora[1], Njenga M John[1], Gidraph G Wairire[6], Ndichu Maingi[1], Raphael G Wahome[1] and Ricky Ireri[5]

Abstract

Background: Peste des petits ruminants (PPR) is a contagious viral disease of small ruminants. Serum samples from sheep ($n = 431$) and goats ($n = 538$) of all ages were collected in a cross-sectional study in Turkana County, Kenya. The objective was to estimate the sero-prevalence of PPR virus (PPRV) infection and associated risk factors in both species.

PPRV competitive enzyme-linked immuno-sorbent assay (c-ELISA) analysed the presence of antibodies in the samples. All analyses were conducted for each species separately. Multivariable logistic regression models were fitted to the data to assess the relationship between the risk factors and PPRV sero-positivity. Mixed-effect models using an administrative sub-location as a random effect were also fitted to adjust for possible clustering of PPRV sero-positivity. Intra-cluster correlation coefficients (ρ) that described the degree of similarity among sero-positive responses for each species in each of the six administrative divisions were estimated.

Results: Goats had a significantly higher sero-prevalence of 40% [95% confidence interval (CI): 36%, 44%] compared to sheep with 32% [95% CI: 27%, 36%] ($P = 0.008$). Combined sero-prevalence estimates were heterogeneous across administrative divisions ($n = 6$) (range 22% to 65%) and even more across sub-locations ($n = 46$) (range 0% to 78%). Assuming that PPRV antibodies are protective of infection, a large pool of PPRV susceptible middle age group (>6 months and < 24 months) in both species was estimated. This was based on the low sero-prevalence in this group in goats (14% [95% CI: 10%, 20%]) and in sheep (18% [95% CI: 13%, 25%]). Regression analysis returned significant risk factors across species: in sheep - vaccination status, age and administrative division; in goats - sex, age, administrative division and sex*age interaction. The intra-sub-location correlation coefficients varied widely across divisions (range <0.001 to 0.42) and across species within divisions.

Conclusions: Biological, spatial and socio-ecological factors are hypothesized as possible explanations for variation in PPRV sero-positivity in the Turkana pastoral ecosystem.

Keywords: PPRV, Sero-prevalence, c-ELISA, Risk factors, Vaccination, Turkana, Kenya

Background

Peste des petits ruminants (PPR) is a highly infectious and often fatal viral disease of sheep, goats and wild small ruminants. The disease is caused by PPR virus (PPRV), classified under genus *Morbillivirus* in the family *Paramyxoviridae* [1]. PPR is transmitted by direct contact with infectious animals shedding the virus in both ocular-nasal discharges and in fecal matter [2]. Fomite contamination with the virus

from infected animals such as feed troughs and bedding is an additional source of infection, albeit, for briefer periods of time [3]. These factors determine the frequency and distribution of the disease in endemic areas. PPR is largely controlled by vaccination [4].

Geographically, the disease has been reported in the Middle East, South Asia, China and sub-Saharan Africa [5]. In the Eastern Africa region, PPR serological evidence has been documented in Uganda, Sudan, Tanzania and Ethiopia [6-9]. In Kenya, the disease was first suspected in 1992 [10] and confirmed by serology and molecular assays from Turkana County [11,12]. The disease has since spread to all arid and semi-arid pastoral districts in Kenya [13].

* Correspondence: simon.kihu@vetworks-ea.org
[1]Faculty of Veterinary Medicine, University of Nairobi, PO Box 29053-00625, Uthiru, Kenya
[2]Vetworks Eastern Africa, PO Box 10431-00200, Nairobi, Kenya
Full list of author information is available at the end of the article

The majority of residents of Turkana County carry out nomadic or semi-nomadic pastoralism as their main socio-economic activity [14]. The main livestock species contributing to livelihoods are goats, sheep, cattle and camels [15]. Livestock diseases, frequent droughts and insecurity arising from livestock raids have been identified as the major constraints limiting livestock production in Turkana County [15,16]. Participatory studies investigating relative incidence of livestock diseases and their impact on livelihoods in Turkana County reported PPR as one of the most important diseases based on morbidity and case fatality rates [15].

In response to the 2006/7 outbreaks of PPR, the Government of Kenya together with development partners conducted vaccination campaigns in Turkana County and other arid and semi-arid pastoral regions of Kenya (Government of Kenya, Veterinary department, 2009 unpublished report). However, no published sero-epidemiological information is available as yet in Kenya. In this study, our first aim was to quantify the prevalence of PPR antibodies in small ruminants in Turkana County. Our second aim was to identify factors that were associated with positive PPR sero-positivity. The purpose of the study was to generate baseline information necessary for designing control strategies.

Methods

Study area

Turkana County is located in the northwestern part of Kenya. The county shares borders internationally with Ethiopia to the north, Sudan to the northwest and Uganda to the west. Internally, the county borders Marsabit, Samburu, and West Pokot and Baringo Counties (Figure 1). The county is characterized by arid and semi-arid lands covered with sparse thorny shrubs. A large proportion of the county's area consists of low-lying plains with isolated rocky mountainous, hilly ranges and several seasonal rivers. The rainfall pattern and distribution are unreliable and erratic over time ranging annually between 120 mm and 430 mm. Temperatures range annually from a low of 24°C to a high of 38°C with a mean of 30°C [17]. Administratively, Turkana County is divided into 17 divisions and 67 sub-locations [14]. Six administrative divisions namely, Loima, Oropoi, Kakuma, Lokichogio, Kibish and Kaaleng which served as the international frontier bordering divisions that reported initial PPR outbreaks in 2006 were purposively selected for this study. These divisions were perceived to be the foci of disease introduction into the county.

Study design, sampling unit, sample size calculation and sampling process

The study design was based on a proportionate stratified random sampling design while the sample frame was based on sheep and goat populations in the six administrative divisions that formed the study area. The sampling unit was an individual animal of specific age and vaccination status belonging to a village herd known locally as an *adakar*. In the Turkana community, an *adakar* entails a cluster of often-related households that pursue similar socio-economic activities such as search for pasture, water and security, under a trusted leader [15]. An *adakar* is, therefore, more or less synonymous to a village flock.

Since there is no serological test available that could differentiate animals vaccinated with homologous PPR vaccine from animals that had recovered from a natural PPR infection, the Turkana pastoral community, through focus group discussions (FGD), was deemed the best source of information regarding vaccination status of sheep and goats to aid in sampling. Together with the age structure, also sourced from FGD, these variables were subsequently used in the sample stratification. Five strata (young kids and lambs <6 months of age; middle-aged >6 months and <24 months of age vaccinated and unvaccinated groups; adults >24 months of age vaccinated and unvaccinated groups) were considered in this study for each of the two species (sheep and goats) investigated. Strata populations for each species were determined from the population of sheep and goats in the county, herd structure in Turkana herds established through participatory epidemiology approaches [19,20] and estimated vaccination prevalence of 14% in Turkana reported in unpublished data of Director of Veterinary services of the Government of Kenya.

For each species (sheep and goat), the stratum sample sizes determination was carried out using the formula by Bennett *et al.* [21] implemented within the ProMESA software program for statistical sampling in animal populations [22]. In determining the sample size, we ignored the sensitivity and specificity of the diagnostic test given their high values of 100% as reported by manufacturers in c-ELISA diagnostic test data control sheet. We assumed the prevalence of PPRV seropositivity was 50% with a relative error of 10%. We chose the 50% sero-prevalence because it provides the largest sample size (for given values of absolute error). The sample size was determined as 384 samples per each species and was then proportionately allocated to each of the strata based on sheep and goat population in each stratum. The strata sample sizes were determined as detailed in the online supplementary file.

The number of households in each *adakar* varies from 40 to 100 with an average of 70 [23]. The average number of sheep and goats per household were estimated at 34 (ranging between 3 and 100) and 54 (ranging between 7 and 167) respectively. We used this information to estimate the number of *adakars* in a sub-location and the population of sheep and goats in an *adakars*. A total

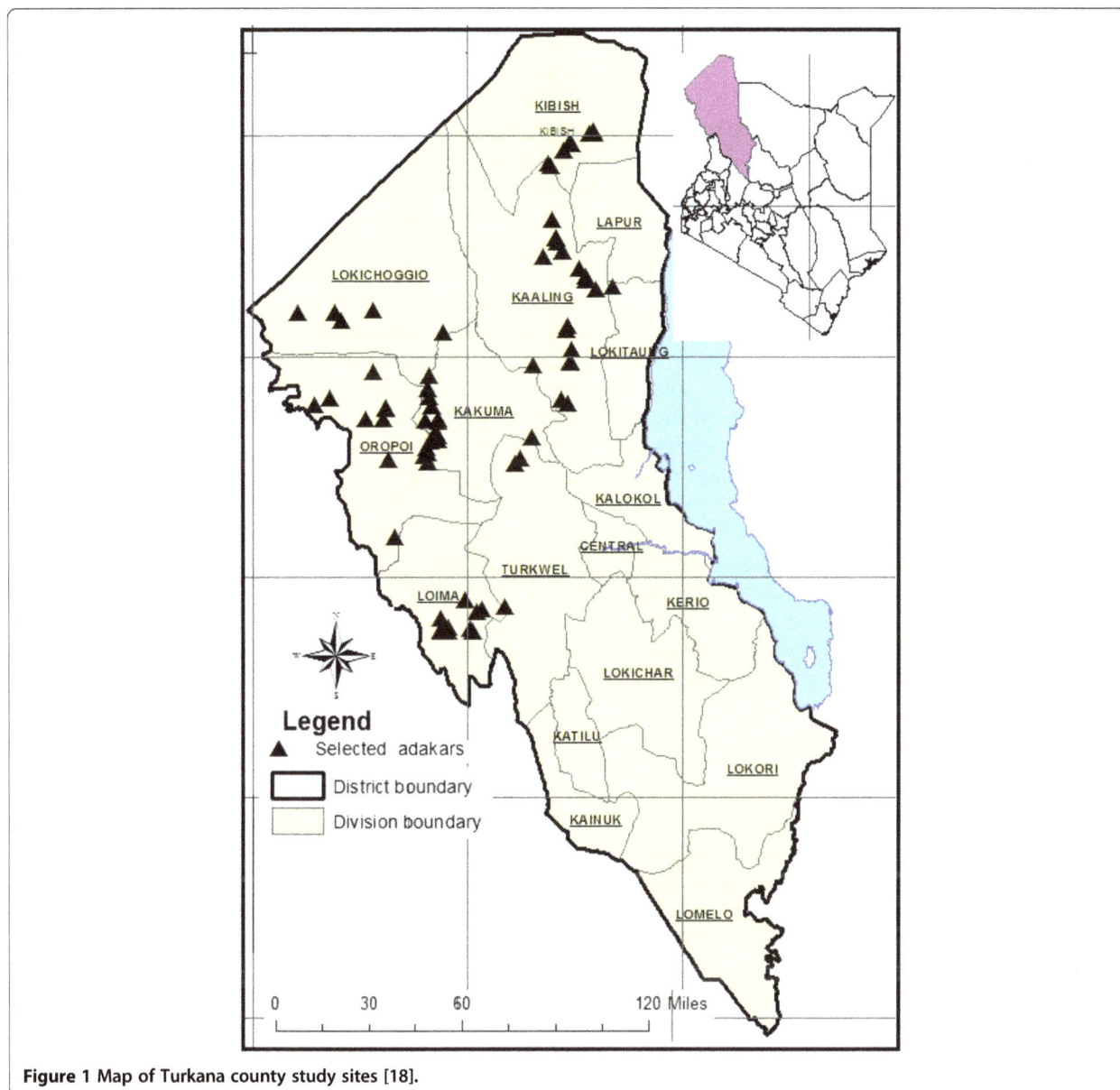

Figure 1 Map of Turkana county study sites [18].

population of 535 *adakars* was estimated in all the sublocations within the six selected administrative divisions. The sheep and goat population for each *adakars* was estimated by dividing the population of sheep and goats in a sub location with number of *adakars* estimated in that sub-location. In this instance, we assumed equal herd sizes in *adakars* in any one sub-location.

All *adakars* in all six study divisions were allocated sequential numbers from 1 to 535. We arbitrarily listed the divisions beginning with Loima, Oropoi, Kakuma, Lokichoggio, Kibish and then Kaaleng divisions. For each division, the five animal strata populations were listed alongside each *adakar*. Cumulative population estimate *per* stratum for all *adakars* was calculated with the

first animal in the stratum being from Loima and last being from Kaaleng. An individual animal was subsequently selected using simple random sampling using the random number function in Microsoft Excel®. Out of the 535 *adakars* estimated in the study area, selected animals fell in 155. Some animals selected were located in inaccessible *adakars* experiencing insecurity from livestock rustling, high mobility of the Turkana pastoralists and impassable roads. The inaccessible areas were in:

1) whole of Oropoi division except Kalobeyei location,
2) Lokichoggio division in such areas as Lorao location and sub locations of Songot and Lokudule and

3) Kaleng division in Nadunga, Kangakipur, Kakelae and Loruth Esekon sub locations.

To compensate, additional random numbers were generated while keeping the stratum proportion rule. Animals were then selected if they fell in safe and accessible *adakars*. The final number of samples collected for each species was slightly higher (431 and 538 sheep and goat samples respectively).

Ethics statement

This field serological study was conducted in manner to ensure quality and integrity of the research. The ethical approval as well as consent of this study was sought from Directorate of Veterinary Services who granted the approval and permission for collection of field laboratory samples on Peste des petits ruminants vide letter referenced "Ref.Meat/Vol.XIV/42 dated 1st July 2011. The Directorate of Veterinary Service belongs to the State department of Livestock development in the Ministry of Agriculture, Livestock and fisheries development of the Government of Kenya. Consent was also sought from Turkana herders for voluntary presentation of their small stock for collection of blood samples which they granted and facilitated the exercise.

Serum collection and storage

During serum collection activity, the pastoral herders were asked to recall and provide information on vaccination status of each of the animals selected for sampling. Blood was collected by jugular-vein puncture using venoject needles and vacutainer tubes (Venoject, UK). The blood was transported to the field laboratories where it was left to clot overnight. The serum was decanted into sterile tubes and centrifuged to remove the remaining red blood cells before being transferred to 2-ml cryovials and stored at -20°C.

Competitive Enzyme Linked Immuno-sorbent Assay (c-ELISA) for antibody detection

The peste des petits ruminants c-ELISA test kit ID Screen® PPRC, product code PPRC 1209, Lot 320 from IDVET innovative Diagnostic, Montpellier, France with an expiry date of July 2013 and assay protocol was supplied by the manufacturer. The test kit was used as per manufacturers recommended protocol to determine the presence of antibodies against PPRV in the samples of sheep and goats sera following the protocol supplied [24].

Statistical analysis

Ascent® Software version 2.6 (Thermo Electron Corporation, Theorem Electron Oy, Vantaa, Finland), a Windows-based Software designed to power all Thermo's Ascent® microplate research instruments, was used to control the Thermo Scientific Multiskan® EX microplate reader used for the c-ELISA. The software's spreadsheet function was used to generate results data that were subsequently exported to Microsoft Excel®, (Microsoft Inc. USA) and frequency plots generated. SPSS statistical software version 17.0 (IBM Corp., Armonk, NY) was used to generate descriptive statistics based on variables investigated.

For each species, the prevalence was estimated as: $p = y/n$, where y denoted the total number of animals positive for PPRV antibodies out of the sample size, n. This formula was used to compute not only the overall sero-prevalence for a species but also divisional-specific sero-prevalence by replacing the numerator and denominator to the relevant number of animals in the respective administrative unit. Differences in the sero-prevalences were tested using the chi-square test.

Univariable models were first run to assess the relationship between PPRV antibody sero-prevalence and individual risk factors for PPRV sero-positivity. The risk factors assessed included sex, age group, vaccination status and administrative division. The significance level was set at $P \leq 0.1$. A multivariable logistic regression model was subsequently built using significant variables in the univariable analysis by extending the univariable model to include other risk factors. In the latter analysis, all the significant risk factors were initially offered to the model. Model building used backwards elimination method to decide on the factors to exclude from the model using the likelihood ratio test ($P < 0.05$). The strength of association between the risk factor and PPRV sero-positivity was estimated using the odds ratios (OR) which were directly derived from the coefficient estimates from the logistic regression models. The odds ratio is a relative measure of risk that describes how much more likely it is that an animal which is exposed to the risk factor under analysis will develop the outcome as compared to an animal which is not exposed. If the odds ratio is 1, the risk factor is unlikely to be associated with the risk of PPRV sero-positivity. For an odds ratio greater or less than 1, the likelihood that the risk factor is associated with risk of sero-positivity increases, and the stronger the association. A plausible interaction – between sex and age - was tested for both species.

The relationship between PPRV infection sero-status and the significant risk variables was finally evaluated by fitting mixed-effect models with the sub-location as a random effect. The latter step was carried out to provide, as much as possible, statistically unbiased estimates of sero-prevalence with associated uncertainty adjusted for clustering of PPRV sero-positivity responses within sub-locations. The intra-cluster correlation coefficient (ρ) is a measure of correlation of observations in a cluster e.g., herds, villages, agro-ecological zones or administrative units. In this study, for each species, ρ for each division were computed indirectly through accounting for heterogeneity of data in sub-locations via the random effect variance. In this instance, the error variance was fixed at $\pi^2/3$ to substitute for the level 1 (animal-level) variance (ε_i) [25]. Thus, for each species and for each division, ρ was calculated as:

$$\sigma^2_{\text{sub-location}}/\left(\sigma^2_{\text{sub-location}} + \pi^2/3\right)$$

where $\sigma^2_{\text{sub-location}}$ is the variance due to sub-location-specific random effects whereas the sum of $\sigma^2_{\text{sub-location}}$ and $\pi^2/3$ is the total variance in the data for each division. Assuming the data is organized as a 2-level hierarchy, the intra-divisional correlation coefficient is the proportion of division-level variance out of the total variance for that division [25]. Coefficients close to zero indicate that responses (in our case PPRV sero-positivity) within clusters are no more similar to each other than responses from different clusters (implying that the response is randomly distributed among clusters) and *vice versa*. To evaluate whether ρ was associated with the magnitude of the serological response of the animals, non-parametric correlations (Spearman correlation coefficient) between ρ and the sero-prevalence was computed.

The sero-prevalence maps were produced using ArcGIS version 9.1 (ESRI, Redlands, California).

Results

Distribution and characteristics of the sampled animals and univariable analyses

Table 1 shows the distribution and characteristics of the sampled animals, sero-positivity results and outcomes of univariable models. The proportion of females in both species was larger compared to the proportion of males. The proportion of middle age groups and adults across the two species was almost similar, constituting >80% of the samples. The majority of sampled animals (>85%) across the species had not been vaccinated against PPR.

PPR serology

PPR antibody sero-prevalence distribution

Goats had a significantly higher apparent PPR sero-positivity of 40% [95% CI: 36%, 44%] compared to that of sheep which was estimated to be 32% [95% CI: 27%, 36%] ($P = 0.008$).

PPR antibody sero-prevalence by sex

Female sheep had a higher PPR antibody sero-prevalence compared to males but this was not significantly different ($P = 0.323$) (Table 1). Female goats had a significantly higher ($P = 0.024$) PPR antibody sero-prevalence compared to male goats (Table 1). Figure 2(A) shows the sero-prevalence differences among sex in the two species and their 95% confidence limits.

PPR antibody sero-prevalence status by age

The PPR antibody sero-prevalence in goats was significantly different ($P < 0.001$) between age groups (Table 1). Similarly, PPR antibody sero-prevalence in sheep was significantly different ($P < 0.001$) between age groups (Table 1). Assuming that PPRV antibodies are protective of infection, our results indicate the presence of a large pool of PPRV susceptible, middle aged animals in the study population. Figure 2(B) shows the sero-prevalence differences among age in the two species and their 95% confidence limits.

PPR antibody sero-prevalence status by vaccination status

The serum samples from both species were stratified by vaccination status and their sero-positivity estimated (Figure 3). Generally, as expected, the vaccinated stock was more likely to be sero-positive compared with the non-vaccinated stock. However, there was a difference in antibody sero-prevalence based on age among non-vaccinated stock across species. For instance, in both species, non-vaccinated middle-age and adults groups differed significantly ($P < 0.05$) (Figure 3).

PPR antibody sero prevalence status by administrative divisions

Table 1 and Figure 4 show the PPR antibody sero-prevalence by geographical divisions. Sero-prevalence estimates for each species were heterogeneous across administrative divisions. These intra-divisional sero-prevalence differences were significant for each species ($P < 0.001$) (Table 1).

Multivariable risk factor analyses for PPR sero-positivity

Multivariable analyses of the sheep data returned age, vaccination status and administrative division as significant factors ($P < 0.05$) (Table 2). Both middle age and adult sheep were less likely to be sero-positive against PPR virus relative to young sheep. Expectedly, being vaccinated was associated with higher odds of being sero-positive against PPR virus. The sex by age interaction term was not significant.

Multivariable logistic regression analyses on the goat data returned sex, age, administrative division and the interaction between age and sex as the only significant risk factors ($P < 0.05$) (Table 2). Unexpectedly, vaccination status was not associated with higher odds of being sero-positive to PPR virus in goats. Geographically, the risk of being sero-positive to PPRV infection in goats decreased from Oropoi, Kibish, Lokichogio, Loima, Kaaleng and Kakuma in that order (Table 2).

Mixed model analyses

Presence of sub-location random effect resulted in widening of confidence intervals for the sheep data (Table 3).

Table 1 Characteristics of the sampled animals, sero-prevalence and outcomes of univariate analyses ($P \leq 0.1$)

Variable	Sheep n = 431					Goats n = 538				
	Frequency	Sero-positive (n)	% Sero-prevalence [95% CI]	Odds ratio [95% CI]	P-value	Frequency	Sero-positive (n)	% Sero-prevalence [95% CI]	Odds ratio [95% CI]	P-value
Sex					0.323					0.024
Male	170	49	29 [22, 36]	1		215	73	34 [28, 41]	1	
Female	261	87	33 [28, 39]	1.2 [0.8, 1.9]		323	141	44 [38, 49]	1.5 [1.1, 2.2]	
Age					0.000					0.000
Young	64	27	42 [30, 55]	1		100	39	39 [30, 49]	1	
Middle age	170	31	18 [13, 25]	0.3 [0.2, 0.6]		211	30	14 [10, 20]	0.2 [0.1, 0.4]	
Adult	197	78	40 [33, 47]	0.9 [0.5, 1.6]		227	144	63 [57, 70]	2.4 [1.5, 4.0]	
Vaccination status					0.000					0.014
No	374	100	27 [22, 32]	1		462	174	38 [33, 42]	1	
Yes	57	36	63 [49, 76]	4.7 [2.6, 8.4]		76	40	53 [41, 64]	1.8 [1.1, 3.0]	
Administrative division					0.000					0.000
Kaaleng	39	6	15 [6, 30]	1		65	19	29 [19, 42]	1	
Kakuma	92	19	21 [13, 30]	1 [0.5, 2.0]		140	31	22 [16, 30]	0.5 [0.3, 1.0]	
Kibish	100	38	38 [28, 48]	0.5 [0.2, 0.8]		98	54	55 [45, 65]	0.6 [0.3, 1.0]	
Loima	50	16	32 [20, 47]	0.4 [0.3, 0.9]		63	24	38 [26, 51]	0.2 [0.1, 0.4]	
Lokichogio	109	29	27 [19, 36]	0.3 [0.1, 0.8]		104	43	41 [32, 51]	0.3 [0.2, 0.7]	
Oropoi	41	28	68 [52, 82]	3.5 [1.6, 7.6]		68	43	63 [51, 75]	1.4 [0.7, 2.6]	

For each risk factor, the odds ratio represented the effect of that level compared to the reference category (with an odds ratio of 1).

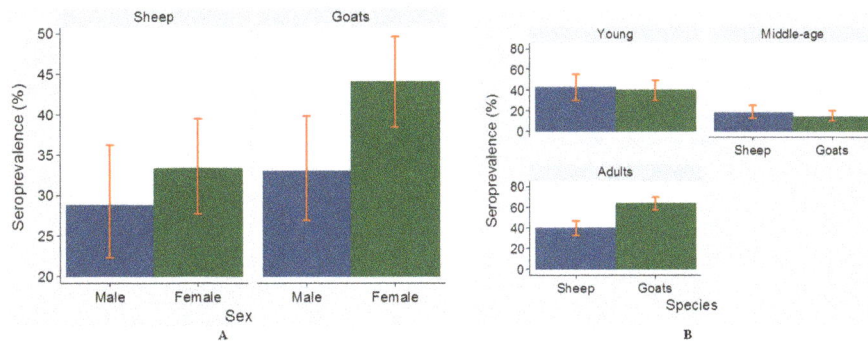

Figure 2 Mean serum antibody prevalence (crude estimates with 95% confidence limits) to PPRV infection in sheep and goats by A sex and B: age groups. (Adult ≥24 months; Middle age > 6 and < 24 months; Young kids & lambs ≤ 6 months).

However, this was not as marked in the goat data. Accordingly, the likelihood ratio test in the sheep model showed that inclusion of sub-location random effect provided a substantially better fit than the fixed-effects logistic regression model at alpha level 0.05 and 0.1 (Table 3). For the goat data, inclusion of sub-location random effect term provided a substantially better fit than the standard multivariate logistic regressions at the alpha level of 0.1 (Table 3). These results implied that whereas the sub-location contributed a relatively large amount to the variation in the sheep data, the contribution in the goat data was modest. This was supported by the findings of the overall intra-cluster correlation coefficient which was larger for sheep (0.16) relative to that for goat data (0.12). For both models, the adjusted estimates (ORs) also differed substantially (increased in magnitude) from the unadjusted estimates presented in Table 2. The predicted PPRV sero-positivity estimates using the regression coefficients from the model were 31% for sheep and 40% for goats.

Divisional-specific intra-cluster correlation coefficient (ρ)

The 6 administrative divisions for which the intra-cluster correlation coefficient (ρ) was calculated had between 3 and 11 sub-locations each (median = 8). These sub-locations, in turn, had between 63 and 140 goats sampled in each (median = 83) and between 39 and 109 sheep sampled in each (median = 71).The estimated ρ are shown in Table 4. The estimated ρ were heterogeneous across the divisions for both species (Table 4). However, for each species, two groups of ρ emerged: three divisions had very low values in both species data (Table 4). Negative Spearman rank correlation coefficients of -0.09 ($P = 0.9$) and -0.43 ($P = 0.4$) in sheep and goats respectively were estimated and these suggested lack of dependence between the two variables (ρ and sero-prevalence).

Discussion

PPR is an emerging and geographically spreading disease of small stock particularly in Africa and Asia. Although

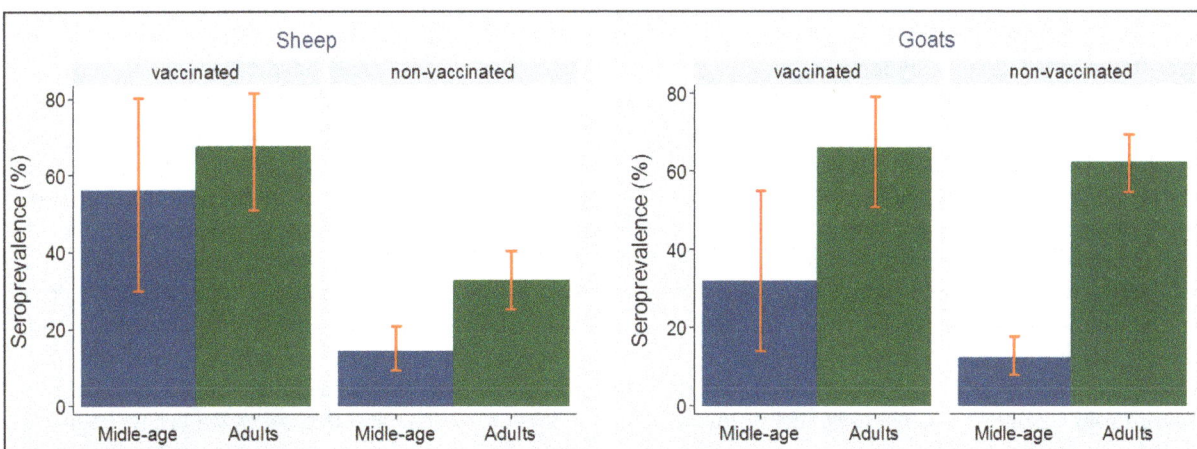

Figure 3 Mean serum antibody prevalence (crude estimates with 95% confidence limits) to PPRV infection in sheep and goats by age groups over vaccination status PPR antibody sero-prevalence by geographical divisions. Note the large difference in sero-positivity among non-vaccinated stock relative to vaccinated stock.

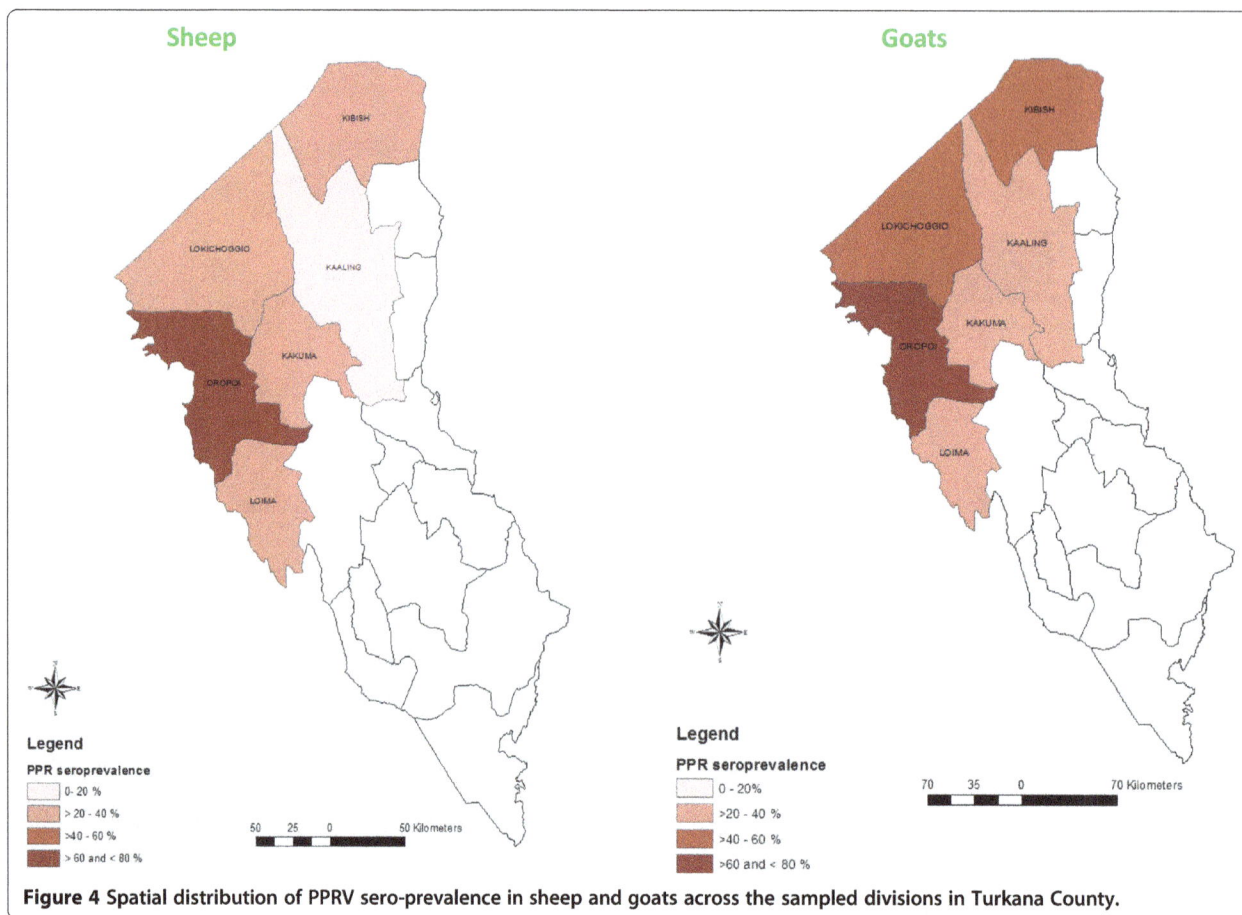

Figure 4 Spatial distribution of PPRV sero-prevalence in sheep and goats across the sampled divisions in Turkana County.

the disease is thought to have been introduced in Kenya in the 1990s, clinical cases were officially reported in Turkana for the first time in 2007 [18]. Epidemiological information about the introduction and factors facilitating the spread of PPR in Turkana County is generally scarce [16,18]. To the best of our knowledge there are no structured, population-based studies of PPR infection in Kenya. This study investigated risk factors for positive serological status in small stock by focusing on a region within the county that served as the international frontier bordering divisions that reported initial PPR outbreaks in 2006. The region was perceived to be the foci of disease introduction into the county.

The study findings shows PPR antibody sero-prevalence was heterogeneous across administrative divisions and even more across the lower administrative unit - the sublocation. Our results further suggest that age and spatial heterogeneity are significant variables associated with PPRV sero-prevalence in both species. Internal correlation of sero-positive samples was not only heterogeneous across divisions but also across species within divisions suggesting an interaction between socio-ecologic and spatial effects in determining the occurrence and distribution of PPRV infection in Turkana County.

The outbreaks in 2006/7 experienced in Turkana were dramatic with high mortality. The national response to the outbreak was mass vaccination initiative that was supported by Government of Kenya and partially by development partners. However, the numbers of small stock vaccinated in Turkana County during the exercise in 2007 were 1,331,681 (*Veterenairies Sans Frontieres* Belgium, 2007 unpublished data on Vaccination and sero-monitoring in Turkana). This number constituted 14% of the total population of 9,512,012 small stocks in Turkana County [14]. Our study, conducted in 2011 established a vaccination prevalence of 14% in goats and 13% in sheep (data not shown). Although the accuracy of this information may have been influenced by recall bias, the Turkana herders in the study area are principally dependent on their livestock for their livelihoods [15]. As such, the community possesses detailed information about disease occurrence [16] and responses down to individual animal. Due to the relative short time that had elapsed between the carrying out of vaccination exercise and this study, we believe at most, the vaccination information of animals at the individual level was accurate. This was corroborated by the high proportion of vaccinated animals from Oropoi division and none from Kaaleng and Kibish divisions in the sample

Table 2 Significant variables in the multivariable (*P* ≤ 0.05) model assessing relationship between PPRV sero-status and variables for sheep and goat data

Variable	Sheep *n* = 431		Goats *n* = 538	
	Odds ratio [95% CI]	Variable likelihood ratio test P-value	Odds ratio [95% CI]	Variable likelihood ratio test P-value
Sex	-			0.0027
Male			1	
Female			0.1 [0.04, 0.51]	
Age		0.000		0.000
Young	1		1	
Middle age	0.2 [0.09, 0.38]		0.05 [0.02, 0.12]	
Adult	0.6 [0.31, 1.13]		0.1 [0.02, 0.65]	
Vaccination status		0.0001	-	
No	1			
Yes	4.5 [2.14, 9.51]			
Administrative division		0.000		0.000
Kaaleng	1		1	
Kakuma	0.9 [0.31, 2.73]		0.7 [0.32, 1.46]	
Kibish	3.8 [1.41, 10.07]		3.5 [1.59, 7.67]	
Loima	2.4 [0.81, 7.30]		1.2 [0.53, 2.87]	
Lokichogio	2.0 [0.75, 5.49]		1.5 [0.68, 3.17]	
Oropoi	8.9 [2.62, 30.12]		6.4 [2.7, 15.0]	
Age*sex interaction	-		2.70 [1.59, 4.58]	0.0002

Hosmer-Lemeshow goodness-of-fit statistic: Sheep model Prob > χ^2 = 0.68; Sheep model Prob > χ^2 = 0.11 indicating that the model fitted the data well; For each risk factor, the odds ratio represented the effect of that level compared to the reference category (with an odds ratio of 1).

(Government of Kenya, Vaccines for the Control of Neglected Animal Diseases in Africa (VACNADA) and Lutheran World Federation/Department for World Service (LWF/DWS) supported - vaccination campaign/treatment report – Turkana West District, 2011; unpublished report). Therefore, the overall PPR antibody profile in this study (goats: 40% and sheep: 32%) was attributed to immunological reactions from both the wild virus and vaccination. In addition, the sero-prevalence reflected wild virus infection as demonstrated by high sero-prevalence levels in non-vaccinated stock in both species. This observation suggested that exposure to wild virus was higher than exposure to vaccine virus probably due to the low coverage of the latter.

The sero-prevalence reported in this study was lower than the overall 55.3% for both sheep and goats in the neighbouring Karamoja, Uganda [6]. Karamoja shares a common boundary complete with social, cultural and environmental similarities with Turkana. Similar differences were reported in Northern Tanzania (49.5% in goats and 39.8% in sheep) [26]. However, these being cross-sectional studies, they can only give an snapshot indicator of the probability of exposure which can vary quite substantially with temporal and seasonal effects [16], host population density, disease control programs and the

social environment that can influence contact rates [6,9,27]. Longitudinal studies are required to better identify the influences of long-term dynamics in PPRV transmission as discussed below.

Age appears to play a significant role in the epidemiology of PPR. Many studies report age as an important risk factor for PPRV sero-positive status [2,9]. In contrast to other studies [9], a linear relationship between age and seropositivity was absent. In our data, the risk of being seropositive in middle aged animals was low compared with younger and older age groups. The high sero-positivity detected in the young stock was likely to be due to maternal antibodies against PPRV [28]. The high sero-positivity in adults may be due to natural exposure to the virus and vaccination. The middle age groups were generally born between 2009 and 2010 when no major vaccination exercise was carried out. We hypothesize that the middle aged groups had encountered limited exposure to both the vaccine and wild virus either as young stock and after losing maternal antibodies. This group, from both species, remained at higher risk of infection for lack of antibody protection. The sero-positives in non-vaccinated middle aged stock most likely resulted from survival from PPRV infections. We are not aware of PPRV properties, e.g. differences in pathogenicity that can contribute to virus

Table 3 Mixed model analyses, variance and summary intra-correlation coefficient (ρ) for exposure to PPRV infection in sheep and goat data

Variable	Sheep n = 431		Goats n = 538	
	Odds ratio [95% CI]	LRT[¥] P-value	Odds ratio [95% CI]	LRT[¥] P-value
Sex	-			0.0023
Male			1	
Female			0.13 [0.04, 0.5]	
Age				0.000
Young	1	0.000	1	
Middle age	0.2 [0.07, 0.35]		0.04 [0.02, 0.12]	
Adult	0.6 [0.3, 1.18]		0.1 [0.02, 0.66]	
Vaccination status			-	
No	1	0.0004		
Yes	4.5 [1.94, 10.6]			
Administrative division				0.0005
Kaaleng	1	0.0036	1	
Kakuma	1.1 [0.27, 4.27]		0.7 [0.27, 1.70]	
Kibish	4.6 [1.25, 16.70]		3.6 [1.39, 9.53]	
Loima	3.1 [0.79, 11.96]		1.2 [0.44, 3.21]	
Lokichogio	3.3 [0.86, 12.64]		1.7 [0.67, 4.52]	
Oropoi	11.7 [2.36, 57.70]		6.8 [2.29, 20.34]	
Age*sex interaction	-		2.8 [1.63, 4.88]	0.0002
Random effect –sublocation variance	0.61 [0.36, 1.04]		0.44 [0.18, 1.1]	

LRT[¥]: Likelihood ratio test.
*denotes age and sex interaction.
Random effect –sublocation: Sheep, likelihood ratio test versus standard logistic regression: chibar2(01) = 10.86; Prob> = chibar2 = 0.0005; ρ = 0.16; Goats, likelihood ratio test versus standard logistic regression: chibar2(01) = 2.07; Prob > =chibar2 = 0.075; ρ = 0.12. "chibar2(01)" test statistic tests whether random effects are greater than zero. The results of this likelihood ratio test shows that inclusion of sub-location random effect provided a substantially better fit than the multivariable logistic regression in Table 2 (at both 0.05 and 0.1 levels of significance (sheep data) and at 0.1 level of significance (goat data).

persistence across population age categories in absence of a definite reservoir as reported in other pathogens [29]. This is an area that requires further investigation.

Biological heterogeneity was evident as goats had a significantly higher percentage of PPRV antibody sero-prevalence compared to sheep. In addition, an interacting effect between sex and age was significant in goats but not in sheep. A closer look at the distribution of sero-positive samples showed that the adult goat population, and more so the females, contributed substantially to the elevated sero-positivity in goats. Female goats are the main source

of breeding stock and rarely leave herds leading to a low demographic turn-over [30]. Thus, it is likely that PPR infection survivors that are immune or vaccinated female adult goats remain in herds for a longer period of time. The same phenomenon also explains the significantly lower sero-positivity in male goats compared to females. Male goats are often culled when young, through sales, as the main source of immediate household income or sacrificed in various cultural ceremonies [31]. Consequently, at any one time, the current population of male goats in herds is likely to be immunologically naïve. On the other hand, sheep succumb easily to drought and other environmental stresses and are also in smaller proportion compared to goats. The Turkana community considers the sheep (both sexes) more for socio-cultural ceremonies rather than of economical purposes [32]. The sheep then experience higher demographic turn-over relative to goats.

The spatial heterogeneity in PPRV sero-positivity increased with decreased spatial scale – i.e. heterogeneity was large for sub-location relative to administrative division. Spatial heterogeneity in PPR sero-prevalence has been reported in many areas where PPR is endemic [2,9].

Table 4 Intra-sublocation correlation coefficients

Division	Sheep	Goats
Kaaleng	0.11	0.15
Kakuma	<0.001	<0.001
Kibish	0.13	<0.001
Loima	<0.001	0.42
Lokichogio	0.29	0.2
Oropoi	<0.001	<0.001

Cross-sectional studies are limited in elucidating the mechanisms behind such heterogeneity. However, at least two hypotheses can be put forward. Firstly, biological interaction between factors that promotes social aggregation and mixing of animals may result in temporal heterogeneity in the local spatial distribution of the host population. Secondly, spatial variability in local factors may affect population parameters related to (1) demographic aspects that may influence births and deaths through density dependence, (2) transmission aspects such as the duration of infectious period, (3) spatial aspects such as movement distance travelled and movement rates which impact on contact patterns between infected and susceptible hosts [33]. Longitudinal analyses of geographic variations in demographic, environmental and socio-economic risk factors are required to explain the spatial production of PPR infections. Nevertheless, Oropoi division reported the highest sero-prevalence in both species because some vaccinations were carried out in early 2011 about three weeks prior to the date on which samples were collected for this study.

Identifying and describing the patterns of correlation was of prime interest in this study in addition to adjusting for effect estimates. Ignoring correlation may cause an error in either over- or under-estimation of the importance of a given risk factor [25]. In our data, accounting for correlation not only widened confidence intervals but also provided larger parameter estimates. The intra sub-location correlation coefficient varied widely across divisions and across species within divisions. These results suggest that a biological interaction between socio-economic and spatial factors may be responsible for PPRV sero-positivity heterogeneity. Waret-Szkuta et al. [9] estimated intra-cluster correlation coefficients for sheep and goats combined as one data and reported similar heterogeneity: two groups of administrative units stood out on the basis of the estimated ρ: a group with very low ρ ($\rho < 0.12$) and a group with very high ρ ($\rho > 0.37$). The authors [9] attributed these differences to biological factors and put forward a hypothesis that the past or recent circulation of PPRV was reflected by a low or a high value of ρ, respectively, along with a low or high sero-prevalence [9]. However, our results are contrary to this hypothesis, given the lack of dependence between sero-prevalence and ρ as confirmed by the negative and non-significant Spearman correlation coefficient. These inconsistencies could have resulted from differences in socio-ecologic factors across regions. In addition their data was country wide with expected high heterogeneity compared to ours which was more local in one ecosystem. However, even within the county of our study, the socio-ecology of disease differs considerably as well; for instance, in terms of socio-aggregation arising from nomadic movement, rustling and trade. Animals in Kakuma, Kibish and Oropoi divisions aggregate more frequently at spatial points relative to animals from other divisions. Kakuma is a livestock market centre attracting a lot of animals while Kibish and Oropoi are extreme dry season grazing zones in north and west frontiers respectively and are prone to persistent livestock rustling. The results also highlight the limitation of using a summary measure of ρ when data on both species is combined or for a spatial scale such as an administrative unit.

Nevertheless, identifying and describing the patterns of correlation in this study provided key insights into the PPRV infection dynamics in Turkana County indicating spatial-scale transmissions should be the focus of preventive programs particularly in sheep population. The ρ estimate in observational studies is very useful in the design and implementation of future studies in the same field. This is because the values obtained could be used as a correction factor for the calculation of sample sizes that are appropriate for a given set of defined study objectives. Studies utilizing simple random sampling require smaller sample sizes that can achieve sufficient statistical power. However, in presence of clustering, the sample sizes calculated under simple random sampling would be inflated by a factor of $1 + \rho(m\text{-}1)$ which is basically the design effect where m is cluster size [25].

Conclusion

This study has shown that, at the time of sampling, there was wide variation in the prevalence of PPRV among the divisions of Turkana County. The study results suggest that the risk of exposure is related to the species, age, sex, vaccination status and spatial location of the animal. Accounting for correlation in estimation of risk factors associated with PPRV sero-prevalence provided more confidence in the precision of estimates and subsequently more reliable information on impact of the factors. The presence of a large pool of small stock in the middle age group could contribute in the persistence of the virus in Turkana ecosystem. Based on our data, our findings indicate that the main group to target for vaccination within the herds would be the middle aged group with bias to goats in high risk administrative divisions when PPR vaccines becomes available. The spatial structure of the host population and the possible spatial variability in local factors affecting population parameters are underlying factors that could contribute to sero-prevalence heterogeneity.

Availability of supporting data

The data sets on sampling supporting the results of this article are available in the LabArchives repository, https://mynotebook.labarchives.com/doc/view/Mi42fDYzMjQ3LzIvRW50cnlQYXJlE5MzgwNzY4Mjd8Ni42?nb_id=ODIyMjEuMXw2MzI0Ny82MzI0Ny9Ob3RlYm9vay8xNTQwMjEyODA1fDIwODcxNS4x&page_num=0.

Abbreviations

CI: Confidence interval; ILRI: International Livestock Research Institute; LWF/ DWS: Lutheran World Federation/ Department for World Service; PPR: Peste des petits ruminants; PPRV: Peste des petits ruminants virus; RUFORUM: The Regional Universities Forum for Capacity Building in Agriculture, a Eastern, Central and Southern Africa; VACNADA: Vaccines for the Control of Neglected Animal Diseases in Africa.

Competing interest

The authors declare that they have no competing interest.

Authors' contributions

SMK, EKN, RI, and CGG collected the data, created the electronic database and cleaned and processed the data for analysis. SMK, JMG, and LCB conceived and performed the data analysis. SMK, JMG drafted the manuscript assisted by CGG, LCB, NMJ and GGW. CGG, LCB, NMJ, GGW, NM. and RGW raised the funding for the study and assisted in its coordination. All authors helped with the interpretation of the results and read and approved the final manuscript.

Acknowledgement

This is to acknowledge RUFORUM (RU/CFP/CGS/TADS/09/1) for financial support and Vetworks Eastern Africa for logistical assistance through this study which was part of corresponding author's PhD research work.

Author details

¹Faculty of Veterinary Medicine, University of Nairobi, PO Box 29053-00625, Uthiru, Kenya. ²Vetworks Eastern Africa, PO Box 10431-00200, Nairobi, Kenya. ³Kenya Agricultural Research Institute -Trypanosomiasis Research Institute, PO Box 362-00902, Kikuyu, Kenya. ⁴International Livestock Research Institute (ILRI), PO Box 30709-00100, Nairobi, Kenya. ⁵Kenya Agricultural Research Institute -Veterinary Research Centre, PO Box 32-00902, Kikuyu, Kenya. ⁶Faculty of Arts, University of Nairobi, PO Box 30197-00100, Nairobi, Kenya.

References

1. Gibbs PJE, Taylor WP, Lawman MP, Bryant J. Classification of the peste des petits ruminants virus as the fourth member of the genus Morbillivirus. Intervirology. 1979;11:268–74.
2. Munir M, Zohari S, Berg M. Molecular Biology and Pathogenesis of Peste des Petits Ruminants Virus. 151. ISSN 2211-7504, ISBN 978-3-642-31450-6, doi:10.1007978-3-64231451-3 Springer Briefs in Animal Sciences; 978-3-642-31450-6. 2013.
3. Lefèvre PC, Diallo A. Peste des petites ruminants. Rev Sci Off int Epiz. 1990;9:951–65.
4. Couacy-Hymann ERF, Bidjeh K, Angba A, Domenech J, Diallo A. Protection of goats against rinderpest by vaccination with attenuated peste des petits ruminants virus. Res Vet Sci. 1995;59:106–9.
5. Shaila MS, Shamaki D, Foryth MA, Diallo A, Goatley L, Kitching RP, et al. Geographical distribution and epidemiology of PPR viruses. Virus Res. 1996;43:149–53.
6. Luka PD, Erume J, Mwiine FN, Ayebazibwe C. Sero-prevalence of Peste des petits ruminants Antibodies in Sheep and Goats after Vaccination in Karamoja, Uganda: Implication on Control. Int J Anim Vet Adv. 2011;3(1):18–22. 2011. ISSN: 2041-2908.
7. Saeed KI, Ali YH, Khalafalla AI, Rahman-Mahasin EA. Current situation of Peste des petits ruminants (PPR) in the Sudan. Trop Anim Health Prod. 2010;42:89–93.
8. Muse EA, Karimuribo ED, Gitao GC, Misinzo G, Mellau LSB, Msoffe PLM, et al. Epidemiological investigation into the introduction and factors for spread of Peste des Petits Ruminants, southern Tanzania. Onderstepoort J Vet Res. 2012;79(2):Art.#457. 6 pages. http://www.ojvr.org/index.php/ojvr/article/viewFile/457/524.
9. Waret-Szkuta A, Roger F, Chavernac D, Yigezu L, Libeau G, Pfeiffer DU, et al. Peste des Petits Ruminants (PPR) in Ethiopia: Analysis of a national serological survey. BMC Vet Res. 2008;4:34. doi:10.1186/1746-6148-4-34.
10. FAO. Peste des petits ruminants (PPR) in Morocco: EMPRES WATCH August 2008. Website: ftp://ftp.fao.org/docrep/fao/011/aj120e/aj120e00.pdf. Accessed on 21st may 2009.
11. Wamwayi HM, Rossiter PB, Kariuki DP, Wafula JS, Barrett T, Anderson J. Peste des petits ruminants antibodies in East Africa. Vet Rec. 1995;136:199–200.
12. ProMed-Mail: Peste des petits ruminants - Kenya (Rift Valley).OIE. 0070117.0226: http://www.oie.int/wahis_2/public/wahid.php/Reviewreport/Review?page_refer=MapEventSummary&reportid=4526.
13. FAO. Trans-boundaryDisease. Bulletin 33, 2009 ftp://ftp.fao.org/docrep/fao/011/i0919e/i0919e00.pdf.
14. 2009 Kenya population and housing census Volume 1 A: Population distribution by administrative units. Kenya National Bureau of Statistics: August 2010
15. Bett B, Jost C, Allport R, Mariner J. Using participatory epidemiological techniques to estimate the relative incidence and impact on livelihoods of livestock diseases amongst nomadic pastoralists in Turkana South District, Kenya. Prev Vet Med. 2009;90:194–203.
16. Kihu SM, Gachohi JM, Gitao CG, Bebora LC, Njenga JM, Wairire GG, et al. Analysis of small ruminants' pastoral management practices as risk factors of Peste des petits ruminants (PPR) spread in Turkana District, Kenya. Res Opin Anim Vet Sci. 2013;3(9):303–14.
17. Savatia, V. Impacts of climate change on water and pasture resulting in cross-border conflicts: a case study of Turkana and Pokot pastoralists of northwestern Kenya. J Meteorol Rel Sci. 2011, 5.
18. Kihu SM, Gitao CG, Bebora LC, Njenga MJ, Wairire GG, Maingi N, et al. Participatory risk assessment of Peste des petit ruminants: Factor analysis of small ruminants pastoral management practices in Turkana district, Kenya. Res Opin Anim Vet Sci. 2012;2(9):503–10.
19. Catley A, Irungu P, Simiyu K, Dadye J, Mwakio W, Kiragu J, et al. Participatory investigations of bovine trypanosomiasis in Tana River District, Kenya. Med Vet Entomol. 2002;16:1–12.
20. Catley A, Mariner J. Where there is no data: participatory approaches to veterinary epidemiology in pastoral areas of the Horn of Africa. IIED.2002, Issue paper No. 110.
21. Bennett S, Woods T, Liyanage W, Smith D. A simplified general method for cluster-sample surveys of health in developing countries. World Health Stat Q. 1991;44:98–106.
22. PROMESA a programme for statistical sampling in animal populations. [http://www.promesa.co.nz/ProMESA_Home.htm]
23. Akabwai D. Extension and livestock development: Experience from among the Turkana pastoralists of Kenya. In: Pastor. Dev. Netw. Pap. 33b. London, UK: ODI (Overseas Development Institute); 1992. p. 14.
24. Libeau G, Prehaud C, Lancelot R, Colas F, Guerre L, Bishop DHL, et al. Development of a competitive ELISA for detecting antibodies to the peste des petits ruminants virus using a recombinant nucleoprotein. Res Vet Sci. 1995;58:50–5.
25. Dohoo I, Martin W, Stryhn H. Veterinary Epidemiologic Research. Prince Edward Island: AVC; 2003. p. 706.
26. Swai ES, Kapaga A, Kivaria F, Tinuga D, Joshua G, Sanka P. Prevalence and distribution of Peste des petits ruminants virus antibodies in various districts of Tanzania. Vet Res Commun. 2009;33:927–36.
27. Kivaria FM, Kwiatek O, Kapaga AO, Swai ES, Libeau G, Moshy W, et al. The incursion, persistence and spread of peste des petits ruminants in Tanzania: Epidemiological patterns and predictions. Onderstepoort J Vet Res. 2013;80(1):Art #593, 10 pages. http://www.ojvr.org/index.php/ojvr/article/view/593.
28. Awa DN, Ngagnou A, Tefiang E, Yaya D, Njoya A. Post vaccination and colostral Peste des petits ruminants antibody dynamics in research flocks of Kirdi goats and Fulbe sheep of North Cameroon. In: Jamin JY, SeinyBoukar L, Floret C (éditeurs scientifiques). Savanes africaines: des espacesen mutation, des acteurs face à denouveauxdéfis. Actes du colloque, mai 2002, Garoua, Cameroun., N'Djamena, Tchad -Cirad Prasac, 2003 Montpellier, France. p 6.
29. Meyers G, Thiel HJ. Molecular characterization of pestiviruses. Adv Virus Res. 1996;47:53–118.
30. Njanja JC. Livestock ercology in Central Turkana. Turkana Resource Evaluation Monitoring Unit (TREMU Technical report No. E-1). Nairobi: UNESCO; 1991.
31. Imana CA. Goat rearing as a livelihood strategy of Turkana Pastoralists in north west Kenya. In: MA thesis. Bloemfontein, South Africa: University of the Free State, Centre for Development Support, UFS; 2008.

32. Wienpahl J. Livestock production and social organization among the Turkana. PhD thesis. University of Arizona, Department of anthropology at the Graduate College; Tucson USA, 1984.

33. Orivea ME, Stearnsa MN, Kellya JK, Barfield M, Smith MS, Holt RD. Viral infection in internally structured hosts. I. Conditions for persistent infection. J Theor Biol. 2005;232:453–66.

15

Expression of genes involved in the T cell signalling pathway in circulating immune cells of cattle 24 months following oral challenge with Bovine Amyloidotic Spongiform Encephalopathy (BASE)

Andrea Trovato[1], Simona Panelli[2], Francesco Strozzi[1], Caterina Cambulli[2], Ilaria Barbieri[3], Nicola Martinelli[3], Guerino Lombardi[3], Rossana Capoferri[2] and John L Williams[1,4]*

Abstract

Background: Bovine Amyloidotic Spongiform Encephalopathy (BASE) is a variant of classical BSE that affects cows and can be transmitted to primates and mice. BASE is biochemically different from BSE and shares some molecular and histo-pathological features with the MV2 sub-type of human sporadic Creutzfeld Jakob Disease (sCJD).

Results: The present work examined the effects of BASE on gene expression in circulating immune cells. Ontology analysis of genes differentially expressed between cattle orally challenged with brain homogenate from cattle following intracranial inoculation with BASE and control cattle identified three main pathways which were affected. Within the immune function pathway, the most affected genes were related to the T cell receptor-mediated T cell activation pathways. The differential expression of these genes in BASE challenged animals at 10,12 and 24 months following challenge, vs unchallenged controls, was investigated by real time PCR.

Conclusions: The results of this study show that the effects of prion diseases are not limited to the CNS, but involve the immune system and particularly T cell signalling during the early stage following challenge, before the appearance of clinical signs.

Keywords: Bovine Amyloidotic Spongiform Encephalopathy (BASE), Transmissible Spongiform Encephalopathies (TSEs), Immune function, Cattle

Background

BSE (Bovine Spongiform Encephalopathy) is a fatal neurodegenerative disorder that affects cattle, which was first identified in 1986 in the UK [1]. Following the first description of BSE, the number of cases rapidly increased and reached epidemic proportions in the UK cattle population. A relatively small number of BSE cases were also found in cattle in other countries. In 1990 the appearance of a new variant of Creutzfeldt Jakob disease (vCJD) in humans was linked to food borne transmission of BSE, which caused major concerns for public health [2].

The key event in the pathobiology of BSE and other Transmissible Spongiform Encephalopathies (TSEs) is the conversion of the cellular prion protein (PrP^c) into an insoluble, protease-resistant isoform, PrP^{res}. This aberrant form of the protein eventually accumulates in the central nervous system (CNS) and is associated with the onset of clinical disease [3]. In the initial phases of classical transmissible prion diseases, such as scrapie and TSE infection via the oral route, PrP^{res} propagates in the peripheral lymphoreticular system before transmission to the CNS [4]. Progression of classical TSE

* Correspondence: john.williams001@adelaide.edu.au
[1]Parco Tecnologico Padano, via Einstein, Lodi 26900, Italy
[4]Present address: School of Animal and Veterinary Sciences, University of Adelaide, Roseworthy, SA 5371, Australia
Full list of author information is available at the end of the article

disease requires the presence of functionally active immune cells, however, the absence of functional lymphocytes does not impair prion pathogenesis and spread to the CNS [5,6]. The pathobiology of spontaneous and atypical prion diseases, however, is not well understood.

The primary biological function of PrP^c, a surface glycoprotein encoded by the PRNP gene, is still unclear. Many studies suggest that it may play a role in the regulation of ion channels and neuronal excitation [7]. PrP may also be linked to immune function [6,8-10] as PrP^c is expressed by several immune cell subsets, including T and B lymphocytes, CD34$^+$ hematopoietic precursors, dendritic cells (DC), natural killer cells (NK), granulocytes and monocytes [11-13]. The highest expression of PrP^c is observed in a sub-population of T lymphocytes, the CD4$^+$ CD25$^+$ FoxP3$^+$ T regulatory cells [14]. PrP^c is implicated in several immune processes, including T cell activation and differentiation, immune memory, monocyte activation, inflammation, DC differentiation and activation, and apoptosis of antigen presenting cells (APC) [8,9,15]. PRNP knock-out mice display impaired renewal of the CD34+ cell precursor pool, an abnormal inflammatory response and phagocytosis, limited capacity of DC to act as APC and impaired T cell activation in response to Concanavalin A (Con-A), which requires a functional T cell receptor (TCR) pathway [8,16]. Other studies have shown that PrP^c interacts with the TCR in the activation of T cells [9,17,18].

All the cases of BSE identified during the major outbreak in the UK were of the same strain type [19]. However, an atypical form of BSE, Bovine Amyloidotic Spongiform Encephalopathy (BASE), was discovered in Italy in 2004 in two old (11 and 15 year old) asymptomatic cows *post mortem* [19]. Other atypical forms of BSE were subsequently reported in France, Germany and Japan [19-22]. The frequency of atypical BSE may be similar to the occurrence of sporadic CJD, which is about 1 per million individuals [23]. BASE can be biochemically differentiated from BSE by the different mobility of PrP fragments on gel electrophoresis. BASE can also be distinguished from BSE histo-pathologically based on differences in the distribution of vacuoles in the brain. BASE shares molecular and histopathological features with the MV2 sub-type of human sporadic CJD (sCJD) [19,22]. BASE has been experimentally transmitted to cattle, primates, and mice [24-26].

In an earlier study [27] we identified genes differentially expressed between healthy cattle and cattle orally challenged with BASE at 12 months post challenge by microarray analysis. The present work examines samples from the same experimental oral challenge of cattle with BASE at additional time points post challenge, prior to the onset of disease, to assess the effects of the challenge on the expression of genes related to the T cell receptor pathway in circulating immune cells.

Methods
Animal resource and RNA preparation
Eleven Holstein heifers of approximately 4 months of age were orally challenged with 50 g brain homogenate from cows inoculated intracranially with BASE (see reference [27]). Challenged animal were regularly clinically monitored and blood (10 ml in EDTA) was collected at 3 month intervals from all animals from 6 months to 24 months post challenge. Ten, age and sex matched Holstein cattle sourced from two commercial farms were used as controls in the analyses. These control animals were deemed free from any obvious disease by veterinary examination.

Animal experimentation was carried out following internal ethical approval of the Istituto Sprimentale Zooprofilattico of Lombardy and Emilia Romagna, and in compliance with the legislation pertinent at the time that the BASE infection and sample collection was carried out, namely European Directive 86/609 and the Italian regulation dl 116/92. Experimental protocols were designed to respect the principle of the 3Rs and to ensure that any suffering was kept to a minimum. BASE challenged animals were inspected daily by qualified veterinary staff for signs of distress, and culling of challenged animals was carried out for sample collection for the parent study using established humane procedures.

Fresh blood was centrifuged at 250 g for 20 minutes, the buffy coat was transferred to a new tube and contaminating red blood cells were lysed with 10 ml of RBC Lysis Solution (5 Prime). RNA was extracted immediately using TRI-reagent (Sigma-Aldrich) following the instructions of the supplier. RNA obtained was quantified using a NanoDrop spectrophotometer (Thermo-Scientific) and quality-checked using a Bioanalyser 2100 (Agilent).

Microarray and pathway analysis at 12 months post-infection
Samples from 5 animals randomly chosen among the 11 challenged animals at 12 months post challenge (MPC), together with samples from five breed, age and sex matched healthy control Holstein cattle which were used in the analysis.

About 1 μg of RNA was amplified and labelled with Cy5-ULS following the manufacturer's protocols (ampULSe Cat. No. GEA-022; Kreatech biotechnology). The purified aRNA was quantified using a NanoDrop spectrophotometer and 4 μg were fragmented to a uniform size, then hybridized to a custom Bovine 90 K array (see [27] for array details). The hybridized arrays were scanned with a GenePix 4000B microarray scanner

(Axon, Toronto, Ca) and images, in TIF format, were exported to the CombiMatrix Microarray Imager Software for hybridization quality verification and spot definition. Data were then extracted, loaded into R using the Limma analysis package and signal intensities were analyzed using the standard procedure of the Bioconductor suite [28]. The list of differentially expressed (DE) genes was generated using the linear modeling analysis in Limma, with an adjusted P-value cut-off equal to 0.01.

A bioinformatics pipeline was created in PERL to connect the gene ID (Ensembl ID, GenBank ID or Uni-Prot ID) with known pathways, using the information available from the Kyoto Encyclopedia of Genes and Genomes (KEGG) database.

Gene expression along the time course of infection

Confirmation and time-course studies were performed by quantitative reverse transcription PCR (qRT-PCR) using samples from four of the five orally challenged cattle used for the array analysis (insufficient material was available from the 5th), and four different negative control Holstein cows obtained from a second BSE negative farm. The kinetics of expression of six selected DE genes (TCR delta chain, TRAT1, CD3E, ZAP70, LAT and LCK) was examined at 10, 12, 24 MPC.

RNA samples were treated with RNase-free DNase (Sigma Aldrich) for 15 minutes at room temperature and then used as a template for first-strand cDNA synthesis using the SuperScript® III First-Strand Synthesis System for RT-PCR (Invitrogen) according to the manufacturer's instruction. Primers for qRT-PCR analysis were designed using Primer Quest (Integrated DNA Technologies) and are shown in Table 1.

Real Time PCR was performed on a Applied Biosystems (ABI) PRISM 7900HT in 10 µl reactions containing 5 µl of Power SYBR®Green (Applied Biosystems), 0.2 µl of each primer at 10 µM and 3.6 µl of water. The thermal program was, 95°C for 10 min, then 40 cycles of amplification including two steps: 15 s at 95°C, 30s at 58°C, 30s at 60°C. Each reaction was performed in triplicate.

Results and discussion
Identification of differentially regulated genes, qRT-PCR validation and pathway analysis

The analysis of gene expression in white blood cells from 5 cattle 12 months after oral challenge with BASE, identified 140 genes differentially expressed (DE) between BASE challenged and control animals, with a $\log_2$ fold change of 1.5 or greater and a p value < 0.01. The majority of DE genes (91) were up-regulated in the BASE animals compared with controls. Gene ontology analysis using the KEGG Database identified 34 genes that fell in 3 pathways each with several genes showing affected expression (Tables 2, 3 and 4). The pathway with the largest number of affected genes was related to immune function (21) followed by signal transduction and cell growth (8) then genes coding for metabolic proteins (5). The microarray data set supporting the results of this article is available in the NCBI GEO data repository with accession number GSE67576, [see http://www.ncbi.nlm.nih.gov/geo/query/acc.cgi?acc=GSE67576].

Table 1 Primer used for qPCR

Gene	Function	Sequence
TCR delta chain	*Antigen receptor of T cells*	Forward 5'TCGCTTGTTTGGTGAAGGA
		Reverse 5'CCCAGGTGAGATGGCAATAG
TRAT1	*TCR associated membrane adapter 1: TCR-mediated T cell activation cascade*	Forward 5'GTGAACAAACTGCAAGACGC
		Reverse 5'CTGGGCTTTCTTCGCTTCC
CD3E	*Marker of thymocytes and peripheral T lymphocytes*	Forward 5'TCTGGGACTCTGCCTCTTATTA
		Reverse 5'CAAACTCTCTAGGGCATGTCAG
LAT	*Linker for activation of T cells, transduction of the activation signal downstream CD3*	Forward 5'GGAGTCGGGAATATGTGAATGT
		Reverse 5'CTGGGAATTCTGGGTGTCAG
ZAP70	*Associated with CD3Z chain; transduction of the activation signal downstream CD3*	Forward 5'CTCATGGCTGACATCGAACT
		Reverse 5'CCACGTCGATCTGCTTCTT
LCK	*lymphocyte-specific protein tyrosine kinase*	Forward 5'GACAGCACCAGAAGCCATTA
		Reverse 5'GCGACCATGAGTGACAATCT
B2MG	*Beta-2-microglobulin precursor*	Forward 5'CAGCGTCCTCCAAAGATTCA
		Reverse 5'ACCCATACACATAGCAGTTCAG
ACTB	*Beta-Actin*	Forward 5'AGTCCTTTGCCTTCCCAAAA
		Reverse 5'AAGCGATCACCTCCCCTGT

B2MG and ACTB were used as internal controls.

Table 2 Differentially expressed Immune related genes

Sequence ID	Gene name and function	Log fold change	P value
ENSBTAG00000005892	ZAP70, Zeta-chain (TCR) associated protein kinase 70 kDa	1.81	0.001924
ENSBTAG00000002259	TCRβ, T Cell Receptor Beta Chain	2.66	0.000014
ENSBTAG00000000431	TCRδ, T Cell Receptor Delta Chain	3.18	0.000025
ENSBTAG00000000183	TRAT1, T cell receptor associated transmembrane adaptor 1	2.26	0.000003
ENSBTAG00000011359	CD7, T Cell Antigen CD7	1.75	0.000607
ENSBTAG00000001002	TCF7, T Cell Specific Transcription factor 7	3	0.000025
ENSBTAG00000015710	CD3E, T Cell surface antigen CD3 epsilon chain	3.21	0.000010
ENSBTAG00000021249	LAT, Linker for activation of T cell	2.79	0.000010
ENSBTAG00000012695	LCK, lymphocyte-specific protein tyrosine kinase	1.54	0.000532
ENSBTAG00000006453	CD3g, , T Cell surface antigen CD3 gamma chain	2.11	0.000058
ENSBTAG00000030425	ID3, inhibitor of DNA binding 3, dominant negative helix-loop-helix protein	1.97	0.000710
ENSBTAG00000005990	S1PR1, sphingosine-1-phosphate receptor 1	1.5	0.001691
ENSBTAG00000020319	ALOX5, arachidonate 5-lipoxygenase	−1.85	0.002847
ENSBTAG00000011990	ALOX12, arachidonate 15-lipoxygenase	−2.15	0.000439
ENSBTAG00000001321	Il1β, Interleukin 1 beta	−1.91	0.000644
ENSBTAG00000019428	CCR1, chemokine (C-C motif) receptor 1	−1.41	0.001837
ENSBTAG00000038042	IL8βR, chemokine (C-X-C motif) receptor 2 (CXCR2)	−1.96	0.004877
ENSBTAG00000003305	NCF1, neutrophilcytosolicfactor 1	−2.04	0.000868
ENSBTAG00000037735	C5L2, G protein-coupled receptor 77 (GPR77)	−1.76	0.000958
ENSBTAG00000027051	PTAFR, platelet-activating factor receptor	−1.41	0.000081
ENSBTAG00000004322	FOS, murine osteosarcoma viral oncogene homolog	−1.57	0.000152

Immune response related genes showing altered expression 12 MPC with BASE

TCR signalling cascade

The pathway with most affected genes at 12 MPC was related to immune function with 21 DE genes, of these 11 belonged to the TCR signalling cascade which regulates the activation of T lymphocytes in response to antigen presented by the Major Histocompatibility Complex (MHC). Three genes involved in this pathway with differential expression (TCRβ, TCRδ, and TRAT1) were missing from the KEGG database for cow and were added manually. The pan-T cell marker, CD7, and the transcription factor TCF7/LEF were also added to the TCR pathway by manual annotation. Ten of the DE genes in the TCR cascade were up-regulated, several of which had the highest log-fold change in expression observed at 12 MPC. One gene, the transcription factor

Fos, was down regulated, and is downstream of the signalling cascade.

Kinetics of expression for genes involved TCR signalling in early phases of BASE infection

As TCR signaling is central to immune function and was affected by BASE challenge, the expression of six genes involved in this pathway (TCRδ, CD3E, ZAP70, TRAT1, LAT, LCK) was analyzed over a time course following BASE challenge (10-12-24 MPC) by qPCR. The qPCR analysis confirmed the micro-array data for TCRδ, CD3E, ZAP70 and TRAT1 which were overexpressed in BASE animals vs controls at 12 MPC (respectively $p < 0.01$; $p < 0.01$; $p < 0.01$; $p < 0.01$). The LAT gene also showed an increase of expression at 12 MPC but the difference compared with controls was not significant.

Table 3 Differentially expressed Metabolic Pathway genes

Sequence ID	Gene name and function	Log fold change	P value
ENSBTAG00000000065	(CRLS1), cardiolipinsynthase 1	1.52	0.0017
ENSBTAG00000031814	SDH, serine dehydratase	−3.55	0.0014
ENSBTAG00000001154	DGAT2, diacylglycerol O-acyltransferase 2	−2.42	0.00044
ENSBTAG00000012855	LPL, lipoproteinlipase	−1.7	0.00045
ENSBTAG00000009733	F16P1, fructose-1,6-bisphosphatase 1 (FBP1)	−1.64	0.00733

Table 4 Other differentially expressed genes

Sequence ID	Gene name and function	Log fold change	P value
ENSBTAG00000013761	STMN1, stathmin 1	1.66	0.00002
ENSBTAG00000008436	CDC25B, Cell division cycle 25B	2.01	0.00003
ENSBTAG00000009663	CSDA, cold shock domain protein A	1.7	0.00015
ENSBTAG00000007336	HCST, hematopoietic cell signal transducer	1.86	0.0003
ENSBTAG00000020350	DUSP2, dualspecificityphosphatase 2	−1.63	0.00264
ENSBTAG00000005947	PLAU, plasminogenactivator, urokinase	−1.61	0.00012
ENSBTAG00000039657	H2A, Histone 2°	−1.5	2.5E-05

Expression of TCRδ, ZAP70 and CD3E was significantly higher in all 4 infected animals examined by qPCR compared with controls at all the time points post challenge. TRAT1 and LAT showed the same trend, with an increase in expression at 10 MPC and 12 MPC. TRAT 1 had statistically significant increased expression at 12 MPC (p < 0.01), then fell to the same level as control samples by 24 MPC. LCK was found to be up-regulated 1.5 fold in the microarray data at 12 MPC but in the qPCR analysis was down-regulated at 12 MPC (p < 0.01), and also had lower expression than controls at 10 and 24 MPC (see Figure 1).

Interestingly, PrP^c has been found to co-precipitate with the TCR [8,18] and with components of the TCR signaling pathway [9], many of which appear among the DE genes identified in the present study (ZAP70, LCK, CD3E, LAT). The physiological function of PrP^C is not fully understood, however, it has been implicated in T cell activation after the binding of the antigen [17]. T cell activation increases PrP^c concentration on the surface of human lymphocytes [9]. In addition antibodies against PrP^c block ConA induced lymphocyte proliferation, which requires a functional TCR complex [16]. How the function of PrP is altered with the change in conformation from PrP^c to PrP^{res} is unclear, although there are some suggestions that there is a gain in function and not simply a loss. PrP^{res} is able to stimulate MAP kinase signaling in neuronal cells whereas PrP^C is not [29]. In, changes in the level of PrP expression are likely to affect cell function e.g. lack of PrP expression on antigen presenting cells affects T cell activation [30], whereas lack of PrP expression on the T cell itself does not inhibit T cell activation. Nevertheless, the level of PrP is increased following activation. Thus perturbed PrP expression or function, as may occur in the change from PrP^C to PrP^{res}, is likely to change the dynamics of T cell activation and expression of genes associated with the T cell receptor complex. In the present study, expression of TCRδ, ZAP 70, CD3E, LCK and TRAT was found to change between 10 and 24 month after the BASE challenge. qPCR analysis suggested that LCK was down regulated during early infection (10–24 MPC), which is of interest as this kinase is a key regulator of the TCR pathway. Following the interaction between the TCR and CD3,

LCK is recruited to the TCR complex, phosphorylates downstream signaling molecules including ZAP70, and activates a phosphorylation cascade that involves LAT and TRAT [31,32]. This suggests that T cell response is indeed affected following BASE challenge.

Genes linked to the inflammatory response

The data presented here also indicate that BASE challenge of cattle is associated with a modified inflammatory response. Expression of ALOX12 and ALOX5, which encode proteins that are key effectors of an inflammatory response were down-regulated at 12 MPC. ALOX12 and ALOX5 have a role in chemotaxis and response in tissue damage [33] and are involved in Arachidonic acid metabolism, which is necessary for Leukotrien production. Leukotriens are key effectors of the inflammatory response [33] and are produced by leukocytes, in particular mast-cells. C5L2 is one of the two receptors for the C5a anaphylotoxin, an extremely potent pro-inflammatory peptide [34], which was also down regulated following BASE challenge. Other pro-inflammatory cytokines or their receptors (IL1β, CCR1, IL8βR and NCF1) were also down-regulated.

Sphingosine 1-phosphate receptor 1 (S1PR1) was up-regulated. S1PR1 is involved in the regulation of inflammatory responses, cell migration and differentiation [35], and the receptor for platelet activating factor (PTARF), a key inflammatory mediator and a pattern recognition receptor involved in the uptake of Gram-positive bacteria [36]. The ID3 gene, which codes for an anti-inflammatory cytokine involved in the TGFβ1 pathway, was also up-regulated. The expression of genes in the TGFβ1 pathway has previously been reported to be up-regulated following prion infection of mice and cattle [37,38]. The results presented here are consistent with previous data, and suggest that prion diseases are associated with an inhibition of inflammation [8]. It is therefore interesting that the expression of IL-8Rβ and NCF1, which are directly linked to chemotaxis of neutrophils, was reduced in BASE challenged animals compared with controls. These results are in agreement with previous studies which proposed that PrP^c has a role in the modulation of inflammation and phagocytosis [8], which was also seen in studies of PrP null mice [8].

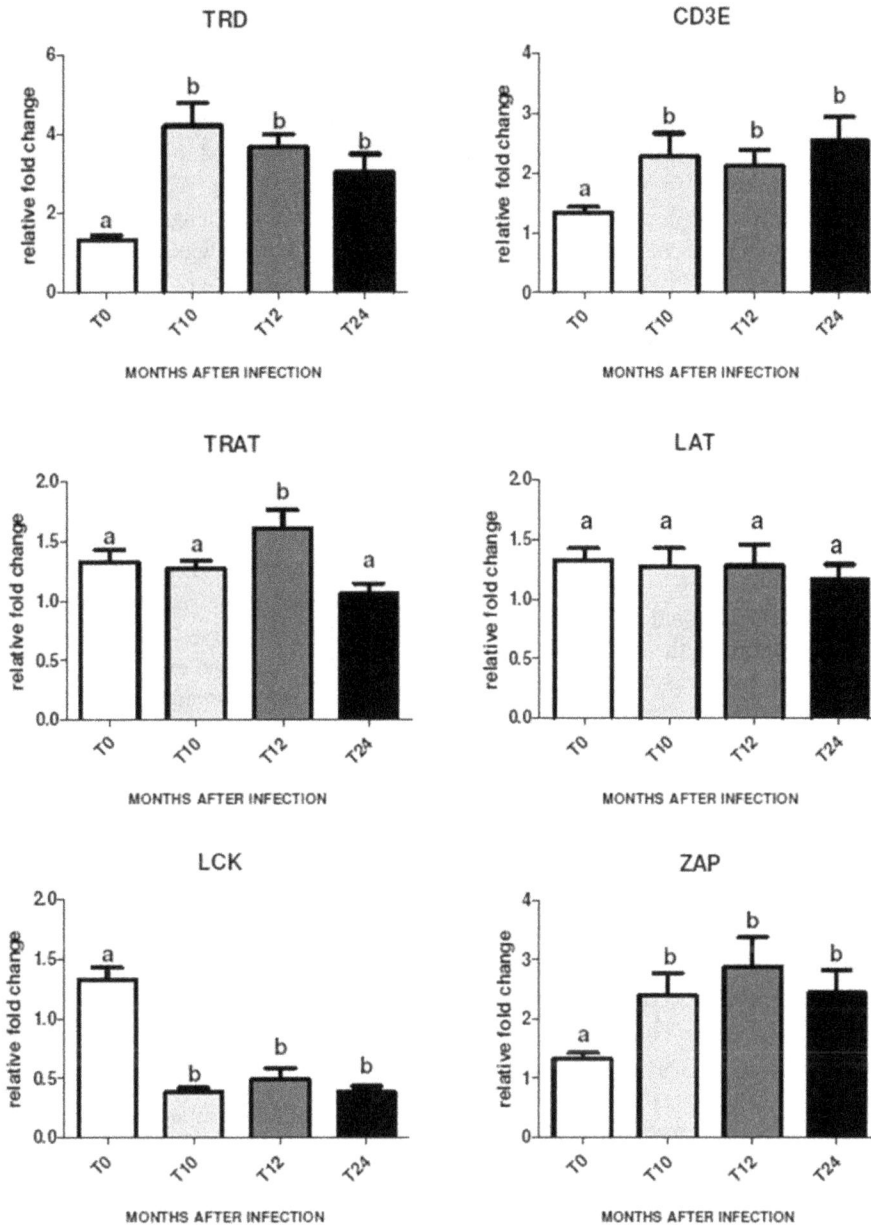

Figure 1 Kinetics of expression for genes involved in the TCR pathway. Results from qPCR analysis of the expression of six genes (TRD, CD3E, TRAT, LAT, LCK, ZAP70) involved in TCR signaling in circulating immune cells, in control animals (T0) and BASE challenged animals at 10-12-24 months post challenge (T10, T12 and T14 respectively). Each column represents the mean ± SEM of at least three separate measurements on 4 individuals. The expression of mRNA normalized to two endogenous reference genes (β-Actin and β-2 Microglobulin), was analyzed by RT-PCR using specific primers as described in Material and Methods. The different *superscripts* indicate significant difference between columns (p < 0.01).

NK-mediated cytotoxicity
HCST, a signal transduction protein involved in NK and T cell activity, especially during anti-viral responses, was up-regulated.

Metabolic and signal transduction genes of WBC affected by BASE at 12 months post-challenge
In addition to immune function related genes, other pathways were affected by BASE infection, including genes involved in energy metabolism and signal transduction, which are discussed here for completeness.

Energy metabolism and storage
Several genes involved in energy metabolism and storage of carbohydrates (F16P1, SDHL) and also genes regulating lipid metabolism and signalling (DGAT2, LIPL), were down regulated in BASE challenged cattle compared with controls at 12 MPC. However, cardiolipin synthase 1

(CRLS1), which is involved in mitochondrial membrane function and is predominantly expressed by tissues with high levels of energy metabolism, was up-regulated. SDHL, which is associated with energy balance, has previously been shown to be affected by TSE diseases. Previous work has shown that proteins related to glucose metabolism have aberrant expression in cerebrospinal fluid of sCJD patients [39]. Patients with sporadic CJD have also been shown to have altered levels of proteins associated with the control of glucose [39] and lipid [37] metabolism. Changes in glucose metabolism are known to trigger apoptotic pathways [39] while changes in lipid metabolism and signalling are one of the early changes apparent in many neurodegenerative diseases, including prion diseases [37]. Therefore this response, while linked to BASE challenge in this study, is not likely to be specific for prion disease.

Cell signalling genes

Two genes involved in signal transduction (STMN1, CDC25B), which code for proteins of the MAP kinase pathway (MAPK), were up-regulated, while a negative regulator of this pathway (DUSP2) was down-regulated in challenged animals at 12 MPC. MAPK pathways are essential for cell survival and were up regulated. It has been suggested that MAPK has a role in the protective response to cellular oxidative stress [40]. Previous studies have reported that MAPK proteins interact with PrP^c [41]. These genes are also known to play an active role in prion disease pathogenesis in nervous tissues and the medulla, with the sequential activation of the various MAPK associated genes during PrP^{res} deposition [37,40]. MAPK pathway genes have been shown to be up regulated in brain tissues of scrapie infected hamster [40] and mice [37], and in the medulla of cattle following oral challenge with BSE [38]. This is consistent with data which showed that PrP^c interacts with MAPK proteins [41].

Genes in other signal transduction pathways also showed changes in expression 12 MPC. CSDA is a member of the highly conserved Cold Shock Domain family of DNA binding proteins which is involved in post-transcriptional control of gene expression [42,43] and was up regulated. The gene coding for histone H2A was down-regulated. Histone 2A is known to co-purify with PrP^{res} extracted from the brains of hamsters infected with experimental scrapie [44].

Coagulation cascade

Expression of the gene coding for thrombin receptor (F2R) was up regulated, while the plasminogen activator urokinase (PLAU), was down-regulated. Expression of genes involved in coagulation have also been shown to be affected in the brain of cattle incubating BSE [38].

The BASE challenged animals used for the expression analysis remained healthy up to the 24 month time-point examined here. The parent study which provided the samples in still in progress, and therefore further information on the health status of the animals is not yet available. Data presented here are consistent with that from the earlier study [27], and all animals studied displayed a consistent change in gene expression in comparison with controls, suggesting that they were responding to the BASE challenge. It should also be noted that while challenged animals were housed in a containment facility, controls were taken from two commercial farms. Hence controls and challenged animals experienced different environments, which may have resulted in differences in expression patterns. DE genes between the challenged animals and controls were consistent between the two control groups, which experienced different management regimes. The DE genes and pathways identified between controls and challenged animals are consistent with those reported in other TSE infection models as discussed above. This give some confidence in these data and that the effects of orally administered BASE on gene expression are similar to other TSEs.

Conclusions

The data presented here on gene expression in circulating immune cells following BASE challenge show that response to BASE has similarities with other prion diseases. PrP^c is known to have a role in the immune system, indeed it is expressed on DC and is important for inducing the T cell proliferative response [30]. Moreover, PrP^c accumulates in the contact point between T cells and DC, and it may have a role in the assembly of the TCR complex [45]. The disease form of this protein (PrP^{res}) has been shown to affect the immune system, e.g. eliciting qualitative differences in the responses of T cells [46]. Moreover, macrophages accumulate PrP^{res}, and may be involved in the transfer of the disease to the CNS [9,47]. The data presented here are consistent with the hypothesis that the effects of TSE diseases are not limited to CNS, but involve the immune system, especially during the early stages following challenge, before the appearance of clinical signs. Our data suggest that BASE challenge affects the TCR signalling pathway, which has also been shown in mouse knock-out experiments [17]. BASE therefore, in common with other prion diseases, seems to be associated with general cellular stress and impaired immune function. These data, from experimentally challenged cattle, suggest that orally administered BASE affects gene expression in circulating immune cells even in the absence of overt disease.

Abbreviations
BASE: Bovine amyloidotic spongiform encephalopathy; BSE: Bovine spongiform encephalopathy; CNS: Central nervous system; DE: Differentially

expressed (genes); MPC: Months post challenge; PCR: Polymerase chain reaction; PrP: Cellular prion protein; sCJD: Sporadic Creutzfeld Jakob disease; TSEs: Transmissible spongiform encephalopathies; TCR: T cell receptor; WBC: White blood cells.

Competing interests
The authors declare that they have no competing interests.

Authors' contributions
AT carried out the confirmation study, participated in the data analysis and writing the manuscript, SP carried out the micro-array study and the initial analysis, FS designed the micro-array and participated in the data analysis, CC designed and carried out qPCR confirmation of some of the differentially expressed genes, IB and NM were responsible for collection and management of biological samples, GL set up the BASE challenge and oversaw the management of animals, RC prepared and managed the RNA samples for analysis, JLW conceived the study, oversaw the work and was responsible for drafting the manuscript. All authors read and approved the final version of the manuscript.

Acknowledgements
This work was supported by grant PRC2005013 from the Italian Health Ministry to G.L. AT was supported by grant PON01_01841 from the Italian Ministry of Science.

Author details
[1]Parco Tecnologico Padano, via Einstein, Lodi 26900, Italy. [2]Istituto Sperimentale Italiano Lazzaro Spallanzani, Loc. La Quercia, 26027 Rivolta d'Adda, Italy. [3]Istituto Zooprofilattico Sperimentale della Lombardia e dell'Emilia Romagna, via Bianchi 9, 25124 Brescia, Italy. [4]Present address: School of Animal and Veterinary Sciences, University of Adelaide, Roseworthy, SA 5371, Australia.

References
1. Wells GA, Scott AC, Johnson CT, Gunning RF, Hancock RD, Jeffrey M, et al. A novel progressive spongiform encephalopathy in cattle. Vet Rec. 1987;121:419–20.
2. Will RG, Ironside JW, Ziedler M, Cousens SN, Estibero K, Alperovich A, et al. A new variant of Creutzfeldt-Jakob disease in the UK. Lancet. 1996;347:921–5.
3. Prusiner SB. Novel proteinaceous infectious particles cause scrapie. Science. 1982;216:136–44.
4. Aucouturier P, Geissmann F, Damotte D, Saborio GP, Meeker HC, Kascsak R, et al. Infected splenic dendritic cells are sufficient for prion transmission to the CNS in mouse scrapie. J Clin Invest. 2001;108:703–8.
5. Aguzzi A, Heppner FL, Heikenwalder M, Prinz M, Mertz K, Seeger H, et al. Immune system and peripheral nerves in propagation of prions to CNS. Br Med Bull. 2003;66:141–59.
6. Nuvolone M, Aguzzi A, Heikenwalder M. Cells and prions: a license to replicate. FEBS Lett. 2009;583:2674–84.
7. Biasini E, Turnbaugh J, Unterberger U, Harris DA. Prion protein at the crossroad of physiology and disease. Trends Neurosci. 2012;35:92–103.
8. Isaacs JD, Jackson GS, Altmann DM. The role of the cellular prion protein in the immune system. Clin Exp Immunol. 2006;146:1–8.
9. Linden R, Martins VR, Prado MAM, Cammarota M, Izquierdo I, Brentani RR. Physiology of the prion protein. Physiol Rev. 2008;88:673–728.
10. Zomosa-Signoret V, Arnaud JD, Fontes P, Alvarez-Maryinez MT, Liautard JP. Physiological role of the cellular prion protein. Vet Res. 2008;39:9–25.
11. Castro-Seoane R, Hummerich H, Sweeting T, Tattum MH, Linehan JM, Fernandez de Marco M, et al. Plasmacytoid dendritic cells sequester high prion titres at early stages of prion infection. PLoS Pathog. 2012;8:201.
12. Starke R, Harrison P, Mackie I, Wang G, Erusalimsky JD, Gale R, et al. The expression of prion protein (PrP(C)) in the megakaryocyte lineage. J Thromb Haemost. 2005;3:1266–73.
13. Dorban G, Defaweux V, Heinen E, Antoine N. Spreading of prions from the immune to the peripheral nervous system: a potential implication of dendritic cells. Histochem Cell Biol. 2010;133:493–504.
14. Isaacs JD, Garden OA, Kaur G, Collinge J, Jackson GS, Altmann DM. The cellular prion protein is preferentially expressed by CD4+ CD25+ Foxp3+ regulatory T cells. Immunology. 2008;125:313–9.
15. Jeon JW, Park BC, Jung JG, Jang YS, Shin EC, Park WP. The soluble form of the cellular prion protein enhances phagocytic activity and cytokine production by human monocytes via activation of ERK and NF-κB. Immune Netw. 2013;13:148–56.
16. Mazzoni IE, Lederbur HC, Paramithiotis E, Cashman N. Lymphoid signal transduction mechanisms linked to cellular prion protein. Cell Biol. 2005;83:644–53.
17. Hu W, Nessler S, Hemmer B, Eagar TN, Kane LP, Rutger-Leliveld S, et al. Pharmacological prion protein silencing accelerates central nervous system autoimmune disease via T cell receptor signalling. Brain. 2010;133:375–88.
18. Mattei V, Garofalo T, Misasi R, Circella A, Manganelli V, Lucania G, et al. Prion protein is a component of the multicellular signaling complex involved in T cell activation. FEBS Lett. 2004;560:14–8.
19. Casalone C, Zanusso G, Acutis P, Ferrari S, Cappucci L, Tagliavini F, et al. Identification of a second bovine amyloidotic spongiform encephalopathy: molecular similarities with sporadic Creutzfeldt-Jakob disease. Proc Natl Acad Sci U S A. 2004;101:3065–70.
20. Béringue V, Bencsik A, Le Dur A, Reine F, Lani TL, Chenais N, et al. Isolation from cattle of a prion strain distinct from that causing bovine spongiform encephalopathy. PLoS Pathog. 2006;2:e112.
21. Biacabe AG, Laplanche JL, Ryder S, Baron T. Distinct molecular phenotypes in bovine prion diseases. EMBO Rep. 2004;5:110–4.
22. Yokoyama T, Mohri S. Prion diseases and emerging prion diseases. Curr Med Chem. 2008;15:912–6.
23. Brown P, McShane LM, Zanusso G, Detwiler L. On the question of sporadic or atypical bovine spongiform encephalopathy and Creutzfeldt-Jakob disease. Emerg Infect Dis. 2006;12:1816–21.
24. Comoy EE, Casalone C, Lescoutra-Etchegarray N, Zanusso G, Freire S, Marcè D, et al. Atypical BSE (BASE) transmitted from asymptomatic aging cattle to a primate. PLoS One. 2008;3:e3017.
25. Fukuda S, Iwamaru Y, Imamura M, Masujin K, Shimizu Y, Matsuura Y, et al. Intraspecies transmission of L-type-like bovine spongiform encephalopathy detected in Japan. Microbiol Immunol. 2009;53:704–7.
26. Lombardi G, Casalone C, D'Angelo A, Gelmetti D, Torcoli G, Torcoli G, et al. Intraspecies transmission of BASE induces clinical dullness and amyotrophic changes. PLoS Pathog. 2008;4:e1000075.
27. Panelli S, Strozzi F, Capoferri R, Barbieri I, Martinelli N, Capucci L, et al. Analysis of gene expression in white blood cells of cattle orally challenged with Bovine Amyloidotic Spongiform Encephalopathy. J Toxicol Environ Health. 2011;74:96–102.
28. Smyth GK. Linear models and empirical Bayes methods for assessing differential expression in microarray experiments. Stat Appl Genet Mol Biol. 2004;3(No. 1):Article 3. Berkeley Electronic Press.
29. Marella M, Gaggioli C, Batoz M, Deckert M, Tartare-Deckert S, Chabry J. Pathological prion protein exposure switches on neuronal mitogen-activated protein kinase pathway resulting in microglia recruitment. J Biol Chem. 2005;280:1529–34.
30. Ballerini C, Gourdain P, Bachy V, Blanchard N, Levavasseur E, Grégoire S, et al. Functional implication of cellular prion protein in antigen-driven interactions between T cells and dendritic cells. J Immunol. 2006;176:7254–62.
31. Davis SJ, van der Merwe PA. Lck and the nature of the T cell receptor trigger. Trend Immunol. 2011;32:1–5.
32. Kirchgessner H, Dietrich J, Scherer J, Isomaki P, Korinek V, Hilgert I, et al. The Transmembrane Adaptor Protein TRIM Regulates T Cell Receptor (TCR) Expression and TCR-mediated signaling via an association with the TCR ζ chain. J Exp Med. 2001;193:1269–83.
33. Stables MJ, Gilroy DW. Old and new generation lipid mediators in acute inflammation and resolution. Prog Lipid Res. 2011;50:35–51.
34. Ward PA. Functions of C5a receptors. J Mol Med. 2009;87:375–8.
35. Van Doorn R, Van Horssen J, Verzil D, Witte M, Ronken E, Van Het Hof B, et al. De Vries HE:Sphingosine 1-phosphate receptor 1 and 3 are upregulated in multiple sclerosis lesions. Glia. 2010;58:1465–6.
36. Fillon S, Soulis K, Rajasekaran S, Benedict-Hamilton H, Radin JN, Orihuela CJ, et al. Murti, Kaushal D, Waaled-Gaber M, Weber JR, Murray PJ. Tuomanen E: Platelet-activating factor receptor and innate immunity: uptake of gram-positive cell wall into host cells and cell-specific pathophysiology J Immunol. 2006;177:6182.
37. Sorensen G, Medina S, Parchaliuk D, Phillipson C, Robertson C, Booth SA: Comprehensive transcriptional profiling of prion infection in mouse reveals networks of responsive genes. BMC Genomics 2008, 3: 9:114.
38. Almeida LM, Basu U, Khaniya B, Taniguchi M, Williams JL, Moore SS. Guan LL:Gene expression in the medulla following oral infection of cattle with

bovine spongiform encephalopathy. J Toxicol Environm Health A. 2011;74:110–26.

39. Gawinecka J, Dieks J, Asif AR, Carimalo J, Heinemann U, Streich J-H, et al. Codon 129 polymorphism specific cerebrospinal fluid proteome pattern in sporadic Creutzfeldt-Jakob disease and the implication of glycolytic enzymes in prion-induced pathology. J Proteome Res. 2010;9:5646–57.

40. Lee HP, Jun YC, Choi JK, Kim JI, Carp RI, Kim YS. Activation of mitogen-activated protein kinases in hamster brains infected with 263K scrapie agent. J Neurochem. 2005;95:584–93.

41. Satoh J, Obayashi S, Misawa T, Sumiyoshi K, Oosumi K, Tabunoki H. Protein microarray analysis identifies human cellular prion protein interactors. Neuropathol Appl Neurobiol. 2009;35:16–35.

42. Mihailovich M, Militti C, Gabaldon T, Gebauer F. Eukaryotic cold shock domain proteins: highly versatile regulators of gene expression. Bioessays. 2010;32:109–18.

43. Saito Y, Nakagami H, Azuma N, Hirata S, Sanada F, Taniyama Y, et al. Critical roles of Cold Shock Domain Protein A as an endogenous angiogenesis inhibitor in skeletal muscle. Antioxid Redox Signal. 2011;15:2109–20.

44. Giorgi A, Di Francesco L, Principe S, Mignogna G, Sennels L, Mancone C, et al. Proteomic profiling of prP27-30-enriched preparations extracted from the brain of hamsters with experimental scrapie. Proteomics. 2009;9:3802–14.

45. Hugel B, Martinez MC, Kunzelmann C, Blattler T, Aguzzi A, Freyssinet JM. Modulation of signal transduction through the cellular prion protein is linked to its incorporation in lipid rafts. Cell Mol Life Sci. 2004;61:2998–3007.

46. Khalili-Shirazi A, Quaratino S, Londei M, Summers L, Tayebi M, Clarke AR, et al. Protein conformation significantly influences immune responses to prion protein. J Immunol. 2005;174:3256–63.

47. Elhelaly AE, Inoshima Y, Ishiguro N. Characterization of early transient accumulation of PrP^{sc} in immune cells. Bioch. and Bioph. Res Comm. 2013;439:340–5.

16

RhoA/ROCK1 regulates Avian Reovirus S1133-induced switch from autophagy to apoptosis

Ping-Yuan Lin[1], Ching-Dong Chang[2], Yo-Chia Chen[1] and Wen-Ling Shih[1,3*]

Abstract

Background: Autophagy is an essential process in the control of cellular homeostasis. It enables cells under certain stress conditions to survive by removing toxic cellular components, and may protect cells from apoptosis. In the present study, the signaling pathways involved in ARV S1133 regulated switch from autophagy to apoptosis were investigated.

Results: ARV S1133 infection caused autophagy in the early to middle infectious stages in Vero and DF1 cells, and apoptosis in the middle to late stages. Conversion of the autophagy marker LC3-I to LC3-II occurred earlier than cleavage of the apoptotic marker caspase-3. ARV S1133 also activated the Beclin-1 promoter in the early to middle stages of infection. Levels of RhoA-GTP and ROCK1 activity were elevated upon ARV S1133 infection, while inhibition of RhoA and ROCK1 reduced autophagy and subsequent apoptosis. Conversely, inhibition of caspase-3 did not affect the level of autophagy. Beclin-1 knockdown and treatment with autophagy inhibitors, 3-MA and Bafilomycin A1, suppressed ARV S1133-induced autophagy and apoptosis simultaneously, suggesting the shift from autophagy to apoptosis. A co-immunoprecipitation assay demonstrated that the formation of a RhoA, ROCK1 and Beclin-1 complex coincided with the induction of autophagy.

Conclusion: Our results demonstrate that RhoA/ROCK1 signaling play critical roles in the transition of cell activity from autophagy to apoptosis in ARV S1133-infected cells.

Keywords: ARV S1133, Autophagy, Apoptosis, RhoA, ROCK1

Background

Avian reoviruses (ARVs) are members of the genus Orthoreovirus, which belongs to the Reoviridae family [1]. ARVs are non-enveloped viruses that contain 10 double-stranded RNA genomic segments and several encoded proteins, including at least 10 structural proteins and 4 nonstructural proteins [2,3]. ARVs cause many poultry diseases, including malabsorption syndrome, chronic respiratory disease and arthritis. In contrast to mammalian reoviruses, ARVs cause massive fusion of host cells but are deficient in hemagglutination activity [4]. The pathogenesis of ARV-induced apoptosis has been studied in ARV-infected chicken tissues, including the intestine,

tendon, liver, and bursa [5]. We previously reported that ARV S1133 induces apoptosis by modulating Src, p53, mitogen-activated protein kinase (MAPK), and protein kinase C δ, and also elicits cytochrome c release from mitochondria to the cytosol [6-8]. ARV S1133 encodes nonstructural protein p10, which mediates cell syncytium formation through the activation of the small GTPase, RhoA, and Rac1 signaling [9]. Autophagy is a basic bulk degradation mechanism that controls the recycling and clearance of intracellular constituents into double-membrane vesicles, and traffic of these vesicles to the lysosomes for continued cell survival [10]. Formation of autophagosomes requires over 15 autophagy-related proteins, including microtubule associated protein 1 light-chain 3, the UNC53-like kinase1 (ULK1) complex, and PI3Ks [11]. Autophagy is tightly regulated by several cellular signaling pathways, and the major negative regulator is the serine/threonine kinase mammalian target of

* Correspondence: wlshih@mail.npust.edu.tw
[1]Department of Biological Science and Technology, Pingtung 91201, Taiwan
[3]Graduate Institute of Biotechnology, National Pingtung University of Science and Technology, 1, Shuefu Rd., Neipu, Pingtung 91201, Taiwan
Full list of author information is available at the end of the article

rapamycin (mTOR); however, the class III PI3K/Beclin-1 pathway positively regulates autophagy [12]. Autophagy has been recognized as a stress response to enable eukaryotic organisms to survive during severe conditions, such as nutrient starvation, oxidative stress, chemicals and infection by intracellular pathogens [13,14].

Previous studies on intestinal epithelial cells, demonstrated that oncogenic Ras increases RhoA activity and promotes the degradation of Beclin-1, leading to the subsequent inhibition of autophagy [15].Under nutrient deprivation conditions, the activation of ROCK1 (Rho-associated, coiled-coil containing protein kinase 1) promotes autophagy by binding to and phosphorylating Beclin-1 at Threonine 119. This threonine phosphorylation inhibits the ROCK1 activity and promotes the association of Beclin-1 with Bcl-2. Thus, ROCK1 is one of the upstream regulators of Beclin-1-mediated autophagy and controls the homeostasis between autophagy and apoptosis [16]. ARV S1133 induces autophagy in both primary chicken embryonic fibroblast cells (CEF) and African green monkey kidney cells (Vero), and infection with this virus increases the number of double-membrane vesicles in these cells through the PI3K/Akt/mTOR pathway [17]. ARV nonstructural protein p17 is an activator of autophagy and regulates the expression of Beclin-1 and LC3 [18]. Thus, ARV S1133 seems to modulate autophagy and apoptosis *via* specific host cell signaling mechanisms. We hypothesized the existence of a switch between the kinetic control of these two kinds of programmed cell death during the ARV S1133 replication cycle. Autophagic cell death could occur in condition which without the involvement of apoptosis or necrosis [19]. Additionally, apoptosis and autophagy can simultaneously occur or exert synergistic effects under the same stress conditions, whereas in certain situations autophagy triggered only when apoptosis is inhibited [20,21]. Some studies have linked these two different types of programmed cell death; however, there exist intricate relationships between them, the significance and precise regulation are controversial [22]. In this study, we investigated the cross-talk between autophagy and apoptosis in ARV S1133-infected cells. We aimed to determine whether a molecular association exists between autophagy and apoptosis, and to elucidate the relationship between these cell death modes.

Results

Kinetics of autophagy and apoptosis in ARV S1133-infected DF1 and Vero cells

To identify the kinetic differences between autophagy and apoptosis, the autophagic and apoptotic cell percentages were first examined simultaneously in ARV S1133-infected cultured cells. The percentages of MDC- and Hoechst 33258-positive DF1 cells infected with ARV S1133 were evaluated by direct counting. Figure 1A shows the changes in the level of cell death during 42 hr of incubation. Autophagic cell death appeared at 6 hpi, increased at 12–18 hpi, decreased at 24 hpi, and disappeared at 30 hpi. However, a large number of apoptotic cells emerged at 18 hpi and continued to accumulate until the end of the observation period. A similar cell death trend was observed in ARV S1133-infected Vero cells (Figure 1B). At the molecular level, we analyzed the expression of microtubule-associated protein1 light chain 3 (LC3) and caspase-3. LC3-I conversion to LC3-II is a reliable marker of autophagosome formation [23,24], and caspase-3 cleavage is a well-established apoptotic index. The fluorescent staining shown in Figure 1C indicates the presence of autophagosomes and apoptotic nuclei. Significant numbers of MDC-labeled fluorescent particles accumulated between 12 hpi and 24 hpi; however this level decreased at 36 hpi. Apoptotic cells with condensed DNA appeared at the middle to late stages of ARV S1133 infection; from 24 hpi to 36 hpi. Figure 2A and B show that LC3 conversion and induced expression of Beclin-1 occurred in the early to middle infectious stages then disappeared gradually in both Vero and DF1 cells; whereas cleaved caspase-3 appeared in the middle of the infectious stage and continued to accumulate in the late stage.

In addition, we investigated whether ARV S1133 affects the expression of Beclin-1, a protein that participates in the regulation of autophagy, by analyzing the transcription of the 5′-flanking regions, from nucleotides –644 to +197, –277 to +197, and –58 to +197, of the *Beclin-1* gene. Our results demonstrated that these 5′-flanking regions constructed with a luciferase reporter were regulated by ARV S1133. Upon ARV S1133 infection, the –644 to +197 regulatory region of the Beclin-1 gene showed a higher luciferase activity than the –277 to +197 control region reporter, and the –58 to +197 region revealed a negligible luciferase response (Figure 2C).

Activation of RhoA signaling by ARV S1133

We next investigated whether the autophagic pathway is regulated by small GTPase by analyzing the possible roles of RhoA signaling in ARV S1133-mediated autophagy and apoptosis. Our results showed that the levels of GTP-bound RhoA and phosphorylated ROCK1, a downstream effector of RhoA, were significantly increased 12 hpi, and this continued until the end of the middle stage (Figure 3A, lanes 3–6). To confirm the activation of ROCK1, the ELISA method was used to quantify the level of active ROCK. The results shown in Figure 3B indicate that the ARV S1133-elicited ROCK activity increased between 12 and 30 hpi. Additionally, the activity of ROCK was fully suppressed in the presence of ROCK inhibitor Y-27632, which further confirmed that the RhoA/ROCK pathway was involved and was active as ARV S1133-infected cells were undergoing autophagy.

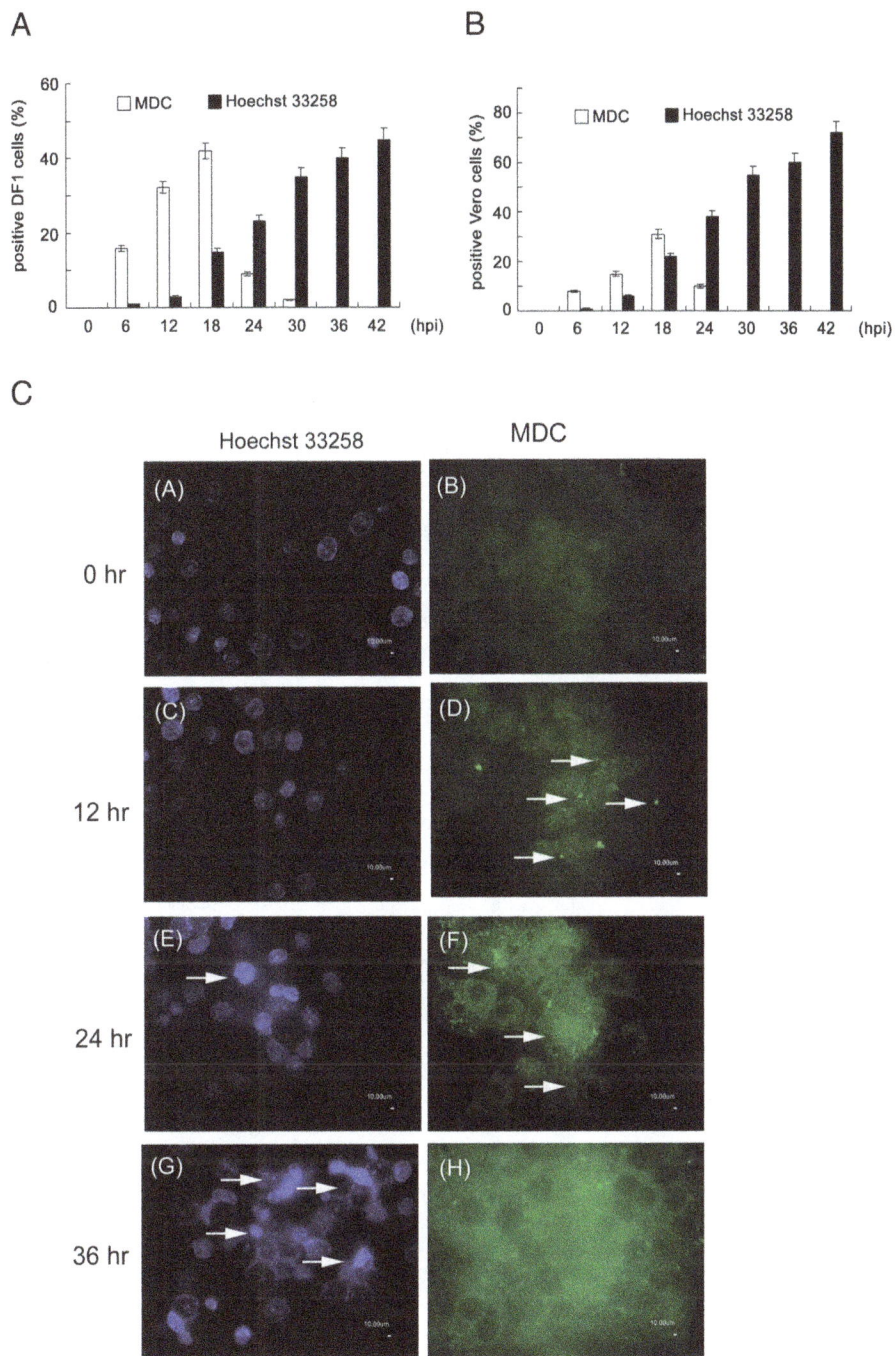

Figure 1 ARV S1133 induces autophagy and subsequent apoptosis in cultured cells. **(A)** DF1 cells infected with ARV S1133 at an MOI of 20. **(B)** Vero cells infected with ARV S1133 at an MOI of 5 for 0–42 hr. At the indicated time points, cells were stained with monodansylcadaverine (MDC) or Hoechst 332588. The percentage of positive cells was calculated for 20 independent fields at a magnification of 200×. **(C)** Vero cells infected with ARV S1133 at an MOI of 5 for 0–36 hr. In Hoechst 33258-stained cells (bright blue), arrows indicate apoptotic nuclei with condensed chromatin. In MDC stained cells, arrows indicate the autophagic vacuoles (×400 magnification, scale bar 10 μm).

RhoA and ROCK1 are required for ARV S1133-induced autophagy and subsequent apoptosis

Dominant negative RhoA-T19N, inhibitors and siRNA techniques were used to elucidate the relationships between previously identified molecules involved in ARV S1133-mediated autophagy and apoptosis. The overexpression of dominant negative RhoA and the inhibition of ROCK by Y-27632 or *ROCK1* siRNA led to a remarkable reduction in MDC positive and LC3-GFP punctuate cells: importantly, pan-caspase inhibitor, Z-VAD-FMK,

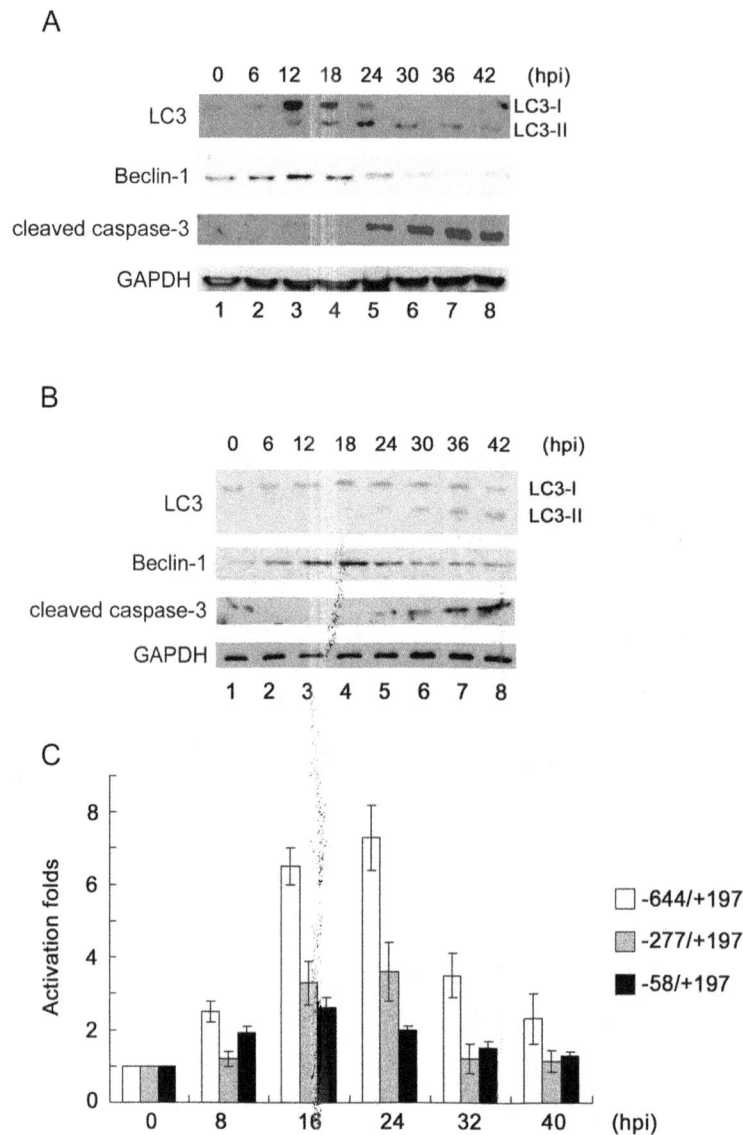

Figure 2 Upregulation of autophagic and apoptotic effectors and the Beclin-1 promoter by ARV S1133. **(A)** Vero cells infected with ARV S1133 at an MOI of 5 **(B)** DF1 cells infected with ARV S1133 at an MOI of 20. At the indicated time points, total cell lysates were collected. 30 μg of the extracted protein was separated by SDS-PAGE and transferred to a PVDF membrane. The expression of specific proteins was detected using the indicated antibodies. **(C)** Luciferase assay. Vero cells were transfected with three luciferase reporters with different lengths of the 5'-end regulatory region of the Beclin-1 gene. Following incubation with ARV S1133 for different time periods, the luciferase and β-galatosidase activities were measured and normalized to the transfection efficiency. The promoter activation levels were calculated against time zero. All experiments were performed three times, each in duplicate. The data are presented as the mean ± standard deviation (SD).

did not affect the percentage of autophagic cells. Autophagy inhibitor Beclin-1 siRNA, 3-Methyladenine (3-MA), and Bafilomycin A1 also reduced the number of cells undergoing autophagy (Figure 4A).

Next, the apoptotic characteristics of the cells were analyzed by Hoechst 33258 staining, the caspase-3 activity was assessed by chemiluminescence ELISA, and apoptotic DNA was measured by ELISA following inhibition of RhoA/ROCK1 signaling, inhibition of autophagy by *Beclin-1* siRNA, and blocking of autophagosome

formation by 3-MA and Bafilomycin A1, which is a known inhibitor of the late phase of autophagy. The results of these three experiments showed that the level of apoptosis was also inhibited when the autophagic process was blocked (Figure 4B). Figure 4C shows the LC3-GFP punctate pattern of ARV S1133-infected Vero cells in the presence of various inhibitors or siRNA. The level of LC3-GFP dots significantly increased in ARV S1133-infected cells (Figure 4C, (B)), as well as in cells in the presence of caspase-3 inhibitor Z-VAD-FMK (Figure 4C, (C)). Upon

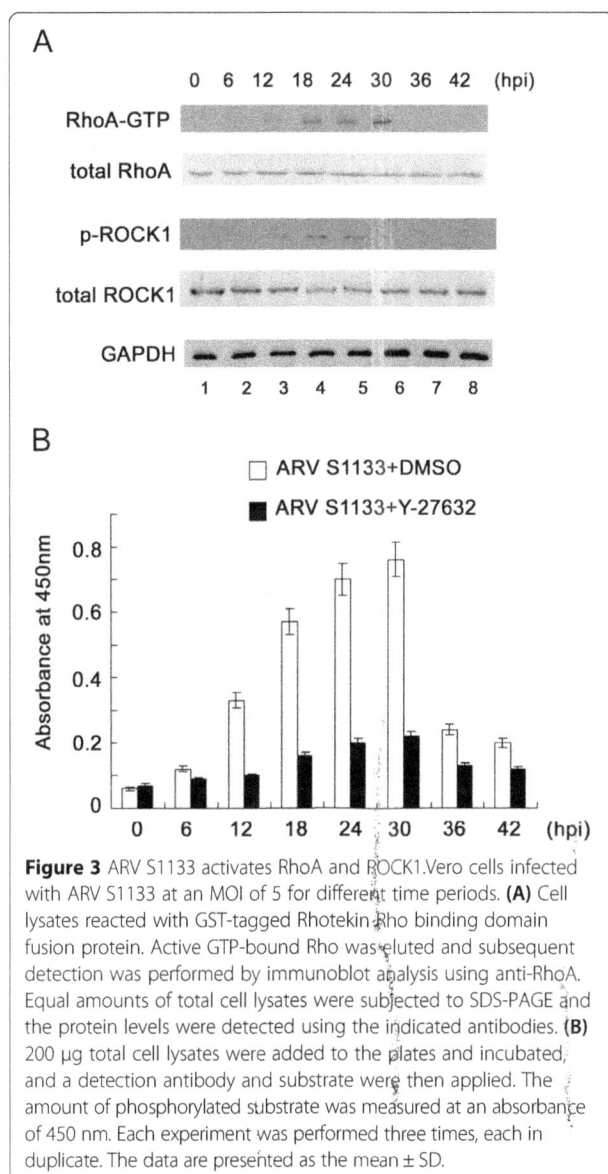

Figure 3 ARV S1133 activates RhoA and ROCK1.Vero cells infected with ARV S1133 at an MOI of 5 for different time periods. **(A)** Cell lysates reacted with GST-tagged Rhotekin Rho binding domain fusion protein. Active GTP-bound Rho was eluted and subsequent detection was performed by immunoblot analysis using anti-RhoA. Equal amounts of total cell lysates were subjected to SDS-PAGE and the protein levels were detected using the indicated antibodies. **(B)** 200 µg total cell lysates were added to the plates and incubated, and a detection antibody and substrate were then applied. The amount of phosphorylated substrate was measured at an absorbance of 450 nm. Each experiment was performed three times, each in duplicate. The data are presented as the mean ± SD.

Functional interaction of RhoA, ROCK1 and Beclin-1 upon ARV S1133 infection

To further understand the molecular mechanisms of ARV S1133-induced autophagy and apoptosis, co-immunoprecipitation followed by Western blotting analysis was utilized to detect the protein complex formation. Cell lysates from ARV S1133-infected cells with or without Y-27632 treatment were immunoprecipitated with anti-ROCK1 (Figure 7A) or anti-Beclin-1 (Figure 7B), then subjected to Western blotting analysis using the indicated various antibodies. ROCK1, Beclin-1 and RhoA formed a complex at 6–12 hpi, which corresponded to autophagy induction. In the presence of the ROCK1 inhibitor, Y-27632, the protein complex was disrupted. Thus, ROCK1 activity is essential for ARV S1133-mediated functional interactions between RhoA, ROCK1 and Beclin-1. It is known that the antiapoptotic protein, Bcl-2, interacts with Beclin-1 in non-stressed, resting cells and prevents autophagosome formation. The Bcl-2-Beclin-1 complex plays a potentially important role in the convergence of the cellular autophagic and apoptotic responses [25]. In non-stimulated Vero cells, Bcl-2 formed a complex with Beclin-1 (Figure 7B, lane 1). 6 h after ARV S1133 infection, this complex was disrupted and Beclin-1 was released, allowing it to participate in autophagy (Figure 7B, panel 3).

Discussion

In this study, we demonstrated that ARV S1133 caused autophagy and apoptosis in Vero and DF1 cells, which was accompanied by the activation of the Beclin-1 promoter in the early to middle stages, and induction of caspase-3 expression in the middle to late stages of infection. Inhibition of autophagy by Beclin-1 knockdown or autophagy inhibitors reduced autophagy and apoptosis simultaneously. In addition, we showed that inhibition of apoptosis did not affect autophagy in ARV-infected Vero cells, and the RhoA/ROCK1 signaling pathway played an important role in the process of switching the cell from autophagy to apoptosis.

Autophagy is a dynamic process by which infected host cells clear invading viruses. A previous study by Chi and colleagues showed that inhibition of autophagy through knockdown of Beclin-1 and LC3 significantly reduced ARV replication [18]. This suggests that in the early stage of viral infection, the induction of autophagy may trigger host cells to avoid apoptotic cell death. In addition to participating in the regulation of autophagy, Beclin-1 has been demonstrated to play important roles in tumor suppression, cell death and development. Moreover, Beclin-1 also interacts with Vps34, the class III phosphatidylinositol 3-kinase (PI-3 K) that mediates autophagy and endocytosis [26]. Many studies have reported that several small GTPases are involved in, and regulate, the

inhibition of the RhoA/ROCK1 pathway, the LC3-GFP positive signals dramatically reduced (Figure 4C, (D)(E)(F)). Inhibition of autophagy mediators by *Beclin-1* siRNA, 3-MA, and Bafilomycin A1, and inhibition of the RhoA/ROCK1 pathway also significantly reduced the number of apoptotic cells, as evidenced by Hoechst 33258 staining and the immunofluorescence assay using an antibody against cleaved caspase-3 (Figure 5). The efficiency of siRNA inhibition and overexpression of dominant negative RhoA were demonstrated by Western blotting analysis (Figure 6). Taken together, these experiments clearly demonstrate that RhoA/ROCK1 signaling plays an important role in the processes of autophagy and apoptosis that occur in the early and late stages of ARV S1133 infection of cultured Vero cells.

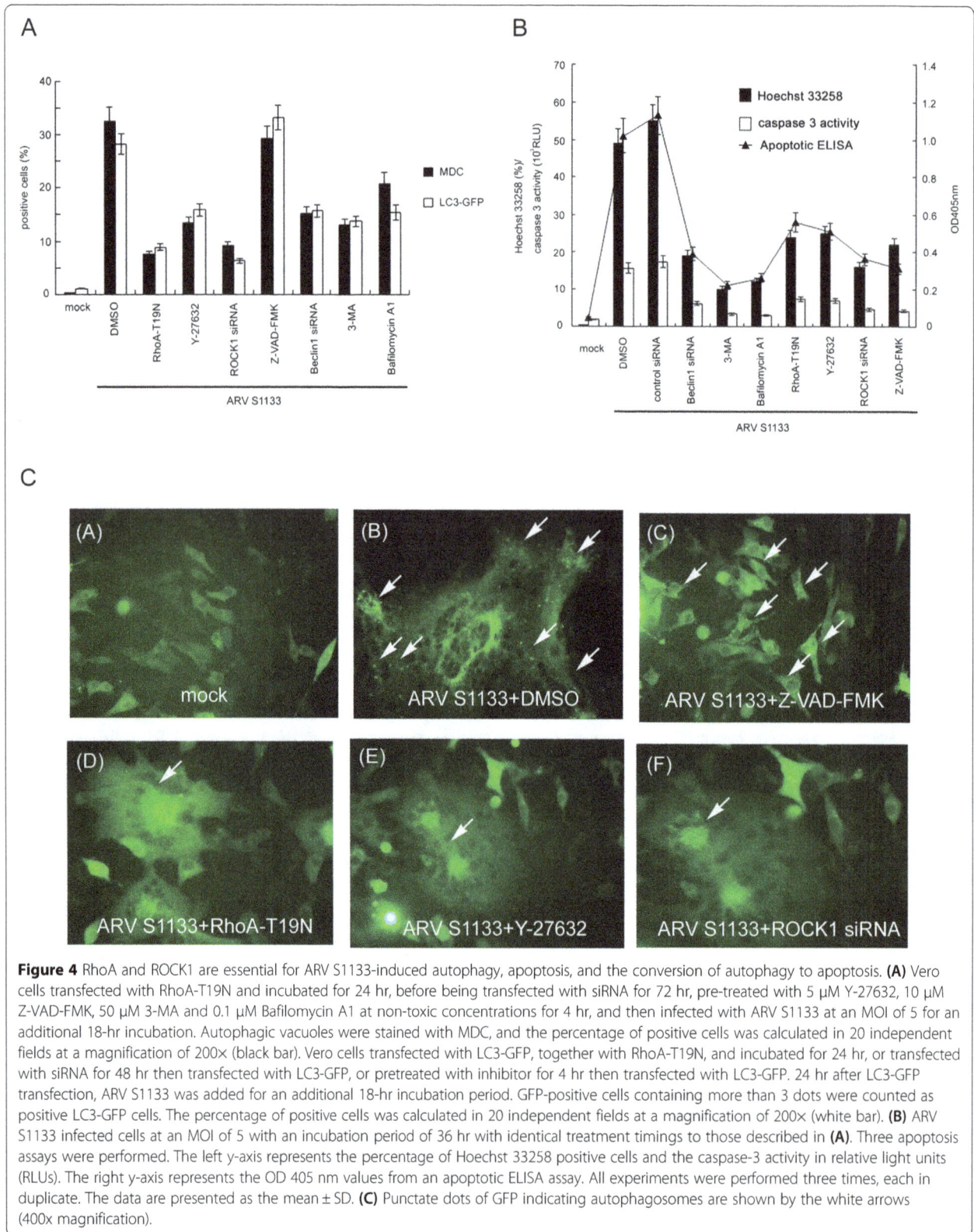

Figure 4 RhoA and ROCK1 are essential for ARV S1133-induced autophagy, apoptosis, and the conversion of autophagy to apoptosis. **(A)** Vero cells transfected with RhoA-T19N and incubated for 24 hr, before being transfected with siRNA for 72 hr, pre-treated with 5 μM Y-27632, 10 μM Z-VAD-FMK, 50 μM 3-MA and 0.1 μM Bafilomycin A1 at non-toxic concentrations for 4 hr, and then infected with ARV S1133 at an MOI of 5 for an additional 18-hr incubation. Autophagic vacuoles were stained with MDC, and the percentage of positive cells was calculated in 20 independent fields at a magnification of 200× (black bar). Vero cells transfected with LC3-GFP, together with RhoA-T19N, and incubated for 24 hr, or transfected with siRNA for 48 hr then transfected with LC3-GFP, or pretreated with inhibitor for 4 hr then transfected with LC3-GFP. 24 hr after LC3-GFP transfection, ARV S1133 was added for an additional 18-hr incubation period. GFP-positive cells containing more than 3 dots were counted as positive LC3-GFP cells. The percentage of positive cells was calculated in 20 independent fields at a magnification of 200× (white bar). **(B)** ARV S1133 infected cells at an MOI of 5 with an incubation period of 36 hr with identical treatment timings to those described in **(A)**. Three apoptosis assays were performed. The left y-axis represents the percentage of Hoechst 33258 positive cells and the caspase-3 activity in relative light units (RLUs). The right y-axis represents the OD 405 nm values from an apoptotic ELISA assay. All experiments were performed three times, each in duplicate. The data are presented as the mean ± SD. **(C)** Punctate dots of GFP indicating autophagosomes are shown by the white arrows (400x magnification).

formation of autophagosomes [27] and apoptotic morphological changes [28]. For example, several Rab proteins have been found to be involved in different stages of autophagy [29]. In the current study, we showed the kinetics of autophagy and apoptosis in ARV S1133-infected DF1 and Vero cells, which are in agreement

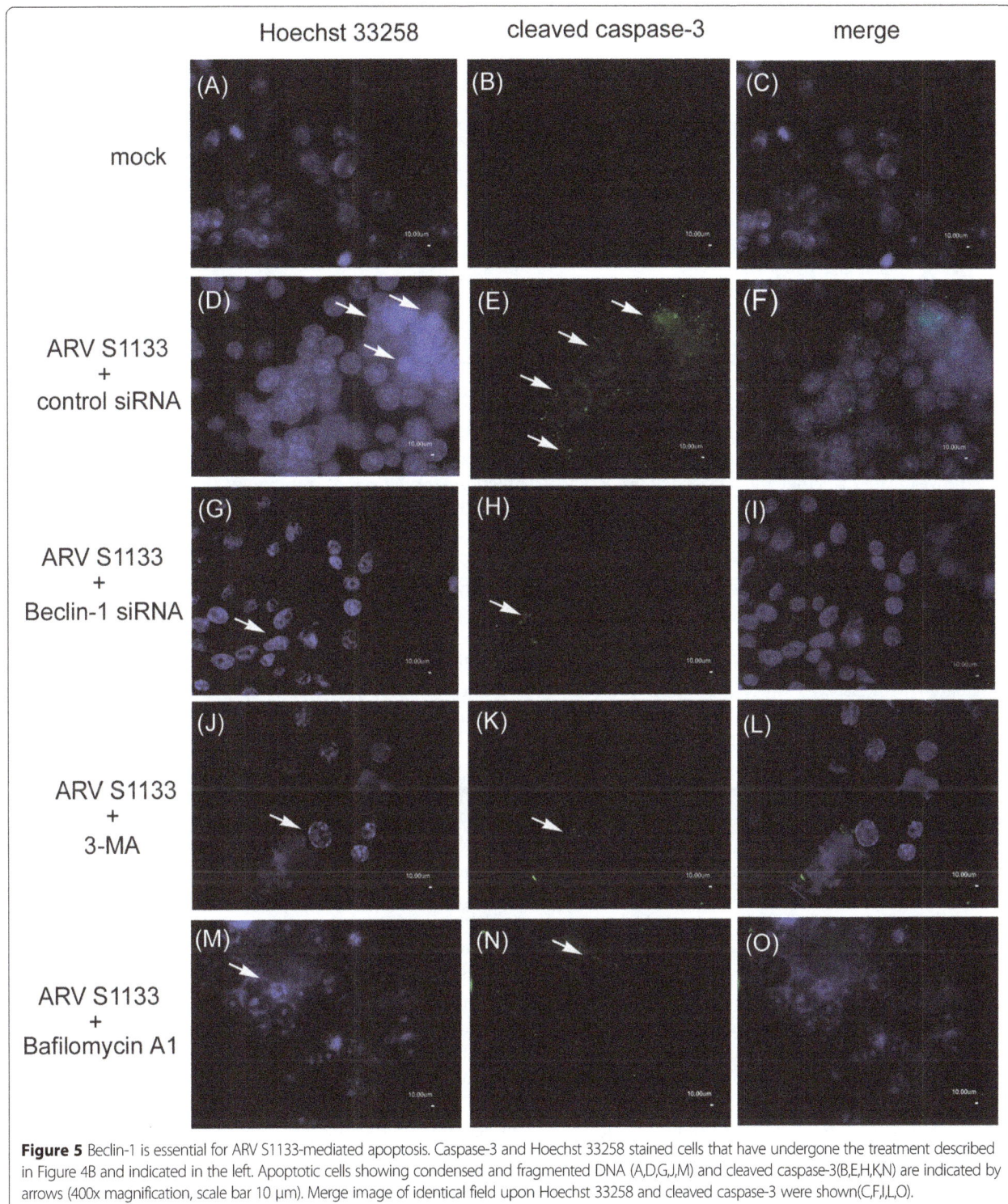

Figure 5 Beclin-1 is essential for ARV S1133-mediated apoptosis. Caspase-3 and Hoechst 33258 stained cells that have undergone the treatment described in Figure 4B and indicated in the left. Apoptotic cells showing condensed and fragmented DNA (A,D,G,J,M) and cleaved caspase-3(B,E,H,K,N) are indicated by arrows (400x magnification, scale bar 10 μm). Merge image of identical field upon Hoechst 33258 and cleaved caspase-3 were shown(C,F,I,L,O).

with those found in previous studies [17,18]. We further identified that ARV S1133 infection induces autophagy and apoptosis sequentially. ROCK1 is an effector of RhoA-GTPase and can be activated by RhoA-GTP under certain conditions [30]. A recent study by Gurkar and coworkers demonstrated that activated ROCK1 induced

by stress increases the binding and phosphorylation of Beclin-1 [16]. The results of our study indicated that the expression of RhoA-GTP is dramatically increased from 12 to 30 hr post-ARV S1133 infection, and the up-regulation of phosphorylated ROCK1 also showed a similar trend. Thus, the results suggest that ARV S1133

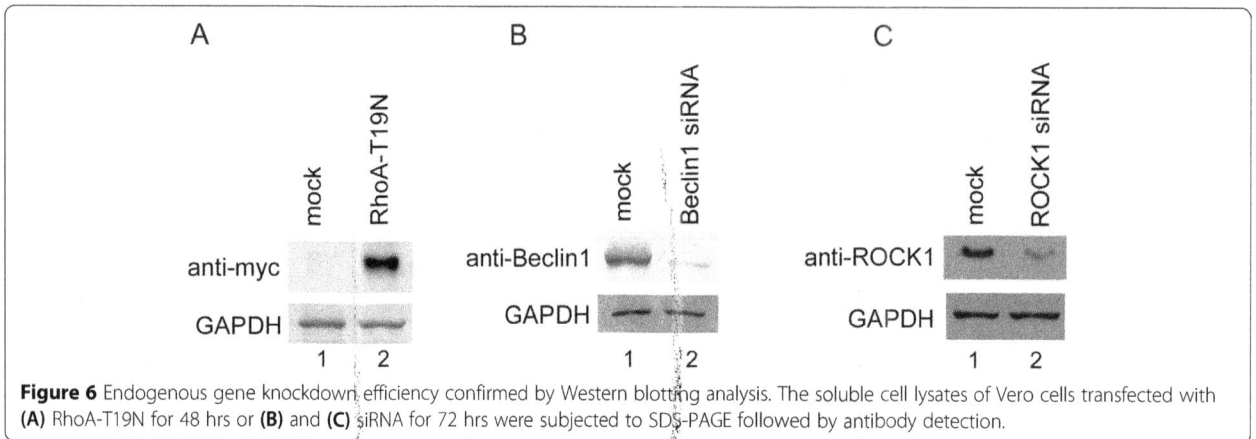

Figure 6 Endogenous gene knockdown efficiency confirmed by Western blotting analysis. The soluble cell lysates of Vero cells transfected with **(A)** RhoA-T19N for 48 hrs or **(B)** and **(C)** siRNA for 72 hrs were subjected to SDS-PAGE followed by antibody detection.

activation of RhoA and its downstream effector ROCK1 are closely correlated with LC3 and Beclin-1 activation, as well as with cells undergoing autophagy.

We also investigated whether the autophagy process is able to regulate apoptosis in Vero cells after ARV S1133 infection. Overexpression of dominant negative RhoA or inhibition of ROCK by a specific inhibitor or siRNA, significantly reduced the number of autophagic cells; while, pre-treating cells with the pan-caspase inhibitor, Z-VAD-FMK, did not have an effect on the inhibition of autophagic activity. The expression of Beclin-1 was downregulated with *Beclin-1* siRNA, blocked autophagosome formation with 3-MA, and inhibited the late phase of autophagy with Bafilomycin A1. Inhibition of Beclin-1 dramatically reduced the level of apoptosis and the caspase-3 activity; suggesting that apoptosis was inhibited when the autophagic process was blocked (Figure 4B). This phenomenon suggests that ARV induces autophagy and apoptosis sequentially, confirming the crosstalk between autophagy and apoptosis proposed by previous researchers [31]. One of the unique aspects of our study was that multiple tools were used, from protein to cell level, to validate the autophagic and apoptotic processes. This helps to reduce bias when analyzing cell death markers after viral infection.

Beclin-1 knockdown or autophagy inhibitor 3-MA and Bafilomycin A1 treatment suppressed ARV S1133-induced autophagy and apoptosis simultaneously, suggesting a switch in cell activity from autophagy to apoptosis.

This indicates that crosstalk between autophagy and apoptosis is present in ARV S1133-infected cells. Several recent studies have also shown that crosstalk between autophagy and apoptosis may occur in cells infected with other viruses, such as the Chikungunya virus [32], enterovirus 71 [33], and ectromelia virus [34]. Although infection with different viruses may share some mechanisms, the relationship between autophagy and apoptosis is complex, as different signaling pathways are involved

in these systems. For example, knockdown of autophagy genes caused enhanced apoptosis and increased viral propagation *in vitro* [32]. However, on enterovirus 71 infection, inhibition of autophagy leads to inhibit the apoptosis that is dependent on the autophagosome processing stage [33].

Our co-immunoprecipitation assay revealed that RhoA, ROCK1, and Beclin-1 formed a complex at a time point coinciding with that of autophagy induction. Taken together, these experiments clearly demonstrate that RhoA/ROCK1 signaling plays an important role in the processes of autophagy and apoptosis that occur in the early and late stages of ARV S1133-infection of Vero cells.

Previous studies have begun to elucidate the mechanisms by which cells switch from autophagy to apoptosis. One key factor is Bcl-2. Bcl-2 has been demonstrated to play a key role in the regulation of both apoptosis and autophagy, by binding to the pro-autophagic protein, Beclin-1, and pro-apoptotic proteins such as Bax [16]. The translocation of Bcl-2 from the endoplasmic reticulum to the mitochondria is an important event that regulates the switch between autophagy and apoptosis [35]. Autophagy-regulating protein 5 (ATG5) also participates in the switch from autophagy to apoptosis. In addition, to initiate autophagosome formation, ATG5 was cleaved by calpain, a calcium-dependent, non-lysosomal cysteine protease. The cleaved ATG5 fragment then translocates to mitochondria and binds to mitochondria-localized anti-apoptotic protein, Bcl-XL, and subsequently induces apoptosis [36-38].

Conclusions

In conclusion, our results demonstrate that RhoA/ROCK1 signaling plays critical roles in the transition from autophagy to apoptosis induced by ARV S1133. The findings indicate that the important signaling molecule, RhoA, and downstream ROCK1 could be linked to the autophagy observed during ARV infection. ARV infection causes economic losses and an effectively to

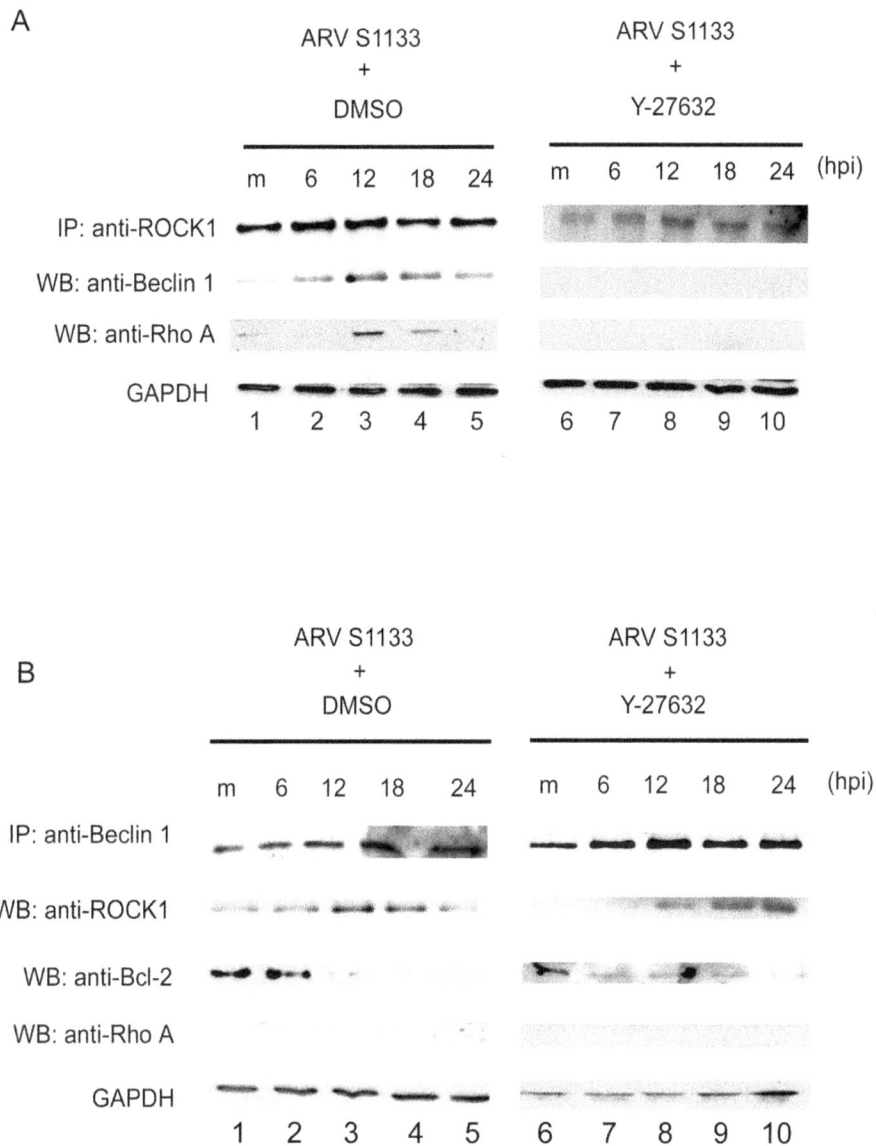

Figure 7 Functional interaction between RhoA, ROCK and Beclin-1 in ARV S1133-infected cells **(A, B)**. Vero cells pretreated with DMSO (left panel) or Y-27632 (right panel) for 4 hr then infected with ARV S1133 at an MOI of 5 for various incubation periods. 500 μg soluble cell lysates were precleared and immunoprecipitated with IP antibodies as indicated. The immunocomplexes were purified by protein A beads and loaded onto an SDS-PAGE gel. The interacting proteins were detected using the Western blotting technique.

control the disease is required. However, the mechanisms behind ARV-induced cell death are still largely unknown. In the present study, the mechanisms involved in the ARV-mediated switch between two different types of cell death were investigated for the first time. Several critical molecules undergoing transcriptional, translational and post-translational modifications following ARV infection were identified through molecular and cellular research approaches. Whether these proposed mechanisms occur in chickens requires further study. Thus, these molecules could be considered as valuable targets for new preventive or therapeutic drugs.

Methods

Cell culture, virus, reagents and antibodies

The method used to culture the DF1 (a spontaneously transformed cell line of chicken embryo fibroblasts) and Vero (a normal African green monkey kidney epithelial cell line) cells followed that described in a previous study [38]. Lipofectamine 2000 (Invitrogen, Carlsbad, CA, USA) was used for RhoA-T19N plasmid transfection. ARV strain S1133 was purified using the CsCl method and quantified as previously described [39]. Anti-ROCK1 antibody was purchased from Millipore (Billerica, MA, USA). Anti-LC3, anti-cleaved caspase-3, anti-Beclin-1, and anti-

GAPDH antibodies were purchased from Cell Signaling Technology Inc. (Beverly, MA, USA). Anti-p-ROCK1 (Thr455/Ser456) was obtained from Bioss (Boston, MA, USA). Y-27632, which selectively inhibits p160ROCK [40], 3-MA, Bafilomycin A1, and Z-VAD-FMK were obtained from Calbiochem (San Diego, CA, USA). Hoechst 33258 and monodansylcadaverine (MDC) were purchased from Sigma. A dominant negative RhoA-T19N plasmid with myc-tag expression was kindly provided by Dr. Jin-Mei Lai (Fu-Jen Catholic University, Taipei, Taiwan).

Western blotting and immunoprecipitation-western blotting analysis

The Western blotting and immunoprecipitation (IP)-Western blotting procedures were carried out as described in previous studies [9,38,39,41]. Briefly, Vero cells were infected with ARV S1133 at a multiplicity of infection (MOI) of 5 for various incubation durations. Soluble total cellular lysates were collected and quantification was performed using a Bio-Rad protein assay dye. For IP-Western blotting, cell lysates were pre-cleared with Protein A beads, and then reacted with the specific antibodies. The precipitated immunocomplex was boiled, separated by SDS-PAGE electrophoresis, and transferred onto a PVDF membrane. The presence of the proteins of interest was verified by specific secondary antibodies conjugated to horseradish peroxidase (HRP). The labeled bands were then detected by adding the enhanced chemiluminescent substrate reagents (Amersham, Buckinghamshire, UK) and exposing the membrane to X-ray film.

Luciferase assay

pGL3-Beclin-1(−644/+197, −277/+197, −58/+197)-luciferase reporter plasmids were kindly provided by Dr. Mujun Zhao (Institute of Biochemistry and Cell Biology, Shanghai, China). pRKbetaGAL containing the CMV promoter-driven β-galactosidase gene was used to normalize the transfection efficiency. A pGL3-Beclin-1-luciferase reporter plasmid and pRKbetaGAL were co-transfected into cultured Vero cells. After 24 hr of incubation, ARV S1133 at an MOI of 5 was added and the mixture incubated for an additional 24 hr. The luciferase activities were quantified using a Luciferase assay system (Promega), and the β-galactosidase activities were quantified using a β-galactosidase Enzyme Assay System (Promega). Luciferase activity was normalized to β-galactosidase activity to calculate the transfection efficiency [42].

RhoA and ROCK activation assay

A nonradioactive Rho activation assay kit and a Rho-associated kinase (ROCK) activity assay kit were purchased from Millipore Corporation and used according to the manufacturer's instructions. Briefly, Vero cells were infected with ARV S1133 at an MOI of 5 for different incubation durations. Cell lysates were harvested and quantified. For the Rho activation assay, lysates were added to Rho assay Reagent (Rhotekin RBD, agarose) and the reaction mixtures were incubated. Finally, Rho was analyzed by Western blotting using an anti-RhoA (clone 55) antibody and by chemiluminescent detection. ROCK inactivates myosin phosphatase through the specific phosphorylation of myosin phosphatase target subunit 1 (MYPT1) at threonine residue 696. The kit provided a plate pre-coated with recombinant MYPT1 that may be phosphorylated upon addition of an active enzyme-containing sample. A detection antibody that specifically detects only MYPT1 phosphorylated at Thr696 and an HRP-conjugated secondary detection antibody is then applied. The amount of phosphorylated substrate is measured by the addition of the chromogenic substrate, tetramethylbenzidine (TMB). The absorbance signal at 450 nm reflects the relative amount of ROCK activity in the sample.

Hoechst 33258 and autophagic vacuoles labeled by MDC

Following the induction of autophagy by ARV S1133 infection, the cells on a coverslip were incubated with 0.1 mM MDC in phosphate-buffered saline or 1 μg/ml Hoechst 33258 at 37°C for 15 minutes [43]. After incubation, the cells were washed and mounted, and then visualized with a fluorescence microscope using an excitation filter of 360 nm and an emission filter of 525 nm for the green MDC fluorescence signal, and was an excitation wavelength of 352 nm and emission filter of 461 nm for the blue Hoechst 33285 fluorescence. MDC-positive autophagosomes revealed a punctate staining structure. The apoptotic cells showed condensed and fragmented DNA characteristics.

siRNA techniques

ROCK1 and Beclin-1 protein knockdowns were performed using ROCK1 siRNA and Beclin-1 siRNA, respectively. Briefly, 5×10^4 Vero cells were seeded in each well of a 6-well plate and cultured for 18 hr. The cells were then transfected with 100 nM specific or control siRNA in the presence of Oligofectamine (Invitrogen). The cells were cultured for an additional 72 hr before viral infection. ROCK1 siRNA (M-003536-02), Beclin-1 siRNA (M-010552-01), and non-targeting control siRNA (D-001210-01) were obtained from Dharmacon.

Caspas-3 activity, caspase-3 staining, and apoptotic cell death ELISA

A caspase-3 activity fluorescence assay kit was purchased from Biovision and an apoptotic cell death ELISA assay kit was obtained from Roche. All procedures were conducted in accordance with the user manuals. For the caspase-3 assay, 1×10^6 Vero cells were resuspended in cold cell lysis buffer before the reaction mix was added. The caspase-3 substrate, DEVD-AFC (Ac-Asp-Glu-Val-Asp-AFC; AFC = 7-Amino-4-trifluoromethylcoumarin), was added and the mixture was incubated at 37°C for 60 min. Finally, the mixture was examined by fluorescence photometry (excitation at 400 nm, emission at 505 nm) in a Modulus Multimode Reader. For the apoptotic cell death ELISA assay, cell lysates were placed in streptavidin-coated wells. The samples contained nucleosomes that reacted with anti-biotin and anti-DNA-peroxidase (POD) antibodies, then the POD activity was determined photometrically using ABTS as the substrate. Measurement of optical density (OD) was performed at 405 nm with ABTS solution as a control. Cells cultured on coverslips were fixed in 4% paraformaldehyde, permeabilized with 0.5% Triton X-100 for 5 min at room temperature, and then reacted with anti-cleaved caspase-3 antibody for 60 min at 37°C. The cells were then washed and incubated with FITC-conjugated secondary antibody. The FITC green fluorescence was visualized using an excitation filter of 360 nm and an emission filter of 525 nm.

Competing interests

The authors declare that they have no competing interests.

Authors' contributions

PYL and CDC performed the cell culture-based analysis and drafted the manuscript. Y C participated in the design and coordination of the study and helped to draft the manuscript. WS, the principle investigator of the study, was responsible for the grant application, interpretation of the results, and manuscript editing. All authors read, commented on, and approved the final manuscript.

Acknowledgements

A grant was obtained from the Ministry of Science and Technology, NSC-101-2313-B-020-025-MY3. We appreciate the assistance of OxBiosci for English editing.

Author details

[1]Department of Biological Science and Technology, Pingtung 91201, Taiwan. [2]Veterinary Medicine, National Pingtung University of Science and Technology, Pingtung, Taiwan. [3]Graduate Institute of Biotechnology, National Pingtung University of Science and Technology, 1, Shuefu Rd., Neipu, Pingtung 91201, Taiwan.

References

1. Hieronymus DR, Villegas P, Kleven SH. Identification and serological differentiation of several reovirus strains isolated from chickens with suspected malabsorption syndrome. Avian Dis. 1983;27(1):246–54.
2. Bodelon G, Labrada L, Martinez-Costas J, Benavente J. The avian reovirus genome segment S1 is a functionally tricistronic gene that expresses one structural and two nonstructural proteins in infected cells. Virology. 2001;290(2):181–91.
3. Varela R, Benavente J. Protein coding assignment of avian reovirus strain S1133. J Virol. 1994;68(10):6775–7.
4. Olland AM, Jane-Valbuena J, Schiff LA, Nibert ML, Harrison SC. Structure of the reovirus outer capsid and dsRNA-binding protein sigma3 at 1.8 A resolution. EMBO J. 2001;20(5):979–89.
5. Lin HY, Chuang ST, Chen YT, Shih WL, Chang CD, Liu HJ. Avian reovirus-induced apoptosis related to tissue injury. Avian Pathol. 2007;36(2):155–9.
6. Ping-Yuan L, Hung-Jen L, Meng-Jiun L, Feng-Ling Y, Hsue-Yin H, Jeng-Woei L, et al. Avian reovirus activates a novel proapoptotic signal by linking Src to p53. Apoptosis. 2006;11(12):2179–93.
7. Liu HJ, Lee LH, Shih WL, Li YJ, Su HY. Rapid characterization of avian reoviruses using phylogenetic analysis, reverse transcription-polymerase chain reaction and restriction enzyme fragment length polymorphism. Avian Pathol. 2004;33(2):171–80.
8. Chulu JL, Lee LH, Lee YC, Liao SH, Lin FL, Shih WL, et al. Apoptosis induction by avian reovirus through p53 and mitochondria-mediated pathway. Biochem Biophys Res Commun. 2007;356(3):529–35.
9. Liu HJ, Lin PY, Wang LR, Hsu HY, Liao MH, Shih WL. Activation of small GTPases RhoA and Rac1 is required for avian reovirus p10-induced syncytium formation. Mol Cells. 2008;26(4):396–403.
10. Deretic V, Delgado M, Vergne I, Master S, De Haro S, Ponpuak M, et al. Autophagy in immunity against mycobacterium tuberculosis: a model system to dissect immunological roles of autophagy. Curr Top Microbiol Immunol. 2009;335:169–88.
11. Ravikumar B, Sarkar S, Davies JE, Futter M, Garcia-Arencibia M, Green-Thompson ZW, et al. Regulation of mammalian autophagy in physiology and pathophysiology. Physiol Rev. 2010;90(4):1383–435.
12. Petiot A, Pattingre S, Arico S, Meley D, Codogno P. Diversity of signaling controls of macroautophagy in mammalian cells. Cell Struct Funct. 2002;27(6):431–41.
13. Kroemer G, Marino G, Levine B. Autophagy and the integrated stress response. Mol Cell. 2010;40(2):280–93.
14. Kiffin R, Bandyopadhyay U, Cuervo AM. Oxidative stress and autophagy. Antioxid Redox Signal. 2006;8(1–2):152–62.
15. Yoo BH, Wu X, Li Y, Haniff M, Sasazuki T, Shirasawa S, et al. Oncogenic ras-induced down-regulation of autophagy mediator Beclin-1 is required for malignant transformation of intestinal epithelial cells. J Biol Chem. 2010;285(8):5438–49.
16. Gurkar AU, Chu K, Raj L, Bouley R, Lee SH, Kim YB, et al. Identification of ROCK1 kinase as a critical regulator of Beclin1-mediated autophagy during metabolic stress. Nat Commun. 2013;4:2189.
17. Meng S, Jiang K, Zhang X, Zhang M, Zhou Z, Hu M, et al. Avian reovirus triggers autophagy in primary chicken fibroblast cells and Vero cells to promote virus production. Arch Virol. 2012;157(4):661–8.
18. Chi PI, Huang WR, Lai IH, Cheng CY, Liu HJ. The p17 nonstructural protein of avian reovirus triggers autophagy enhancing virus replication via activation of phosphatase and tensin deleted on chromosome 10 (PTEN) and AMP-activated protein kinase (AMPK), as well as dsRNA-dependent protein kinase (PKR)/eIF2alpha signaling pathways. J Biol Chem. 2013;288(5):3571–84.
19. Shen HM, Codogno P. Autophagic cell death: Loch Ness monster or endangered species? Autophagy. 2011;7(5):457–65.
20. Fan YJ, Zong WX. The cellular decision between apoptosis and autophagy. Chin J Cancer. 2013;32(3):121–9.
21. Amelio I, Melino G, Knight RA. Cell death pathology: cross-talk with autophagy and its clinical implications. Biochem Biophys Res Commun. 2011;414(2):277–81.
22. Ouyang L, Shi Z, Zhao S, Wang FT, Zhou TT, Liu B, et al. Programmed cell death pathways in cancer: a review of apoptosis, autophagy and programmed necrosis. Cell Prolif. 2012;45(6):487–98.
23. Kabeya Y, Mizushima N, Ueno T, Yamamoto A, Kirisako T, Noda T, et al. LC3, a mammalian homologue of yeast Apg8p, is localized in autophagosome membranes after processing. EMBO J. 2000;19(21):5720–8.
24. Mizushima N, Yamamoto A, Matsui M, Yoshimori T, Ohsumi Y. In vivo analysis of autophagy in response to nutrient starvation using transgenic mice expressing a fluorescent autophagosome marker. Mol Biol Cell. 2004;15(3):1101–11.
25. Erlich S, Mizrachy L, Segev O, Lindenboim L, Zmira O, Adi-Harel S, et al. Differential interactions between Beclin 1 and Bcl-2 family members. Autophagy. 2007;3(6):561–8.
26. Zhong Y, Wang QJ, Li X, Yan Y, Backer JM, Chait BT, et al. Distinct regulation of autophagic activity by Atg14L and Rubicon associated with Beclin 1-phosphatidylinositol-3-kinase complex. Nat Cell Biol. 2009;11(4):468–76.
27. Bento CF, Puri C, Moreau K, Rubinsztein DC. The role of membrane-trafficking small GTPases in the regulation of autophagy. J Cell Sci. 2013;126(Pt 5):1059–69.
28. Coleman ML, Olson MF. Rho GTPase signalling pathways in the morphological changes associated with apoptosis. Cell Death Differ. 2002;9(5):493–504.

29. Ao X, Zou L, Wu Y. Regulation of autophagy by the Rab GTPase network. Cell Death Differ. 2014;21(3):348–58.

30. Matsui T, Amano M, Yamamoto T, Chihara K, Nakafuku M, Ito M, et al. Rho-associated kinase, a novel serine/threonine kinase, as a putative target for small GTP binding protein Rho. EMBO J. 1996;15(9):2208–16.

31. Maiuri MC, Zalckvar E, Kimchi A, Kroemer G. Self-eating and self-killing: crosstalk between autophagy and apoptosis. Nat Rev Mol Cell Biol. 2007;8(9):741–52.

32. Joubert PE, Werneke SW, de la Calle C, Guivel-Benhassine F, Giodini A, Peduto L, et al. Chikungunya virus-induced autophagy delays caspase-dependent cell death. J Exp Med. 2012;209(5):1029–47.

33. Xi X, Zhang X, Wang B, Wang T, Wang J, Huang H, et al. The interplays between autophagy and apoptosis induced by enterovirus 71. PLoS One. 2013;8(2), e56966.

34. Martyniszyn L, Szulc-Dabrowska L, Boratynska-Jasinska A, Struzik J, Winnicka A, Niemialtowski M, et al. Crosstalk between autophagy and apoptosis in RAW 264.7 macrophages infected with ectromelia orthopoxvirus. Viral Immunol. 2013;26(5):322–35.

35. Leber B, Andrews DW. Closing in on the link between apoptosis and autophagy. F1000 Biol Rep. 2010;2:88.

36. Shi M, Zhang T, Sun L, Luo Y, Liu DH, Xie ST, et al. Calpain, Atg5 and Bak play important roles in the crosstalk between apoptosis and autophagy induced by influx of extracellular calcium. Apoptosis. 2013;18(4):435–51.

37. An CH, Kim MS, Yoo NJ, Park SW, Lee SH. Mutational and expressional analyses of ATG5, an autophagy-related gene, in gastrointestinal cancers. Pathol Res Pract. 2011;207(7):433–7.

38. Lin PY, Liu HJ, Chang CD, Chang CI, Hsu JL, Liao MH, et al. Avian reovirus S1133-induced DNA damage signaling and subsequent apoptosis in cultured cells and in chickens. Arch Virol. 2011;156(11):1917–29.

39. Wang CY, Wang HC, Li JM, Wang JY, Yang KC, Ho YK, et al. Invasive infections of Aggregatibacter (Actinobacillus) actinomycetemcomitans. J Microbiol Immunol Infect. 2010;43(6):491–7.

40. Uehata M, Ishizaki T, Satoh H, Ono T, Kawahara T, Morishita T, et al. Calcium sensitization of smooth muscle mediated by a Rho-associated protein kinase in hypertension. Nature. 1997;389(6654):990–4.

41. Shih WL, Liao MH, Lin PY, Chang CI, Cheng HL, Yu FL, et al. PI 3-kinase/Akt and STAT3 are required for the prevention of TGF-beta-induced Hep3B cell apoptosis by autocrine motility factor/phosphoglucose isomerase. Cancer Lett. 2010;290(2):223–37.

42. Lin PY, Lee JW, Liao MH, Hsu HY, Chiu SJ, Liu HJ, et al. Modulation of p53 by mitogen-activated protein kinase pathways and protein kinase C delta during avian reovirus S1133-induced apoptosis. Virology. 2009;385(2):323–34.

43. Biederbick A, Kern HF, Elsasser HP. Monodansylcadaverine (MDC) is a specific in vivo marker for autophagic vacuoles. Eur J Cell Biol. 1995;66(1):3–14.

17

Vertical transmission of honey bee viruses in a Belgian queen breeding program

Jorgen Ravoet[1*], Lina De Smet[1], Tom Wenseleers[2] and Dirk C de Graaf[1]

Abstract

Background: The Member States of European Union are encouraged to improve the general conditions for the production and marketing of apicultural products. In Belgium, programmes on the restocking of honey bee hives have run for many years. Overall, the success ratio of this queen breeding programme has been only around 50%. To tackle this low efficacy, we organized sanitary controls of the breeding queens in 2012 and 2014.

Results: We found a high quantity of viruses, with more than 75% of the egg samples being infected with at least one virus. The most abundant viruses were Deformed Wing Virus and Sacbrood Virus (≥40%), although Lake Sinai Virus and Acute Bee Paralysis Virus were also occasionally detected (between 10-30%). In addition, Aphid Lethal Paralysis Virus strain Brookings, Black Queen Cell Virus, Chronic Bee Paralysis Virus and *Varroa destructor* Macula-like Virus occurred at very low prevalences (≤5%). Remarkably, we found *Apis mellifera carnica* bees to be less infected with Deformed Wing Virus than Buckfast bees (p < 0.01), and also found them to have a lower average total number of infecting viruses (p < 0.001). This is a significant finding, given that Deformed Wing Virus has earlier been shown to be a contributory factor to winter mortality and Colony Collapse Disorder. Moreover, negative-strand detection of Sacbrood Virus in eggs was demonstrated for the first time.

Conclusions: High pathogen loads were observed in this sanitary control program. We documented for the first time vertical transmission of some viruses, as well as significant differences between two honey bee races in being affected by Deformed Wing Virus. Nevertheless, we could not demonstrate a correlation between the presence of viruses and queen breeding efficacies.

Keywords: Honey bee, Eggs, Viruses, Negative-strand detection, Vertical transmission

Background

In view of the spread of varroasis – a mite infestation of the honey bee – over Europe and the problems which this disease has brought about in the beekeeping sector, the Member States of the European Union have been encouraged to set up national programmes aimed at improving the general conditions for the production and marketing of apicultural products. In Belgium, such apicultural programmes now exist for many years and particularly in the Flemish region, a lot of effort has been put in the restocking of hives. Within this programme, a limited number of recognized breeders are provided with the possibility to travel to a land mating yard in Belgium (Kreverhille) and island mating yards in Germany

(Spiekeroog, Norderney) and the Netherlands (Ameland, Marken) with selected virgin queens. When these fertilized queens perform well they become the new breeding queens two years later, and are distributed on a large scale among the other beekeepers. Overall, this programme enjoyed a high participation rate amongst the beekeepers, but failed to a certain extent in terms of the efficacy of the queen breeding programme. This is evident from the fact that in the past four years, between 5,948 and 6,195 larvae were grafted, but only 61.4-70.8% could be raised to newborn queens and from these only 75.0-79.9% became egg-laying. Thus overall, the success ratio of the queen breeding programme has been only 49.1-53.1%, a fairly low number [1].

One of the measures that were taken to tackle this low breeding efficacy was the publication and distribution of a technical brochure describing the proper way to introduce a new queen into a bee colony. Since the problems

* Correspondence: Jorgen.Ravoet@UGent.be
[1]Laboratory of Molecular Entomology and Bee Pathology, Ghent University, Krijgslaan 281 S2, B-9000 Ghent, Belgium
Full list of author information is available at the end of the article

persisted, we subsequently organized sanitary controls of the breeding queens in 2012 and 2014. This measure was taken given that honey bees can be exposed to several single stranded RNA viruses and transmission can occur both horizontally and vertically (reviewed by Chen et al. [2,3]). In horizontal transmission, viruses are transmitted among individuals of the same generation. Vertical transmission occurs from mothers to their offspring and can have two main causes: (I) infected sperm originating from the drones and (II) contaminated eggs originating from infected spermatheca and/or ovaries of the queen. The reproducing individuals, the queen and the drones, have a protective status in the colony because they are fed by the nurse bees. Nevertheless, both castes are susceptible to parasites. Several viruses were already demonstrated in individual queens and drones [4-9]. The presence of viruses in reproductive tissues of queens and drones were also investigated [10-14].

A non-destructive method to investigate whether vertical transmission occurs relies on examination of freshly laid eggs. In this study, we focused on a number of commonly occurring bee viruses [3] e.g. Deformed Wing Virus (DWV), but also on a set of viruses that were recently discovered in the USA such as Lake Sinai Virus (LSV) [15], and which we discovered to be present in Belgian apiaries as well [16]. Moreover, using the Bee-Doctor diagnostic tool [17] which is based on the multiplex ligation-dependent probe amplification technology, we were also able to screen in parallel for the negative-strand intermediate.

Both *Apis mellifera carnica*-breeders and Buckfast-breeders participated in our study. *Apis mellifera carnica* or the carniolan honey bee is the subspecies of the European honey bee native to the Balkan Peninsula and represents the majority of Belgian bee populations due to massive import. This race is favoured for several reasons, e.g. non-aggressiveness and honey yield. The Buckfast bee is a combination race, a cross of various *Apis mellifera* subspecies and was developed in the United Kingdom during several decades.

Methods

Flemish honey bee queen breeders were instructed to collect 10 eggs from worker cells from the same honey bee colony, per sample. In the summer of 2012, 35 queen breeders collected a sample from one colony each. In 2014, a further 43 egg samples were obtained. This set originated from 11 queen breeders, who surveyed each several colonies, varying from one to nine. This resulted in a total of 78 egg samples used in this study. The eggs were preserved at −20°C, transported to the laboratory on dry ice and then stored at −80°C until the RNA was isolated, using the RNeasy Lipid Tissue (Qiagen). The eggs were homogenised in the presence of zirconium beads

and 0.5 ml QIAzol lysis reagent (Qiagen). Using random hexamer primers, 200 ng RNA was retro-transcribed with the RevertAid H Minus First Strand cDNA Synthesis Kit (Thermo Scientific).

The eggs were examined by RT PCR assays for the presence of viruses of the Acute Bee Paralysis Virus (ABPV) complex [18], Aphid Lethal Paralysis Virus strain Brookings (ALPV) [16], Black Queen Cell Virus (BQCV) [19], Chronic Bee Paralysis Virus (CBPV) [20], DWV [21], LSV [16], Sacbrood Virus (SBV) [19] and *Varroa destructor* Macula-like Virus (VdMLV) [11]. Samples positive for the ABPV complex were re-analysed with specific primers for ABPV [22], Israeli Acute Bee Paralysis Virus [23] and Kashmir Bee Virus [22]. We used honey bee β-actin [24] as a control gene to monitor the efficiency of the PCR reaction and its previous steps. All PCR reaction mixtures contained: 2 μM of each primer; 1 mM MgCl$_2$; 0.2 mM dNTPs; 1.2 U Hotstar Taq DNA polymerase (Qiagen) and 2 μl cDNA product. Positive samples of each detected virus, except CBPV and VdMLV, were analysed for their negative-strand. This was detected with the BeeDoctor tool [17] in its uniplex modus, using 3 μl RNA.

PCR products were separated by electrophoresis using 1.4% agarose gels or 4% high resolution agarose gels for the MLPA PCR products, stained with ethidium bromide and visualised under UV light. Amplicons of each virus were sequenced on an ABI 3130XL platform with M13 primers after cloning with the TOPO TA Cloning Kit for sequencing (Invitrogen). DNA sequences were analysed using Geneious R7 to confirm the identity.

The incidence of the screened viruses (percentage infected) as well as the total virus load (total number of detected viruses) in *carnica* and Buckfast bees was compared using binomial and Poisson generalized linear mixed models with function glmer in package lme4 v. 1.1-7 in R v. 3.1.1. In these analyses, race and year were coded as fixed factors and breeder was coded as a random factor, and significance was assessed using Wald tests. Least square means on average infection percentages and total virus load and 95% Wald confidence limits were calculated using the effects package v. 3.0-3. Finally, a linear regression analysis was used to test the effect of virus load (total number of infecting viruses) on the percentage of queens that were born from grafted larvae, the percentage of queens that went on to lay out of all larvae that were grafted and the percentage of all queens that were born that went on to lay. This analysis was performed in GraphPad Prism 6.

Results and discussion

In this study, we found a high prevalence of different honey bee viruses in eggs used in queen breeding operations (Additional file 1: Table S1). Although we investigated representative samples consisting of ten eggs per sample, false negatives can be present. Over two sampling years, 75% (58/78) of the egg samples were infected with at least one virus whereof 32% (25/78) of the samples were infected with a single virus and 42% (33/78) were infected with multiple viruses (Figure 1).

The most abundantly detected viruses were DWV (40%, 31/78) and SBV (42%, 33/78). LSV and ABPV were moderately detected in 28% (22/78) and 14% (11/78) of the samples. The other viruses ALPV, BQCV, CBPV and VdMLV had only low prevalences, respectively 5% (4/78), 5% (4/78), 1% (1/78) and 3% (2/78). Remarkably, *carnica* had a significantly lower infection rate with DWV than Buckfast [binomial GLMM, $z = -3.048$, $p = 0.002$, 30% mean infection rate in *carnica* ([20%, 43%] 95% C.L.) vs. 73% mean infection rate in Buckfast ([49%, 88%] 95% C.L.)] (Figure 2) as well as a significantly lower total virus load (total number of detected viruses) per sample [Poisson GLMM, $z = -3.911$, $p = 9.10^{-5}$, average of 1.1 infecting viruses in *carnica* ([0.8, 1.4] 95% C.L.) vs. an average of 2.3 infecting viruses in Buckfast ([1.7, 3.2] 95% C.L.)]. No significant differences were found in the incidence of the other viruses screened (binomial GLMM, $p > 0.05$).

Our results, however, did not indicate a correlation between the virus burden (total number of infecting viruses) and queen breeding efficacy (Additional file 2: Figure S1). It might be the case though that variation in beekeeping management skills required for successful queen breeding [1] hides any effect of virus burden on queen breeding efficacy. Given the important effects that some of the viruses detected here have on honey bee health, including a large effect on winter mortality [25-28], delayed negative effects on honey bee health are likely, particularly given the implied vertical transmission to offspring workers. Indeed, this study is the first to document vertical transmission for ALPV, LSV and VdMLV. This is

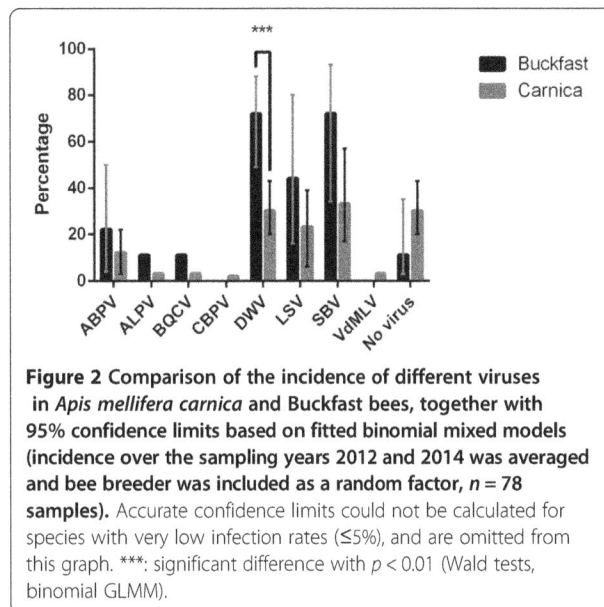

Figure 2 Comparison of the incidence of different viruses in *Apis mellifera carnica* and Buckfast bees, together with 95% confidence limits based on fitted binomial mixed models (incidence over the sampling years 2012 and 2014 was averaged and bee breeder was included as a random factor, n = 78 samples). Accurate confidence limits could not be calculated for species with very low infection rates (≤5%), and are omitted from this graph. ***: significant difference with $p < 0.01$ (Wald tests, binomial GLMM).

another confirmation that these viruses can infect honey bees, especially given that the negative strand was previously detected [15,16]. Moreover, BQCV lethally affects developing queen larvae and pupae. After death of the pupae, the wall of the queen cell eventually colours dark [3]. This virus is reported to be a common cause of queen larvae mortality [29] and is correlated with the queenless condition of an apiary [26].

Furthermore, we have detected the negative-strand of SBV. Although this might indicate that SBV replicates in eggs, it is also possible that this originates from transovum transmission, such as surface contamination with sperm containing negative-strand RNAs. Replication of SBV was previously reported in adults and larvae of European (*A. mellifera*) and Asian honey bees (*Apis cerana*) [30-32]. This virus is frequently found in adult bees that are covertly infected. A Belgian screening of adult forager bees revealed a prevalence of 19% [17], but this varies greatly in other European countries [22,33,34]. Larvae can be overtly infested, which then results in a failure to pupate and eventually death [3]. Nonetheless, problems with this virus are seldom reported by beekeepers, in contrast to the Asian serotypes that infect *A. cerana* [35,36]. Although SBV is mainly horizontally transmitted, its detection in eggs demonstrated that vertical transmission also occurs. It can be expected that a replicating virus in honey bee eggs can have consequences for the development into a queen, resulting in a clinical relevance for queen breeding, and can also have knock-on effects after being transmitted to the offspring workers or drones [3].

A broad virus screening of honey bee eggs was not yet performed. Nevertheless, few studies reported the presence of viruses [6-8,19,37] but only limited numbers of colonies were screened. However, our study of fertilised

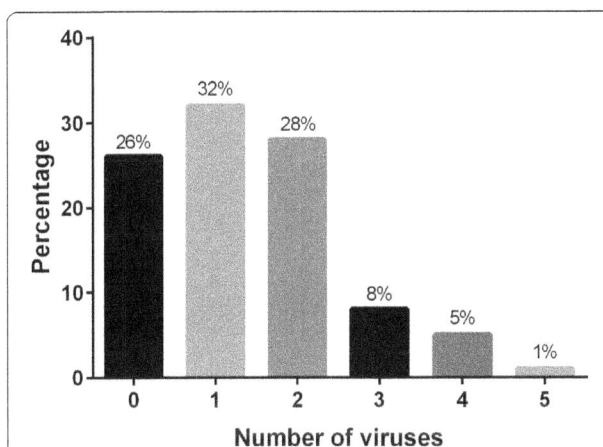

Figure 1 Number of detected viruses and their prevalences. The samples used in our study were co-infected with a number of viruses, ranging from 1 to 5. In almost 26% of the samples were no viruses detected.

eggs does not allow us to pinpoint the infection source, queen or drone, which could be important for eventual remedial actions. Because surface-sterilisation was not applicable in our study design, we could not distinguish between viruses on the surface of the eggs (transovum transmission) or within the eggs (transovarian transmission). Because of the possible transovum transmission, the emerging larvae will not necessarily be infected with viruses as previously demonstrated [6]. Nevertheless, these larvae are exposed to horizontal transmission via feeding (reviewed by Chen *et al.* [2]).

Conclusions

A survey of viruses in honey bee eggs in the context of a queen breeding program demonstrated high incidences of two viruses (DWV and SBV) and moderate to low incidences of a further six viruses (ABPV, ALPV, BQCV, CBPV, LSV and VdMLV). Vertical transmission (transovum or transovarian) of some viruses (ALPV, LSV, VdMLV) was demonstrated for the first time as well as negative-strand detection of SBV. We could not demonstrate a correlation between the presence of viruses and the low queen breeding efficacies. Remarkably, we found *Apis mellifera carnica* bees to be less infected with Deformed Wing Virus (p < 0.01) than Buckfast bees, and also found them to have a lower average total number of infecting viruses (p < 0.001). This is a significant finding, given that Deformed Wing Virus has earlier been shown to be a contributory factor to winter mortality, and offers interesting perspectives for breeding virus-resistant bees. However, we cannot make general conclusions about the virus-resistant state of *carnica* race compared to Buckfast race solely based on our data. Concluding, further sanitary screenings in the context of queen breeding seems advisory, especially because BQCV infection is a common cause of queen larval death [29].

Ethics statement

The study involved the European honey bee (*Apis mellifera*), which is neither an endangered nor a protected species.

Additional files

Additional file 1: Table S1. Overview of the detected viruses in honeybee egg samples, subdivided per year. For each sample is the corresponding apiary, bee race and total virus burden shown. The virus prevalence per sampling year and the overall occurrence are indicated.

Additional file 2: Figure S1. Linear regression analysis of the effect of virus loads (total number of detected viruses) on queen breeding efficacies: effect on (A) the percentage of queens that were born from grafted larvae, (B) the percentage of queens that went on to lay out of all larvae that were grafted and (C) the percentage of all queens that were born that went on to lay.

Competing interests
The authors declare that they have no competing interests.

Authors' contributions
DCdG designed the study. JR carried out all the experimental work. TW performed the statistical analyses. JR, DCdG and TW drafted the manuscript. All authors read and approved the final manuscript.

Acknowledgements
This study was supported by the Research Foundation of Flanders (FWO-Vlaanderen G.0628.11). We would like to the participating beekeepers for supplying the honey bee egg samples.

Author details
[1]Laboratory of Molecular Entomology and Bee Pathology, Ghent University, Krijgslaan 281 S2, B-9000 Ghent, Belgium. [2]Laboratory of Socioecology and Social Evolution, KU Leuven, Naamsestraat 59, B-3000 Leuven, Belgium.

References
1. Buchler R, Andonov S, Bienefeld K, Costa C, Hatjina F, Kezic N, et al. Standard methods for rearing and selection of *Apis mellifera* queens. J Apicult Res. 2013;52:1–30.
2. Chen YP, Evans JD, Feldlaufer M. Horizontal and vertical transmission of viruses in the honeybee, *Apis mellifera*. J Invertebr Pathol. 2006;92:152–9.
3. Chen YP, Siede R. Honey bee viruses. Adv Virus Res. 2007;70:33–80.
4. Retschnig G, Williams GR, Mehmann MM, Yanez O, de Miranda JR, Neumann P. Sex-specific differences in pathogen susceptibility in honey bees (*Apis mellifera*). PLoS One. 2014;9:e85261.
5. Chen YP, Pettis JS, Feldlaufer MF. Detection of multiple viruses in queens of the honey bee *Apis mellifera* L. J Invertebr Pathol. 2005;90:118–21.
6. Chen YP, Pettis JS, Collins A, Feldlaufer MF. Prevalence and transmission of honeybee viruses. Appl Environ Microbiol. 2006;72:606–11.
7. Chen YP, Higgins JA, Feldlaufer MF. Quantitative real-time reverse transcription-PCR analysis of deformed wing virus infection in the honeybee (*Apis mellifera* L.). Appl Environ Microbiol. 2005;71:436–41.
8. Shen MQ, Cui LW, Ostiguy N, Cox-Foster D. Intricate transmission routes and interactions between picorna-like viruses (Kashmir bee virus and sacbrood virus) with the honeybee host and the parasitic varroa mite. J Gen Virol. 2005;86:2281–9.
9. Gregorc A, Bakonyi T. Viral infections in queen bees (*Apis mellifera carnica*) from rearing apiaries. Acta Vet Brno. 2012;81:15–9.
10. Francis RM, Nielsen SL, Kryger P. Patterns of viral infection in honey bee queens. J Gen Virol. 2013;94:668–76.
11. Gauthier L, Ravallec M, Tournaire M, Cousserans F, Bergoin M, Dainat B, et al. Viruses associated with ovarian degeneration in *Apis mellifera* L. queens. PLoS One. 2011;6:e16217.
12. Fievet J, Tentcheva D, Gauthier L, de Miranda J, Cousserans F, Colin ME, et al. Localization of deformed wing virus infection in queen and drone *Apis mellifera* L. Virol J. 2006;3:16.
13. Yue C, Schroder M, Bienefeld K, Genersch E. Detection of viral sequences in semen of honeybees (*Apis mellifera*): evidence for vertical transmission of viruses through drones. J Invertebr Pathol. 2006;92:105–8.
14. Yanez O, Jaffe R, Jarosch A, Fries I, Moritz RFA, Paxton RJ, et al. Deformed wing virus and drone mating flights in the honey bee (*Apis mellifera*): implications for sexual transmission of a major honey bee virus. Apidologie. 2012;43:17–30.
15. Runckel C, Flenniken ML, Engel JC, Ruby JG, Ganem D, Andino R, et al. Temporal analysis of the honey bee microbiome reveals four novel viruses and seasonal prevalence of known viruses, Nosema, and Crithidia. PLoS One. 2011;6:e20656.
16. Ravoet J, Maharramov J, Meeus I, De SL, Wenseleers T, Smagghe G, et al. Comprehensive bee pathogen screening in Belgium reveals Crithidia mellificae as a new contributory factor to winter mortality. PLoS One. 2013;8:e72443.
17. De Smet L, Ravoet J, de Miranda JR, Wenseleers T, Mueller MY, Moritz RFA, et al. BeeDoctor, a versatile MLPA-based diagnostic tool for screening bee viruses. PLoS One. 2012;7:e47953.
18. Francis RM, Kryger P. Single assay detection of Acute Bee Paralysis Virus, Kashmir Bee Virus and Israeli Acute Paralysis Virus. J Apic Sci. 2012;56:137–46.
19. Singh R, Levitt AL, Rajotte EG, Holmes EC, Ostiguy N, van Engelsdorp D, et al. RNA viruses in hymenopteran pollinators: evidence of inter-Taxa virus

transmission via pollen and potential impact on non-Apis hymenopteran species. PLoS One. 2010;5:e14357.

20. Blanchard P, Olivier V, Iscache AL, Celle O, Schurr F, Lallemand P, et al. Improvement of RT-PCR detection of chronic bee paralysis virus (CBPV) required by the description of genomic variability in French CBPV isolates. J Invertebr Pathol. 2008;97:182–5.

21. Forsgren E, de Miranda JR, Isaksson M, Wei S, Fries I. Deformed wing virus associated with Tropilaelaps mercedesae infesting European honey bees (*Apis mellifera*). Exp Appl Acarol. 2009;47:87–97.

22. Tentcheva D, Gauthier L, Zappulla N, Dainat B, Cousserans F, Colin ME, et al. Prevalence and seasonal variations of six bee viruses in *Apis mellifera L.* and Varroa destructor mite populations in France. Appl Environ Microbiol. 2004;70:7185–91.

23. Palacios G, Hui J, Quan PL, Kalkstein A, Honkavuori KS, Bussetti AV, et al. Genetic analysis of Israel acute paralysis virus: Distinct clusters are circulating in the United States. J Virol. 2008;82:6209–17.

24. Scharlaken B, de Graaf DC, Goossens K, Peelman LJ, Jacobs FJ. Differential gene expression in the honeybee head after a bacterial challenge. Dev Comp Immunol. 2008;32:883–9.

25. Berthoud H, Imdorf A, Haueter M, Radloff S, Neumann P. Virus infections and winter losses of honey bee colonies (*Apis mellifera*). J Apicult Res. 2010;49:60–5.

26. Nguyen BK, Ribiere M, van Engelsdorp D, Snoeck C, Saegerman C, Kalkstein AL, et al. Effects of honey bee virus prevalence, Varroa destructor load and queen condition on honey bee colony survival over the winter in Belgium. J Apicult Res. 2011;50:195–202.

27. Genersch E, von der Ohe W, Kaatz H, Schroeder A, Otten C, Buchler R, et al. The German bee monitoring project: a long term study to understand periodically high winter losses of honey bee colonies. Apidologie. 2010;41:332–52.

28. Highfield AC, El NA, Mackinder LC, Noel LM, Hall MJ, Martin SJ, et al. Deformed wing virus implicated in overwintering honeybee colony losses. Appl Environ Microbiol. 2009;75:7212–20.

29. Anderson DL. Pathogens and queen bees. Australasian Beekeeper. 1993;94:292–6.

30. Bailey L. Multiplication of Sacbrood Virus in the adult honeybee. Virology. 1968;36:312.

31. Mussen EC, Furgala B. Replication of Sacbrood Virus in larval and adult honeybees, *Apis mellifera*. J Invertebr Pathol. 1977;30:20–34.

32. Bailey L. The multiplication and spread of sacbrood virus of bees. Ann Appl Biol. 1969;63:483–91.

33. Antunez K, Anido M, Garrido-Bailon E, Botias C, Zunino P, Martinez-Salvador A, et al. Low prevalence of honeybee viruses in Spain during 2006 and 2007. Res Vet Sci. 2012;93:1441–5.

34. Forgach P, Bakonyi T, Tapaszti Z, Nowotny N, Rusvai M. Prevalence of pathogenic bee viruses in Hungarian apiaries: situation before joining the European Union. J Invertebr Pathol. 2008;98:235–8.

35. Liu X, Zhang Y, Yan X, Han R. Prevention of Chinese sacbrood virus infection in Apis cerana using RNA interference. Curr Microbiol. 2010;61:422–8.

36. Roberts JM, Anderson DL. A novel strain of sacbrood virus of interest to world apiculture. J Invertebr Pathol. 2014;118:71–4.

37. Yue C, Schroder M, Gisder S, Genersch E. Vertical-transmission routes for deformed wing virus of honeybees (*Apis mellifera*). J Gen Virol. 2007;88:2329–36.

18

Another potential carp killer?: Carp Edema Virus disease in Germany

Verena Jung-Schroers[1][*][†], Mikolaj Adamek[1][†], Felix Teitge[1], John Hellmann[1], Sven Michael Bergmann[2], Heike Schütze[2], Dirk Willem Kleingeld[3], Keith Way[4], David Stone[4], Martin Runge[5], Barbara Keller[5], Shohreh Hesami[6], Thomas Waltzek[6] and Dieter Steinhagen[1]

Abstract

Background: Infections with carp edema virus, a pox virus, are known from Japanese koi populations since 1974. A characteristic clinical sign associated with this infection is lethargy and therefore the disease is called "koi sleepy disease". Diseased koi also show swollen gills, enophthalmus, and skin lesions. Mortality rates up to 80 % are described. For a long period of time, disease outbreaks seemed to be restricted to Japan. However, during the last years clinical outbreaks of koi sleepy disease also occurred in the UK and in the Netherlands.

Case presentation: In spring 2014 koi from different ponds showing lethargic behavior, skin ulcers, inflammation of the anus, enophthalmus, and gill necrosis were presented to the laboratory for diagnosis. In all cases, new koi had been purchased earlier that spring from the same retailer and introduced into existing populations. Eleven koi from six ponds were examined for ectoparasites and for bacterial and viral infections (cyprinid herpesviruses in general and especially koi herpesvirus (KHV) known formally as *Cyprinid herpesvirus 3* (CyHV–3); and Carp Edema Virus). In most of the cases parasites were not detected from skin and gills. Only opportunistic freshwater bacteria were isolated from skin ulcers. In cell cultures no cytopathic effect was observed, and none of the samples gave positive results in PCR tests for cyprinid herpesviruses. By analyzing gill tissues for CEV in seven out of eleven samples by a nested PCR, PCR products of 547 bp and 180 bp (by using nested primers) could be amplified. An outbreak of Koi Sleepy Disease was confirmed by sequencing of the PCR products. These results confirm the presence of CEV in German koi populations.

Conclusion: A clinical outbreak of "koi sleepy disease" due to an infection with Carp Edema Virus was confirmed for the first time in Germany. To avoid transmission of CEV to common carp testing of CEV should become part of fish disease surveillance programs.

Keywords: Carp Edema Virus, Koi sleepy disease, *Cyprinus carpio*

Background

Virus infections are responsible for serious diseases associated with high morbidity and mortality in fish [1–3]. In common carp and ornamental koi (*Cyprinus carpio*), *Cyprinid herpesvirus 3* (CyHV–3, KHV), is considered as major viral pathogen. It causes a notifiable disease (KHVD) for OIE [4] and EU [5] which is associated with skin lesions and gill necrosis [2]. Since its first appearance in the late 1990s it seriously affects carp aquaculture, wild carp, and koi trade worldwide. In addition, infections with carp edema virus (CEV), a poxvirus, are known to cause health problems in koi apparently with geographically restricted incidence [6, 7]. CEV infections have been observed in Japan since 1974, mainly in spring and autumn at water temperatures between 15 °C and 25 °C, when koi are moved from earthen ponds to freshwater containing cement-lined ponds [6]. In adult fish, lethargic behavior is a characteristic clinical sign associated with this infection and therefore the disease was named "koi sleepy disease" (KSD). Other typical pathological symptoms include swollen gills [6], enophthalmus and skin lesions, often

* Correspondence: verena.jung-schroers@tiho-hannover.de
[†]Equal contributors
[1]Fish Disease Research Unit, University of Veterinary Medicine, Hannover, Germany
Full list of author information is available at the end of the article

around the mouth, and at the base of the fins [7]. Mortality rates up to 80 % were observed, without the presence of parasites, fungi, or high levels of fish pathogenic bacteria in diseased koi [3]. For decades KSD outbreaks seemed to be restricted to Japan, but during the last years CEV infections associated with clinical outbreaks of KSD occurred in defined koi populations in the UK [7] and in the Netherlands [8]. In the present study, a clinical outbreak of KSD due to an infection with CEV was confirmed in spring 2014 for the first time in koi in Germany. The outbreak originated from one source, involved several koi populations in different ponds and confirmed the pathogenic nature of the virus.

Case presentation

In spring 2014 several koi hobbyists presented koi showing similar clinical signs to the consulting service of the Fish Disease Research Unit at the University of Veterinary Medicine in Hannover, Germany. In most cases the koi displayed the following clinical signs: lethargy, ulcerations on the mouth, or on the lateral side of the body, a reddened inflamed anus (Fig. 1), enophthalmus and gill swelling, or gill necrosis (Fig. 2) affecting up to one third of the gill tissue. In one pond all koi died within three days without showing disease symptoms. In all ponds the water temperature ranged between 17 °C and 22 °C. A failure of the filter systems was excluded as cause of death, as water analyses showed no alterations. In all cases new koi had been purchased in spring 2014 from the same retailer. In affected ponds newly purchased koi as well as koi kept already for a couple of years developed clinical symptoms. Other fish species, like goldfish, and sturgeons, kept in the same ponds were not affected. Hence an infectious agent was suspected to be responsible for the disease outbreaks.

In total 11 fish from 6 ponds were examined. Fresh smears of gills and skin of all koi were inspected microscopically for ectoparasites. Bacteriological examinations were performed by routine cultivation methods by taking

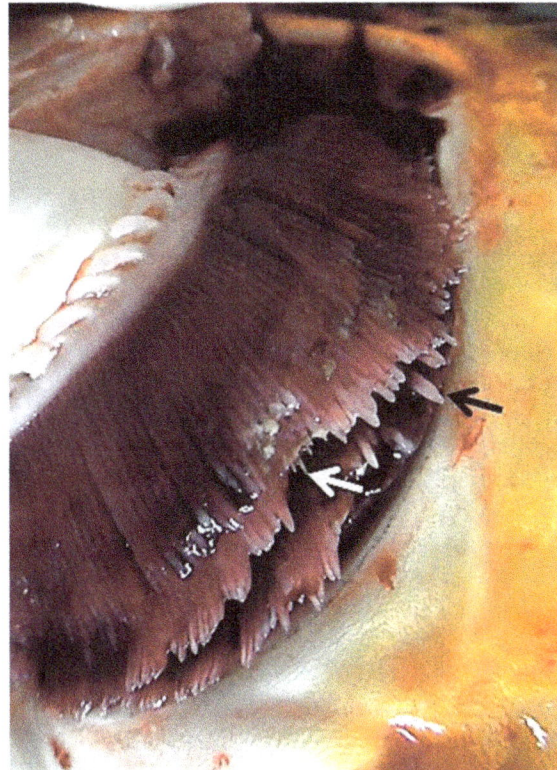

Fig. 2 Gills of CEV-infected Koi. Swelling of the primary filaments (black arrow) and necrosis of gill tissue (white arrow) can be seen

swabs from skin ulcerations and from internal organs. Gill tissues from humanely euthanized koi were fixed in 4 % buffered formalin, embedded into paraffin, cut, and stained with hematoxylin and eosin (HE staining) for histological evaluation [9]. For virological examination, samples of gills, kidney, gut, and brain were collected. Samples from 3 fish from different ponds were inoculated on Fathead Minnow (FHM) cells at 22 °C and on Common Carp Brain (CCB) cells at 25 °C for two passages of each 7 to 10 days according to standard procedures [10]. From all fish, DNA was isolated from tissue pools as well as from separate gill samples by DNA isolation kits (Qiagen, Germany, Macherey & Nagel, Germany). Samples were analysed for the presence of DNA sequences specific for cyprinid herpesviruses in general by an end point PCR described by Engelsma et al. [11] using KAPA2G Robust Hot Start PCR kit (Peqlab, Germany). For CyHV−3 samples were tested by real time PCR according to Gilad et al. [12] using Quantitect Multiplex qPCR Mix (Qiagen, Germany). DNA from gills was examined for the presence of CEV specific DNA sequences by end point PCR described by Oyamatsu et al. [13].

In 10 cases parasites could not be detected in skin and gill smears. A moderate to high amount of opportunistic freshwater bacteria, in particular *Aeromonas* spp., could be isolated from skin, while in samples taken from

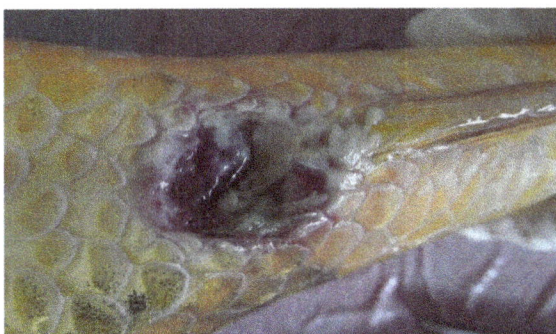

Fig. 1 Koi of this study showing an ulcerative inflammation of the anus. The koi was CEV-infected

internal organs no bacterial growth was found. In the histological examination gill tissue of diseased fish showed hyperplasia and clubbing of primary gill filaments, thickening, and edema of epithelial cells in secondary filaments and a detachment of epithelial cells (Fig. 3).

Cytopathic effect was not observed in any of the virus isolations. In PCR analyses none of the samples gave positive results for cyprinid herpesviruses, including CyHV–3. By analysing gill tissues for CEV, 7 out of 11 samples showed PCR products of 547 bp and 180 bp (by using nested primers) which were sequenced (LGC Genomics, Berlin, Germany). In the German reference laboratory for koi herpesvirus disease at the Friedrich Loeffler-Institut the sequences were compared to sequences obtained from positive CEV material from the OIE reference laboratory in Weymouth (CEFAS, UK), the Wildlife, and Aquatic Veterinary Disease Laboratory in Gainesville, Florida (WAVDL, USA), and to the sequence published in the PhD Thesis of Oyamatsu [14]. Nucleotide comparisons with the original sequence from Oyamatsu [14] revealed greater than 96 % sequence identity, confirming CEV was detected in this study (Additional file 1). The received sequence was added to gene bank (Gene Bank ID: KM283182). Furthermore, transmission electron microscopy studies performed at WAVDL have revealed that samples from koi positive for CEV by PCR also yield poxvirus-like virions (Fig. 4) within infected gill epithelial cells as has been repeatedly reported [3, 6, 15].

The disease induced by CEV occurs at a temperature range similar to KHVD and also develops similar clinical signs [16]. In particular gill and skin alterations, delineated as characteristic in outbreaks of KHVD [2], were also recorded from clinical KSD [6, 15]. In the cases described here, most affected koi showed profound gill necrosis. In the few PCR positive fish that displayed

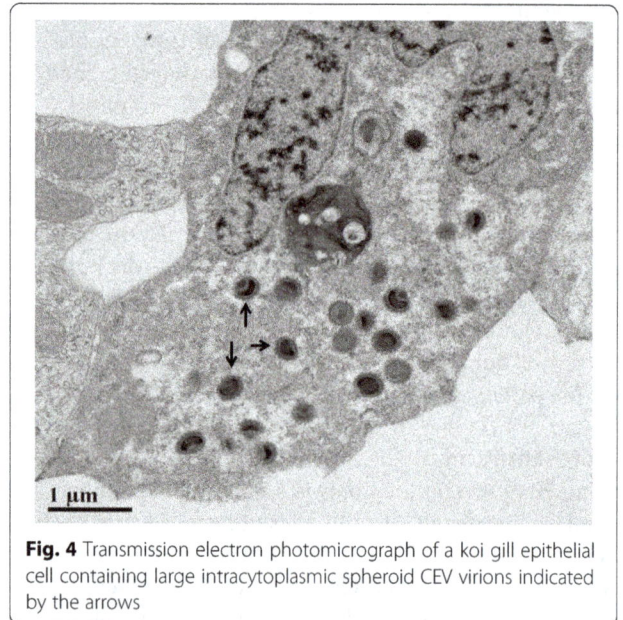

Fig. 4 Transmission electron photomicrograph of a koi gill epithelial cell containing large intracytoplasmic spheroid CEV virions indicated by the arrows

normal gills during gross examinations, histological changes were noted including hyperplasia of gill tissue consistent with previous reports on CEV [6, 7]. Additionally an inflammation of the anus was detected in many cases. The similarity of the clinical signs of KHVD and KSD complicate diagnosis. During the past years in our practice several cases of mortality in koi associated with gill necrosis were observed without detection of CyHV–3 or a severe gill infection with parasites or bacteria. Some of those cases could be related to an infection with CEV, but this would need testing to confirm.

An infection with a CEV-like virus was also detected in stocks of clinically healthy koi imported from Israel and Japan to the UK [7]. Hence, trading clinically healthy but CEV infected koi might promote spread of KSD, not only to ornamental koi but also to European carp aquaculture. A CEV-like virus was already detected in cultured common carp undergoing mortality and displaying clinical disease in the UK in March 2012 [7].

Conclusion

This is the first report of CEV detection related to KSD outbreaks in Germany. It further confirms the presence of Carp Edema Virus in European koi populations. We recommend to include the CEV PCR into routine diagnostics.

Fish health services of continental Europe should be aware of the presence of CEV in Europe which may result in high losses in carp aquaculture. Action should be taken to prevent transmission of CEV from koi to common carp. Infections with CEV might be treated as an emerging disease in Germany. Therefore it is considered, if, and what kind of action according to EU directive 2006/88/EG is necessary in the case of koi sleepy

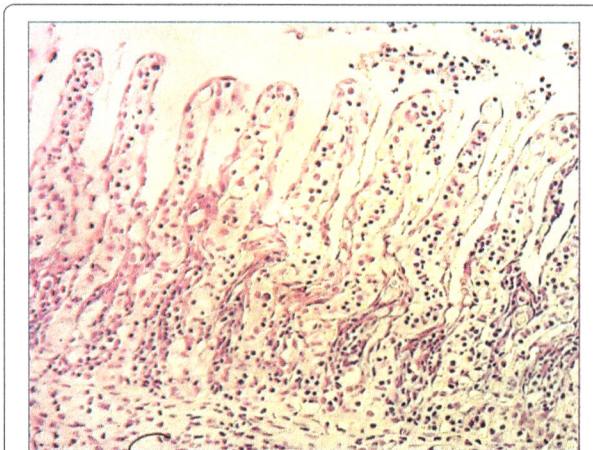

Fig. 3 Histopathology of gill tissue of a CEV-infected koi showing cell edema and detachment of epithelial cells. HE staining at 400 × magnification

disease outbreaks. European countries should avoid the spread of CEV infections in Europe like it happened with KHVD, where surveillance programs were established too late to prevent spread of the disease. Therefore, testing koi, and carp for CEV should become part of fish disease surveillance programs of national and regional fish disease laboratories.

Additional file

Additional file 1: Comparison of the sequence obtained in this study to the sequence published in the PhD Thesis of T. Oyamatsu (Reference 14).

Competing interests

The authors declare that they have no competing interests.

Authors' contributions

VJS performed clinical examinations, collected samples, advices the owners, was responsible for contacting the reference laboratory and the veterinary agency and wrote the manuscript. MA was responsible for the molecular examinations and assisted in writing the manuscript. FT and JH performed clinical examinations and collected samples. SMB, HS, KW, TW, SH, and DSto analyzed the sequences and confirmed the diagnosis. TW and SH performed the transmission electron microscopy. DWK was responsible for contacting the ministry. MR performed the testing for CyHV–3 infection. BK performed cell culture examinations. DSth was responsible for contacting researchers and assisted in writing the manuscript. VJS, MA, SMB, HS, KW, DSto, DWK, and DSth were involved in a case advisory board. All authors read and approved the final manuscript.

Author details

[1]Fish Disease Research Unit, University of Veterinary Medicine, Hannover, Germany. [2]Friedrich-Loeffler-Institut, Federal Research Institute for Animal Health, Institute of Infectology, Greifswald, Germany. [3]Lower Saxony State Office for Consumer Protection and Food Safety, Veterinary Task-Force, Hannover, Germany. [4]Centre for Environment, Fisheries, and Aquaculture Science (CEFAS), Weymouth, Dorset, UK. [5]Lower Saxony State Office for Consumer Protection and Food Safety, Food and Veterinary Institute Braunschweig/Hannover, Hannover, Germany. [6]Department of Infectious Diseases and Pathology, University of Florida, College of Veterinary Medicine, Gainesville, FL, USA.

References

1. Amita K, Oe M, Matoyama H, Yamaguchi N, Fukuda H. A survey of koi herpesvirus and carp edema virus in colorcarp cultured in Niigata Prefecture. Japan Fish Pathol. 2002;37(4):197–8.
2. Hedrick RP, Gilad O, Yun S, Spangenberg JV, Marty GD, Nordhausen RW, et al. A herpesvirus associated with mass mortality of juvenile and adult koi, a strain of common carp. J Aquat Anim Health. 2000;12(1):44–57.
3. Oyamatsu T, Hata N, Yamada K, Sano T, Fukuda H. An etiological study on mass mortality of cultured colorcarp juveniles showing edema. Fish Pathol. 1997;32(2):81–8.
4. OIE: Aquatic Animal Health Code, Chapter 10.6. Koi Herpesvirus Disease. 2012;1–6.
5. Council Directive 2006/88/EC of 24 October 2006 on animal health requirements for aquaculture animals and products thereof, and on the prevention and control of certain diseases in aquatic animals. 2006;1–56.
6. Miyazaki T, Isshiki T, Katsuyuki H. Histopathological and electron microscopy studies on sleepy disease of koi Cyprinus carpio koi in Japan. Dis Aquat Organ. 2005;65(3):197–207.
7. Way K, Stone D. Emergence of Carp edema virus-like (CEV-like) disease in the UK. CEFAS Finfish News. 2013;15:32–4.
8. Haenen O, Way K, Stone D, Engelsma M. "Koi Sleepy Disease" voor het eerst in Nederland aangetoond in koikarpers. Tijdschr Diergeneeskd. 2014;4:26–9.
9. Romeis B. Mikroskopische Technik, 16th edition edn: R. Oldenbourg Verlag München Wien; 1968.
10. Freshny RI. Culture of Animal Cells, A manual of basic technique. 3 ednth ed. New York: Wiley-Liss; 1994.
11. Engelsma MY, Way K, Dodge MJ, Voorbergen-Laarman M, Panzarin V, Abbadi M, et al. Detection of novel strains of cyprinid herpesvirus closely related to koi herpesvirus. Dis Aquat Organ. 2013;107(2):113–20.
12. Gilad O, Yun S, Zagmutt-Vergara FJ, Leutenegger CM, Bercovier H, Hedrick RP. Concentrations of a Koi herpesvirus (KHV) in tissues of experimentally infected Cyprinus carpio koi as assessed by real-time TaqMan PCR. Dis Aquat Organ. 2004;60(3):179–87.
13. Oyamatsu T, Matoyama H, Yamamoto K, Fukuda H. A trial for detection of carp edema virus by using polymerase chain reaction. Aquac Science. 1997;45(2):247–51.
14. Oyamatsu T. 1996. コイの浮腫症に関する研究. 東京水産大学博士学位論文 平成8年度 (1996) 資源育成学 課程博士 甲第142号; Study on edema disease of carp. Dissertation (1996) No. 142:1–109. Tokyo University of Fisheries [In Japanese].
15. Ono SI, Nagai A, Sugai N. A histopathological study on Juvenile Colorcarp, Cyprinus-Carpio showing edema. Fish Pathol. 1986;21(3):167–75.
16. Gilad O, Yun S, Adkison MA, Way K, Willits NH, Bercovier H, et al. Molecular comparison of isolates of an emerging fish pathogen, koi herpesvirus, and the effect of water temperature on mortality of experimentally infected koi. J Gen Virol. 2003;84:2661–8.

19

Rapid and specific detection of porcine parvovirus using real-time PCR and High Resolution Melting (HRM) analysis

Hai-Qiong Yu[1†], Xian-Quan Cai[2*†], Zhi-Xiong Lin[1], Xiang-Li Li[3], Qiao-Yun Yue[2], Rong Li[2] and Xing-Quan Zhu[4*]

Abstract

Background: Porcine parvovirus (PPV) is the important causative agent for infectious infertility, which is a fairly tough virus that multiplies normally in the intestine of pigs without causing clinical signs in the world.

Results: We developed an assay integrating real-time PCR and high resolution melting (HRM) analysis for the detection of PPV. Primers targeting the VP gene were highly specific, as evidenced by the negative amplification of closely related viruses, such as porcine circovirus 2 (PCV2), porcine reproductive and respiratory syndrome virus (PRRSV), pseudorabies virus (PRV), classical swine fever virus (CSFV), or Japanese encephalitis virus (JEV). The performance of unlabeled real time PCR was compared to TaqMan real time PCR, and the detection limits of the two methods were nearly equal. Moreover, there was good correlation between Cp and diluted genomic DNA when tested with the two methods. The assay has the accuracy of 100% in reference to labeled real time PCR, when it was tested on 45 clinical samples.

Conclusions: The present study demonstrated that the established assay integrating real-time PCR and HRM is relatively cost-effective and more stable, which provides an alternative tool for rapid, simple, specific and sensitive detection of PPV.

Keywords: Porcine parvovirus (PPV), High resolution melting (HRM), Real-time PCR

Background

Porcine parvovirus (PPV) is a major cause of reproductive failure in pigs. The PPV is a very resistant virus that can survive without a host for several months, which makes it difficult to remove the virus from the pig herd and its environment [1]. PPV does not cause clinical signs at any other time than during pregnancy, when it may cross the placenta and infect developing embryos and fetuses, resulting in resorption and mummification, abortion, stillbirth, neonatal death and reduced neonatal vitality [2]. PPV has been reported in many countries. Furthermore, although PPV has little if any effect on mature boars, they may act as non-infected carriers [3].

Several methods have been developed for rapid detection of PPV, including specific PCR, ELISA and LAMP [4-6]. Real-time PCR applications can be completed rapidly since no post-amplification modifications were required [7,8]. The analysis of amplified products by means of probes or melt curve analysis is furthermore highly accurate compared to analysis on agar gels. However, the probe-based real time PCR requires synthesis of the probe, which will increase the cost, and the probe is prone to degradation. Recently, high-resolution melting (HRM) for high-throughput analysis of many pathogens has been developed, for example, for variation scanning [9], genotyping [10] and species determination [11]. As different amplicons produce distinct melting curves, these can easily be compared to a reference melting curve to determine the identity of the amplicon [12]. Here, we developed a real-time PCR assay coupled with HRM analysis for the rapid and specific detection of PPV.

* Correspondence: caixianquan@126.com; xingquanzhu1@hotmail.com
†Equal contributors
2Technical Center, Zhongshan Entry-Exit Inspection and Quarantine Bureau, Zhongshan, Guangdong Province 528403, PR China
4State Key Laboratory of Veterinary Etiological Biology, Lanzhou Veterinary Research Institute, Chinese Academy of Agricultural Sciences, Lanzhou, Gansu Province 730046, PR China
Full list of author information is available at the end of the article

Methods

Ethics statement

This study was performed in strict accordance with the recommendations of the Animal Ethics Procedures and Guidelines of the People's Republic of China. The protocol was approved by the Animal Ethics Committee of Lanzhou Veterinary Research Institute, Chinese Academy of Agricultural Sciences (Permit No: LVRIAEC2013-010). Every effort was made to minimize suffering of the examined pigs.

Genomic DNA extraction

A total of 45 pig tissue samples (liver, lung, spleen and kidney), suspected of being infected with PPV from different pig farms in Guangdong Province, China, were collected by The Center of Quality Test and Supervision for Breeding Swine (Guangzhou). The pigs suffered from a variety of clinical signs such as respiratory diseases, systemic diseases, diarrhea, or reproductive disorders. The ages of the pigs sampled ranged from neonatal to adult. One gram of the tissue was minced and diluted 1:10 in Dulbecco's Modified Eagle Medium (DMEM). Homogenization was carried out in a Stomacher 80. 60 μL extraction buffer and 10 μl proteinase K were added to 100 μl tissue homogenate supernatant, or cell culture inoculated with reference virus or closely related viruses. The mixture was incubated at 50°C for 2 h, DNA extractions were carried out with phenol/chloroform (1:1), refrigerated and centrifuged at 10000 rpm. Precipitation was performed with 95% ethanol for 18 h at -20°C and pellets were diluted in 25 μl sterile distilled water.

Real time PCR detection of PPV with HRM analysis

Unlabelled real-time PCR amplification was performed in Lightcycler 480 (Roche, USA). A pair of primers designed targeting the VP1 gene, which is very important for PPV positioning within the host nucleus (sense: 5'-TCACCAAACAATTAATAATAGC-3'; PPV; antisense: 5'- GGTTCATCATCATTATATTGTG-3') was synthesized by Takara Biotechnology (Dalian, China). The total reaction volume was 20 μl, consisted of 1 × HRM master mix (Roche, USA), 0.35 μM of each primer and 1 μl DNA as template. The PCR was carried out with initiation at 94°C for 10 min, followed by 10 cycles of 94°C, 30 s; annealing temperature step downs every 2 cycles of 1.0°C (from 63°C to 54°C). The annealing temperature for the final 25 cycles was 59°C with denaturation and extension phases as above. When PCR amplification was completed, HRM analysis was performed by lowering the temperature to 60°C for 5 min, followed by increasing the temperature ramping from 60°C to 95°C at 0.11°C/s, 25 acquisitions/°C. In this process, the PCR amplicons were allowed to denature and re-anneal in fluorescence with changes in temperature (dF/dT). The HRM profile was then analyzed using HRM analysis software, as reported previously [13].

Real time PCR detection of PPV using TaqMan probe

The primers and probe were synthesized by Takara Biotechnology (Dalian, China) according to previous studies [7] targeting the VP2 gene as follows: (sense: 5-CCAA AAATGCAAACCCCAATA-3, antisense: 5-TCTGGCG GTGTTGGAGTTAAG-3), which amplified a fragment of 194 bp in length. The TaqMan probe, FAM- CTT GGAGCCGTGGAGCGAGCC-TAMRA, was used to detect any amplification. The real-time PCR amplification was carried out in a reaction mix of 20 μl TaqMan reaction mix consisted of 2.0 μl of 10× buffer, 0.4 μl of 10 mM dNTP, 3.6 μl of 25 mM MgCl$_2$, 0.2 μl of 10 μM fluorogenic FAM-labeled PPV probe, 0.4 μl of 10 μM forward primer, 0.4 μl of 10 μM reverse primer, and 1 μl of DNA solution. The thermal conditions were as follows: one cycle at 94°C for 5 min; followed by 45 cycles at 94°C for 5 s, 60°C for 15 s. PCR amplification was performed by using the same thermal cycler LC 480 (Roche, USA).

Results

Specificity of the detection assay and confirmation of amplicon identity

The specificity of the primers was determined by performing PCR using pure genomic DNA from closely related viruses, including porcine circovirus 2 (PCV2), porcine reproductive and respiratory syndrome virus (PRRSV), pseudorabies virus (PRV), classical swine fever virus (CSFV), or Japanese encephalitis virus (JEV). No fluorescence signal was detected from all the 'heterologous control samples', as mentioned above. Moreover, A BLAST search of the chosen primers resulted in a hit of the target sequence in PPV, suggesting the specificity of the primers. To ensure the accuracy of the method, all amplicons were sequenced and proved highly homologous to corresponding sequences.

Detection limit and correlation between Cp and diluted DNA

In order to evaluate the detection limit and correlation of the real-time PCR coupled with HRM analysis, the sensitivity of the real-time PCR was compared with a TaqMan real time PCR reported previously [7], serial dilutions of plasmid between 10^7 copies and 10^1 copies per reaction or 10-fold diluted genomic DNA was tested. Standard curves were generated using the protocol described above. The assay approaches the sensitivity of TaqMan real time PCR (Figure 1).

One pg genomic DNA and plasmid DNA of 10^1 copies can be detected easily by both methods. The amplification curve evenly raised when applied with 0.1 pg viral DNA,

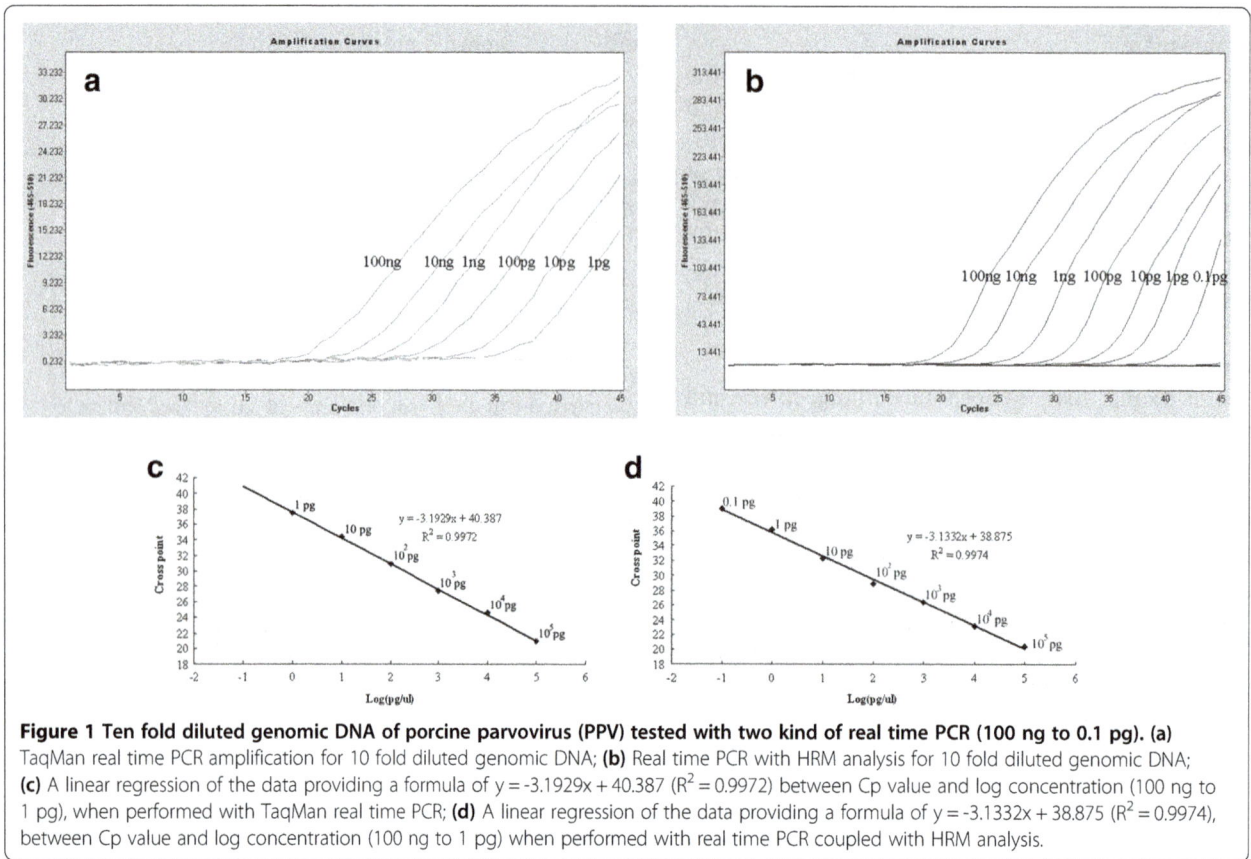

Figure 1 Ten fold diluted genomic DNA of porcine parvovirus (PPV) tested with two kind of real time PCR (100 ng to 0.1 pg). (a) TaqMan real time PCR amplification for 10 fold diluted genomic DNA; **(b)** Real time PCR with HRM analysis for 10 fold diluted genomic DNA; **(c)** A linear regression of the data providing a formula of y = -3.1929x + 40.387 (R² = 0.9972) between Cp value and log concentration (100 ng to 1 pg), when performed with TaqMan real time PCR; **(d)** A linear regression of the data providing a formula of y = -3.1332x + 38.875 (R² = 0.9974), between Cp value and log concentration (100 ng to 1 pg) when performed with real time PCR coupled with HRM analysis.

but the melting curve shape of low amount DNA (0.1 pg) is obviously different with other dilutions (Figure 2b), and the Tm of 0.1 pg PPV DNA is 81.28°C while Tm of others dilutions is 80.76 ± 0.06°C. A good correlation was acquired. The formula between Cp value and concentration (100 ng to 1 pg) is y = -3.1929x + 40.387 (R² = 0.9972), when performed with TaqMan real time PCR (Figure 1c), while it is y = -3.1332x + 38.875 (R² = 0.9974), when performed with real time PCR coupled with HRM analysis (Figure 1d).

Testing of clinical samples

Forty-five clinical pig samples were tested using both the real time PCR coupled with HRM analysis and TaqMan real time PCR. Results of the two assays were 100% consistent, and both methods showed that 12 of the examined samples were positive, while 33 were negative.

HRM analysis

Constant HRM profiles with distinct Tm peaks were persistently obtained for all field samples and 10 diluted

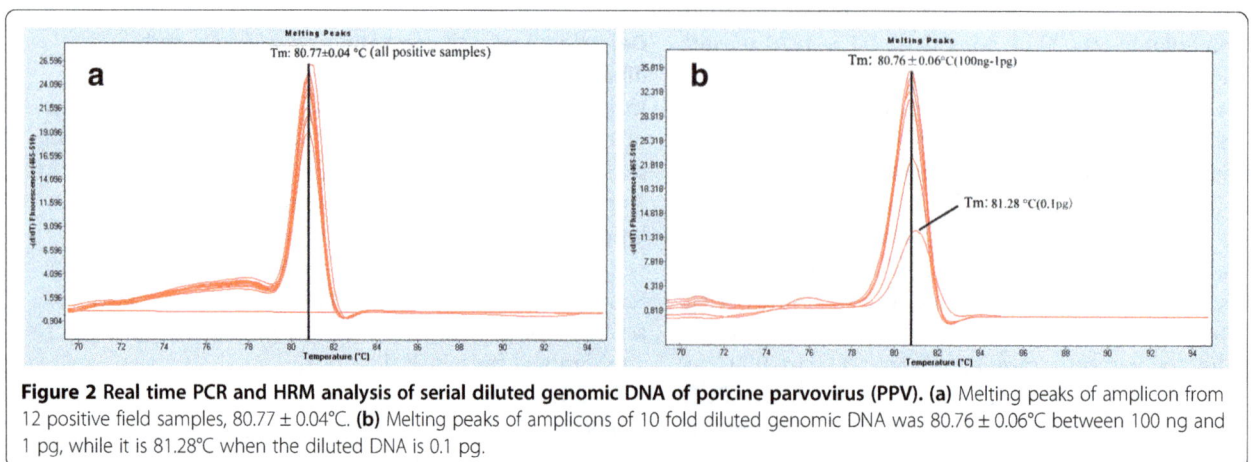

Figure 2 Real time PCR and HRM analysis of serial diluted genomic DNA of porcine parvovirus (PPV). (a) Melting peaks of amplicon from 12 positive field samples, 80.77 ± 0.04°C. **(b)** Melting peaks of amplicons of 10 fold diluted genomic DNA was 80.76 ± 0.06°C between 100 ng and 1 pg, while it is 81.28°C when the diluted DNA is 0.1 pg.

standard DNA. As shown in Figure 2, there is only one kind of characteristic profiles. The amplification products from all 12 positive samples had a Tm of 80.77 ± 0.04°C, and the 10 diluted standard DNA (100 ng - 1 pg) had a Tm of 80.76 ± 0.06°C. To ensure the accuracy of the method, the amplified products were sequenced. The results showed that all sequences were uniform with the HRM analysis results. The HRM analysis with different concentrations of the template appeared to be reliable, while the profile is unsatisfactory when the concentrations was 0.1 pg such as obviously different melting curve (Figure 2c), which is consistent with a previous report [13].

Discussion

Diagnosis of PPV infection is very important for effective treatment and controlling the spread of infections. Here, we developed an unlabelled real-time PCR coupled with HRM assay targeting the VP1 gene which has been proven critical to replication efficiency in cell culture [14]. The data showed that there is a 26.7% positivity of all tested samples, which is lower than that of a previous study (41.6%) [5]. The reason may attribute to diverse regions and different sample sizes.

Melt curve analysis (MCA) is well known for identification of amplicons, but classical MCA can only distinguish gross differences (0.5°C) between PCR products [15], which will possibly make mistakes when tested with closely related viruses. HRM curve analysis allows for the detection of subtle sequence variations between products and provides a much more accurate comparison between amplicons [16]. Important to note is that this feature is mainly due to the binding characteristics of new generation dyes such as LC Green, which will saturates the molecule preventing dye relocation during the melting process. However, classical MCA was commonly applied with non-saturating dyes such as SYBR Green I.

To date, various detection and diagnostic techniques for detection of PPV have been developed [4-8]. There are, however, many drawbacks to these methods, for example, crude or recombinant antigens have been reported, however, the specificity and sensitivity of these methods are still in great need of improvement. TaqMan real-time PCR requires expensive probe, and LAMP has high risk of contamination.

Here, a touchdown PCR protocol was used that covers a range of annealing temperature between 63°C and 54°C. With touchdown PCR, a relatively high annealing temperature was used in the early cycles of PCR to ensure high accuracy of priming and amplification. Decreasing the annealing temperature in later cycles guarantees adequate amounts of PCR amplicons. With the help of saturates dyes such as LC green, the fluorescence of unlabelled real time PCR was nearly 10-fold

stronger than TaqMan real time PCR (Figure 1b). It is well known that positive results should be proven by the obviously rising curve and exact temperature of melting (Tm) when tested with HRM. As shown in Figure 1, there is an ascending curve with 0.1 pg viral DNA, but the Tm of 0.1 pg PPV DNA is 81.28°C, while Tm of other dilutions is 80.76 ± 0.06°C. Hence, our results is not enough to prove that 0.1 pg PPV DNA can be accurately detected by HRM, so we could not conclude that it is more sensitive than TaqMan real time PCR. Less sensitivity of TaqMan real time assay was previously reported, because only single point mutation in TaqMan probe will decrease the sensitivity by 47% [17], other reasons for example, inefficiency of 5' exonuclease, and repeatedly thawing of probe may also contribute to it.

Conclusions

The present study demonstrated that the real-time PCR platform coupled with HRM is an alternative tool for rapid, simple, specific and sensitive detection of PPV, which reduces turnaround time of the assay to almost 1 h, eliminates the risk of contamination, and saves expense. These features make it advantages for use in laboratories, and therefore could be a useful tool for determining the infected individuals.

Competing interests
The authors declare that they have no competing interests.

Authors' contributions
HQY, XQC and XQZ conceived and designed the study. HQY, XQC, ZXL and XLL performed the experiments and analyzed the data. QYY and RL helped in the study design and manuscript revision. HQY, XQC and XQZ wrote the manuscript. All authors read and approved the final manuscript.

Acknowledgements
Project support was provided by the Science & Technology Program of Zhongshan (Grant No. 20123A299), the Science & Technology Program of Guangdong Inspection and Quarantine Bureau (Grant No. 2011GDK053 and 2014GDK50) and the Science Fund for Creative Research Groups of Gansu Province (Grant No. 1210RJIA006).

Author details
[1]Technical Center, Guangdong Entry-Exit Inspection and Quarantine Bureau, Guangzhou, Guangdong Province 510630, PR China. [2]Technical Center, Zhongshan Entry-Exit Inspection and Quarantine Bureau, Zhongshan, Guangdong Province 528403, PR China. [3]Zhongshan Torch Polytechnic College, Zhongshan, Guangdong Province 528403, PR China. [4]State Key Laboratory of Veterinary Etiological Biology, Lanzhou Veterinary Research Institute, Chinese Academy of Agricultural Sciences, Lanzhou, Gansu Province 730046, PR China.

References
1.   Mengeling WL, Lager KM, Zimmerman JK, Samarikermani N, Beran GW. A current assessment of the role of porcine parvovirus as a cause of fetal porcine death. J Vet Diagn Invest. 1991;3:33–5.
2.   Hälli O, Ala-Kurikka E, Nokireki T, Skrzypczak T, Raunio-Saarnisto M, Peltoniemi OA, et al. Prevalence of and risk factors associated with viral and bacterial pathogens in farmed European wild boar. Vet J. 2012;194:98–101.

3.   Cságola A, Lőrincz M, Cadar D, Tombácz K, Biksi I, Tuboly T. Detection, prevalence and analysis of emerging porcine parvovirus infections. Arch Virol. 2012;157:1003–10.

4.   Soares RM, Durigon EL, Bersano JG, Richtzenhain LJ. Detection of porcine parvovirus DNA by the polymerase chain reaction assay using primers to the highly conserved nonstructural protein gene, NS-1. J Virol Methods. 1999;78:191–8.

5.   Roić B, Cajavec S, Toncić J, Madić J, Lipej Z, Jemersić L, et al. Prevalence of antibodies to porcine parvovirus in wild boars (Sus scrofa) in Croatia. J Wildl Dis. 2005;41:796–9.

6.   Chen HT, Zhang J, Yang SH, Ma LN, Ma YP, Liu XT, et al. Rapid detection of porcine parvovirus DNA by sensitive loop-mediated isothermal amplification. J Virol Methods. 2009;158:100–3.

7.   Chen HY, Li XK, Cui BA, Wei ZY, Li XS, Wang YB, et al. A TaqMan-based real-time polymerase chain reaction for the detection of porcine parvovirus. J Virol Methods. 2009;156:84–8.

8.   Song C, Zhu C, Zhang C, Cui S. Detection of porcine parvovirus using a TaqMan-based real-time pcr with primers and probe designed for the NS1 gene. Virol J. 2010;7:353.

9.   Nissen PH, Christensen SE, Ladefoged SA, Brixen K, Heickendorff L, Mosekilde L. Identification of rare and frequent variants of the CASR gene by high-resolution melting. Clin Chim Acta. 2012;413:605–11.

10. Zianni MR, Nikbakhtzadeh MR, Jackson BT, Panescu J, Foster WA. Rapid discrimination between *Anopheles gambiae*s.s. and *Anopheles arabiensis* by High-Resolution Melt (HRM) analysis. J Biomol Tech. 2013;24:1–7.

11. Tajiri-Utagawa E, Hara M, Takahashi K, Watanabe M, Wakita T. Development of a rapid high-throughput method for high-resolution melting analysis for routine detection and genotyping of noroviruses. J ClinMicrobiol. 2008;47:435–40.

12. Cousins MM, Swan D, Magaret CA, Hoover DR, Eshleman SH. Analysis of HIV using a High Resolution Melting (HRM) diversity assay: automation of HRM data analysis enhances the utility of the assay for analysis of HIV incidence. PLoS One. 2012;7:e51359.

13. Cai XQ, Yu HQ, Ruan ZX, Yang LL, Bai JS, Qiu DY, et al. Rapid detection and simultaneous genotyping of *Cronobacter* spp. (formerly *Enterobacter sakazakii*) in powdered infant formula using real-time PCR and high resolution melting (HRM) analysis. PLoS One. 2013;8:e67082.

14. Fernandes S1, Boisvert M, Tijssen P. Genetic elements in the VP region of porcine parvovirus are critical to replication efficiency in cell culture. J Virol. 2011;85:3025–9.

15. Zheng LL, Wang YB, Li MF, Chen HY, Guo XP, Geng JW, et al. Simultaneous detection of porcine parvovirus and porcine circovirus type 2 by duplex real-time PCR and amplicon melting curve analysis using SYBR Green. J Virol Methods. 2013;187:15–9.

16. Yuan J, Haroon M, Lightfoot D, Pelletier Y, Liu Q, Li XQ. A high-resolution melting approach for analyzing allelic expression dynamics. Curr Issues Mol Biol. 2009;11 Suppl 1:i1–9.

17. Richardson J, Molina-Cruz A, Salazar MI, Black W4th. Quantitative analysis of dengue-2 virus RNA during the extrinsic incubation period in individual *Aedes aegypti*. Am J Trop Med Hyg. 2006;74:132–41.

20

Development of vaccine-induced immunity against TRT in turkeys depends remarkably on the level of maternal antibodies and the age of birds on the day of vaccination

Marcin Smialek[*], Daria Pestka, Bartlomiej Tykalowski, Tomasz Stenzel and Andrzej Koncicki

Abstract

Background: Avian Metapneumovirus (aMPV) infections are a huge economical issue for the poultry industry worldwide. Although maternal antibodies do not protect turkey poults against turkey rhinotracheitis (TRT), almost no studies have been conducted so far regarding the impact of these antibodies on vaccine induced immunity development against aMPV infection. We conducted four experiments on commercial turkeys aimed at comparing local humoral and cell mediated immune response of maternally delivered anti-aMPV antibody positive (MDA+; Experiment I and II) and negative (MDA-; Experiment III and IV) turkeys following vaccination with an attenuated live aMPV subtype A vaccine at the day of hatch (Experiment I and III) or at two weeks of age (Experiment II and IV).

Results: Regardless of the birds' age, vaccination of MDA- turkeys resulted in strong stimulation of CD8$^+$ T lymphocytes in the Harderian gland and tracheal mucosa, whereas vaccination of MDA+ birds stimulated mainly CD4$^+$ T cells in those structures. An increase in the level of anti-aMPV IgY antibodies was noted in the serum (but not in tracheal washings) as early as 7 days after vaccination, but only in birds possessing low levels (MDA+ birds vaccinated at 2 weeks of age) or no maternal anti-aMPV antibodies at the time of vaccination. In MDA+ turkeys vaccinated at hatch, the decrease in serum levels of maternal anti-aMPV antibodies proceeded faster (in comparison to control group), which, together with faster viral clearance, indicates that maternal antibodies can inhibit vaccine virus replication and influence the development of vaccine-induced immunity.

Conclusion: This study provides the first documented evidence that the frequency of TRT outbreaks in the field and/or failure of TRT vaccination could be correlated with differences in the immunological status and/or age of vaccinated turkeys.

Keywords: Avian metapneumovirus, Turkeys, Vaccination, Humoral immunity, Cell mediated immunity, Maternally derived antibodies

Background

The avian metapneumovirus (aMPV), a member of the family *Paramyxoviridae*, genus *Metapneumovirus* [1], is a strongly infectious RNA virus that causes turkey rhinotracheitis (TRT) in flocks of turkeys and the swollen head syndrome (SHS) in chickens. aMPV infections cause massive financial losses in the poultry industry worldwide. aMPV was first identified in South Africa in 1978 [2], and since then, it has spread to numerous countries, excluding Australia and Canada. aMPV has been classified into 4 subtypes (A–D) based on its nucleotide sequence and antigen structure [3-5].

In most immunoprophylaxis programs, one-day-old turkey poults are administered live attenuated vaccines against TRT by coarse spray to provide the earliest possible protection of the upper respiratory tract against aMPV infections [6]. Despite the above, TRT outbreaks in the field are noted very frequently [7-9].

* Correspondence: marcin.smialek@uwm.edu.pl
Department of Poultry Diseases, Faculty of Veterinary Medicine, University of Warmia and Mazury, Oczapowskiego 13/14, 10-719 Olsztyn, Poland

Humoral immunity is strongly stimulated by vaccination or aMPV infection [7,10-13], but antibodies do not play a key role in protection against TRT and should not be considered as indicators of immunity against aMPV infections [7,9,11,12,14-16]. It has been shown, however, that high antibody titers suppress aMPV replication in the upper respiratory tract, thus alleviating the clinical course of TRT [6,11,12,14]. In one-day-old turkey poults, most of which originate from parent flocks vaccinated against TRT, the possible influence of maternal antibodies on the development of vaccine-induced immunity against aMPV is questionable.

Cell-mediated immunity (CMI) is increasingly often considered as the decisive factor in protection against TRT. Unfortunately, little is known about local CMI mechanisms in turkeys' upper respiratory tract during infections and after vaccination against TRT. These mechanisms seem to play a particularly important role because aMPV infects the host through mucosal sites in the upper respiratory tract. Liman and Rautenschlein [7] demonstrated a significant increase in the percentage of $CD4^+$ T lymphocytes with concurrent upregulation of IL-6 and/or IFN-γ in the Harderian gland (HG) after vaccination or infection with aMPV/A or B. Conversely, Cha [17] reported an increase in the percentage of $CD8^+$ T cells, but not in $CD4^+$ T cells, in the upper respiratory tract after aMPV/C inoculation. The cited results indicate that CMI actively participates in protection against aMPV infections and that local CMI mechanisms may be related to age and the aMPV subtype.

In view of the diverse immunopathogenesis of TRT, the aim of this study was to describe selected parameters of local CMI and humoral immunity in the upper respiratory tract of turkeys immunized against TRT with live attenuated aMPV/A vaccines. The specific goal of the study was to characterize the development of vaccine-induced immunity in variously-aged birds and in turkeys with, or without maternal anti – aMPV antibodies on the day of vaccination.

Methods

The experimental procedures and animal handling procedures were conducted with the approval of the Local Ethic Committee for Animal Experiments in Olsztyn, Poland (resolution No. 37/2011).

Turkeys and vaccination

The experiments were carried out on 568 commercial Hybrid Converter turkeys of both sexes. The birds were not vaccinated at hatchery, and the absence of aMPV genetic material in samples collected at hatch was confirmed by nested RT-PCR. The MDA+ group comprised 284 turkeys that were positive for maternally derived antibodies and were obtained from a parent flock

vaccinated against TRT (3 times with live aMPV/A vaccine and twice with inactivated vaccine). MDA+ birds were provided by the Grelavi S.A. hatchery (a Hendrix Genetics Company) in Kętrzyn, Poland. The MDA- group consisted of 284 turkeys that were negative for maternally derived antibodies and originated from a parent flock not vaccinated against TRT (reproductive flock from Canada). MDA- birds were provided by the Gerczak Nord-Pol Hatchery in Laseczno, Poland.

Turkeys were housed in isolated units maintained at a biosafety PCL 3 facility. Water and feed were given to birds *ad libitum*. Birds were vaccinated with aMPV/A strain BUT1 #8544 of lyophilized attenuated commercial vaccine. Each bird was inoculated with 10^4 of tissue culture infectious doses ($TCID_{50}$) per bird oculonasally. Unvaccinated birds received sterile vaccine diluent.

Experimental design
Experiment I

Experiment I was carried out on 160 one-day-old MDA+ turkeys. The birds were randomly divided into vaccinated (MDA+0/V) and unvaccinated (MDA+0/NV) groups. Before vaccination, samples were collected from 24 randomly selected turkeys for further analysis. The day of vaccination (hatch day) was termed zero day of life (DOL), and the results for samples collected on this day were marked as zero day post-vaccination (DPV).

Birds of both groups were raised to 14 DOL, and further samples were collected on 3, 7 and 14 DPV (from 20–24 birds in each group in each sampling).

In each sampling, choanal swabs (e-Swab, Copan Diagnostics, Canada) were collected from 5 birds for RT-PCR analysis (swabs were stored at –76°C until further analysis) and blood samples were collected from 15 birds. The birds were euthanized, and HG and trachea (TC, cut from the larynx to the cranial aperture of body cavity) were collected. HG and TC were pooled from 4–6 birds per sample (the number of birds per sample were equal in each sampling), which produced 4 samples of each organ for flow cytometry analysis. Tracheal washings were collected from 10 birds in each group by passing 1 ml of phosphate-buffered saline (PBS, pH 7.2, Sigma Aldrich, Germany) through the lumen of the trachea with a 2 ml syringe. The trachea was massaged gently to intensify the washing effect. Following centrifugation, the supernatant and serum samples were stored at –20°C for further use.

Experiment II

The experimental design was identical to that of Experiment I. The experiment was carried out on 124 MDA+ turkeys raised until 14 dol. On 14 DOL, samples were collected from 20 birds, and the remaining turkeys were divided randomly into vaccinated (MDA+14/V) and unvaccinated (MDA+14/NV) groups. Similarly to Experiment I, the results reported for samples that were collected before vaccination (14 DOL) represent 0 DPV, and further samples were collected on 3 (17 DOL), 7 (21 DOL) and 14 (28 DOL) DPV (from 16–20 birds in each group in each sampling).

Experiment III

Experiment III was carried out on 160 one-day-old MDA- turkeys. The experimental design and schedule, the day of vaccination and the sample collection protocol were identical to those described in Experiment I. Turkeys were divided into two groups of vaccinated (MDA-0/V) and unvaccinated (MDA-0/NV) birds.

Experiment IV

Experiment IV was carried out on 124 fourteen-day-old MDA- turkeys. The experimental design and schedule, the day of vaccination and the sample collection protocol were identical to those described in Experiment II. Turkeys were divided into two groups of vaccinated (MDA-14/V) and unvaccinated (MDA-14/NV) birds.

Isolation and determination of mononuclear cell counts

HG were homogenized in a manual Dounce tissue grinder in 3 ml of complete cell culture medium (RPMI – 1640, 10% Fetal Bovine Serum (FBS), 1% MEM Non-essential Amino Acids solution, 1% Penicillin – Streptomycin, 1% HEPES, 1% Sodium pyruvate, Sigma Aldrich, Germany) and filtered (70 μm mesh). After centrifugation in culture medium at 450 g for 10 min at 20°C, the supernatant was discarded and cell pellets were resuspended in 3 ml of 40% Percoll density gradient and gently layered on 3 ml of 60% Percoll. Percoll concentrations were obtained by combining 100% Percoll solution (Percoll with 10% Hank's balanced salt solution, Sigma Aldrich, Germany) with the appropriate amount of culture medium. Mononuclear cells were collected from the interphase after density centrifugation (20 min, 1900 g, 20°C) and washed twice in PBS with 5% FBS.

TC were cut into 2–3 mm pieces and placed in 100 ml an Erlenmeyer flask with 25 ml of DL-Dithiothreitol solution (RPMI – 1640, 5% FBS, 1% HEPES, 2 mM DL-Dithiothreitol, Sigma Aldrich, Germany) and incubated at room temperature for 5 min to remove epithelial cells with intraepithelial lymphocytes. TC were filtered (70 μm mesh), and flasks were rinsed with RPMI – 1640 before collagenase treatment. TC were placed in 25 ml of Collagenase type IV solution (RPMI – 1640, 1% HEPES, 1% Penicillin – Streptomycin, 200 Collagen Digestion Units/ml, Sigma Aldrich, Germany) and incubated at 38°C for 35 min to isolate lamina propria lymphocytes. TC were filtered (70 μm mesh) after incubation. Filtrates from both incubations were washed three times in culture medium. Final pellets of intraepithelial lymphocytes were merged with lamina propria lymphocytes from the same sample, they were washed and resuspended in 3 ml of 40% Percoll. The isolation procedure was identical to that involving HG. The obtained HG and TC mononuclear cells were resuspended in 1 ml of PBS, and the absolute lymphocyte counts (ALC)/ml were calculated for each sample with the Vi-cell XR (Beckman Coulter, USA) cell counter and cell viability analyzer.

Flow cytometry and dual platform analysis

2.5×10^5 (or 1.25×10^5, depending on the ALC) of viable mononuclear cells from HG or TC were stained with monoclonal Mouse anti-Chicken CD4 - FITC (clone 2–35) and CD8 - PE (clone 11–39) for T lymphocytes, or polyclonal Goat anti-Chicken IgM - FITC for B cells (AbD Serotec, UK), incubated for 30 min on ice and washed twice in PBS. The cells were analyzed with the FACSCanto II (BD, USA) flow cytometer.

Data acquisition was performed in FACSDiva Software 6.1.3. (BD, USA). Cells were analyzed and immunophenotyped in the FloJo 7.5.5 (Tree Star, USA). Relative cell counts (RCC) of T and B lymphocytes in HG and TC were established in the above environment.

Absolute cell counts (ACC) of T and B cells were calculated by dual platform analysis with the use of the following formula: ACC = (ALC * RCC)/100%. Data were expressed as the mean ACC of CD4$^+$ and CD8$^+$ T lymphocytes or the mean x-fold change in ACC of IgM$^+$ B lymphocytes in vaccinated groups relative to control groups.

Enzyme-linked immunosorbent assay (ELISA)

Sera and tracheal washings were tested for specific IgY anti-aMPV antibodies with the APV Ab ELISA kit (IDEXX Laboratories, USA). Sera of MDA- birds were diluted 100-fold rather than 500-fold (manufacturer's recommendations) to enhance detection of low antibody levels. 100-fold dilution, as a comparative to 500-fold, was also used in analyses of MDA+14/V and NV serum. Tracheal washings were incubated undiluted. Successive steps of the procedure were performed according to the manufacturer's recommendations. ELISA was carried out with the use of the Eppendorf epMotion 5075 LH automated pipetting station (Eppendorf, Germany), BioTek ELx405 automatic plate washer (BioTek, USA) and BioTek ELx800 plate reader (BioTek, USA). The sample to positive (S/P)-ratio was calculated based on the ODs and used to express the mean (S/P)-ratio +/– SD per group and per DPV.

Nested RT-PCR

Nested RT-PCR was performed in accordance with the protocol described in a previous study [18] with minor modifications. RNA was extracted from choanal swabs with the RNeasy Mini Kit (Qiagen, Germany) according to the manufacturer's recommendations. The concentrations and purity of extracted RNA were evaluated with the NanoDrop 2000 spectrophotometer (ThermoScientific, USA). Samples ranging from 1.8 to 2.0 of the OD 260/280 ratio were used for further analysis. RT was performed with the EnhancedAvian HS RT-PCR Kit (Sigma-Aldrich, USA) according to the manufacturer's recommendations. PCR was performed with the use of the HotStarTaq Plus Master Mix (Qiagen, Germany) and the vapo.protect (Eppendorf, Germany) thermocycler. The first PCR was carried out with 10 μl of HotStarTaq *Plus* DNA, 0.1 μl of 100 μM primers G1+A and G6, 6.8 μl of RNase-free water and 3 μl of cDNA. Nested PCR was performed with 10 μl of HotStarTaq *Plus* DNA, 0.1 μl of 100 μM primers G8+A and G5, 2 μl of CoralLoad PCR, 5.8 μl RNase-free water and 2 μl of the amplicon from the first PCR. Primer sequences and product sizes for every PCR are summarized in Table 1. Both PCRs had the following thermal profile: 95°C for 5 min, 30 cycles of 94°C for 1 min, 54°C for 45 s, 72°C for 45 s, and final elongation at 72°C for 10 min.

Nested PCR amplicons were analyzed in 2% agarose gel with 0.5 μl/ml of ethidium bromide dye (Sigma-Aldrich, USA). Electrophoresis results were visualized with GelDoc XR+ (Bio-Rad, USA).

Statistical analysis

The flow cytometry results were processed by Student's t-test for independent samples in Graphpad Prism 6 software (San Diego, USA) and results of serological examination by non-parametric Mann–Whitney U-test in Statistica PL V10. Differences were considered statistically significant at $p \leq 0.05$ and highly significant at $p \leq 0.01$.

Results

Absolute lymphocyte count

No statistical differences in absolute lymphocyte counts in HG and TC were observed between vaccinated and unvaccinated birds in all experiments, excluding ALC in TC in the MDA-14/V group. In this group, ALC in TC on 14 DPV increased significantly in comparison with control group (data not shown).

Table 1 Sequences of the oligonucleotide primers used in nested RT-PCR analysis and expected PCR product size

Primer	Sequence	Product size
G1+A	5'-GGGACAAGTATCTCTATG-3'	444 bp
G6	5'-CTGACAAATTGGTCCTGATT-3'	
G8+A	5'-CACTCACTGTTAGCGTCATA-3'	268 bp
G5	5'-CAAAGArCCAATAAGCCCA -3'	

Flow cytometry analysis of T cells

In Experiment I, a highly significant and significant increase in CD4+ T ACC was noted in the MDA+0/V group on day 7 and 14 PV in HG and TC, respectively, in comparison with virus-free birds (Figure 1A). In Experiment II, CD4+ T ACC did not increase significantly in vaccinated birds, but a brief increase of this parameter was reported in HG on 7 DPV in the MDA+14/V group. A significant decrease in CD4+ T ACC was observed in the MDA+14/V group on 7 DPV in TC in comparison with control (Figure 1B). The noted decrease was short-lived and no significant differences in the value of analyzed parameter were reported between groups in Experiment II on day 14 PV.

In Experiment III, significant increase in CD4+ T ACC was noted on 14 DPV in HG in the MDA-0/V group, whereas a significant decrease in this parameter was observed in TC on 7 DPV in comparison with unvaccinated birds (Figure 1C). In Experiment IV, a statistical increase in CD4+ T ACC on day 7 PV and a highly significant increase on day 14 PV were reported in HG of MDA-14/V birds, whereas a significant decrease in CD4+ T ACC in TC was observed on day 3 PV in comparison with unvaccinated turkeys (Figure 1D).

In Experiments I and II, no significant differences in T CD8+ ACC were observed in neither HG nor TC (Figures 2A and B). The number of these cells increased briefly in vaccinated birds (in particular in HG), but the observed changes were not statistically significant.

In Experiment III, a highly significant increase in CD8+ T ACC was reported in HG of MDA-0/V birds on days 7 and 14 PV, and a highly significant decrease in the analyzed parameter was observed in TC on 7 DPV in comparison with unvaccinated birds (Figure 2C). The recorded decrease in CD8+ T cell count was short-lived, and on 14 DPV, a highly significant increase in this parameter was reported in TC of vaccinated turkeys in comparison with virus-free birds.

The most prominent infiltration of CD8+ T cells induced by the vaccine virus was observed in Experiment IV. In the MDA-14/V group, a highly significant increase in CD8+ T ACC was noted in TC on days 7 and 14 PV and in HG on 7 DPV in comparison with control. T CD8+ cell counts in HG decreased significantly on 14 DPV (Figure 2D).

In Experiments III and IV, significant differences were also observed in double-positive CD4+CD8+ T ACC (data not shown). In Experiment III, a significant decrease in the absolute counts of double-positive T cells was reported in the MDA-0/V group in TC on day 7 PV. In Experiment IV, a highly significant increase in double-positive T ACC was noted in both HG and TC on 14 DPV. No statistical differences in CD4+CD8+ T

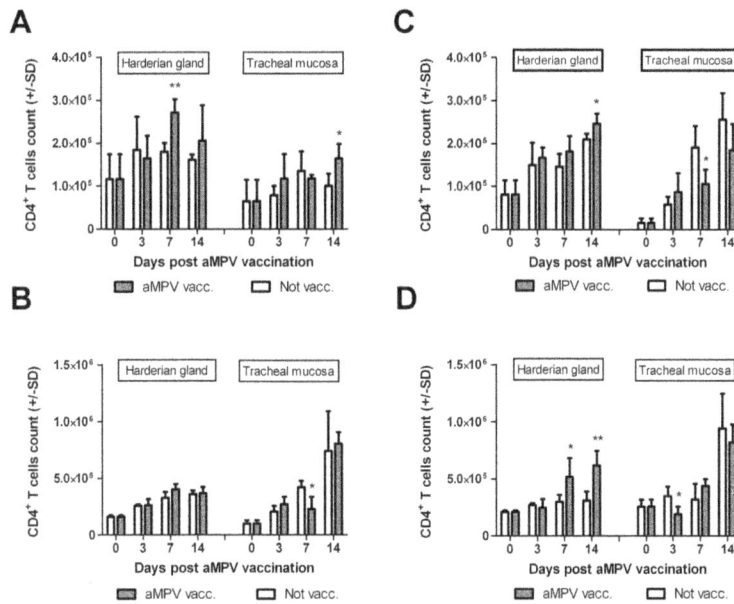

Figure 1 Summary of CD4+ ACC in HG and TC (n = 4) at different days post aMPV/A vaccination. Results for vaccinated (aMPV vacc.) and not vaccinated (Not vacc.) groups in different experiments **(A)** Experiment I; groups MDA+0/V and MDA+0/NV; **(B)** Experiment II; groups MDA+14/V and MDA+14/NV; **(C)** Experiment III; groups MDA-0/V and MDA-0/NV **(D)** Experiment IV; groups MDA-14/V and MDA-14/NV. Results for every experiment are presented as mean CD4+ ACC ± SD. */**Significant differences at different DPV (T-test, *as p < 0,05, **as p < 0,01).

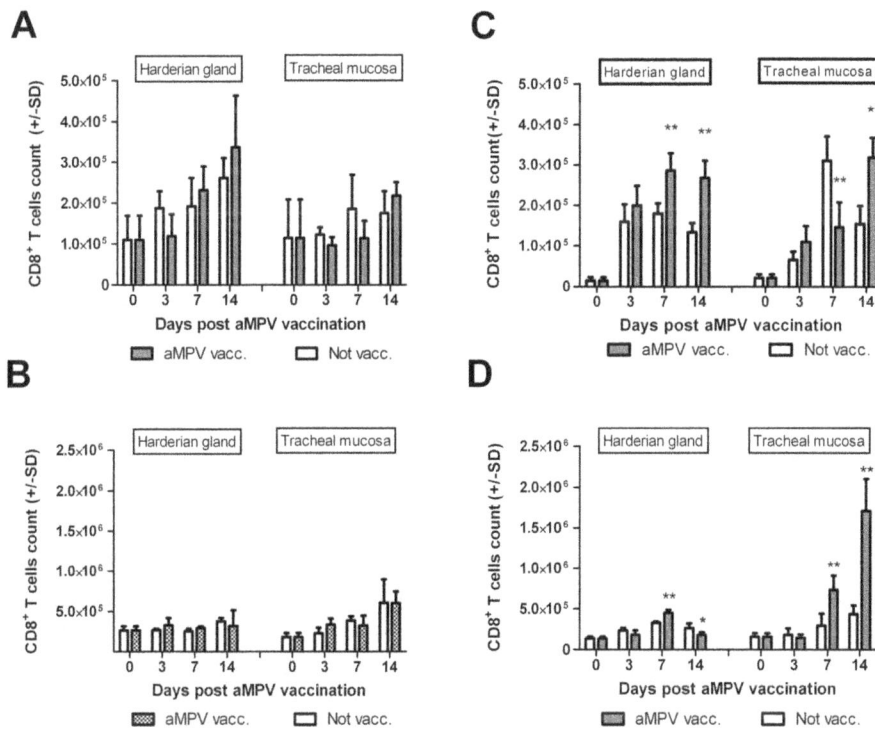

Figure 2 Summary of CD8+ ACC in HG and TC (n = 4) at different days post aMPV/A vaccination. Results for vaccinated (aMPV vacc.) and not vaccinated (Not vacc.) groups in different experiments **(A)** Experiment I; groups MDA+0/V and MDA+0/NV; **(B)** Experiment II; groups MDA+14/V and MDA+14/NV; **(C)** Experiment III; groups MDA-0/V and MDA-0/NV **(D)** Experiment IV; groups MDA-14/V and MDA-14/NV. Results for every experiment are presented as mean CD8+ ACC ± SD. */**Significant differences at different DPV (T-test, *as p < 0,05, **as p < 0,01).

ACC were observed between MDA+ vaccinated groups and unvaccinated birds (data not shown).

Flow cytometry analysis of B cells

In Experiment I, a significant decrease in B IgM^+ ACC in TC was observed in MDA+0/V on 7 DPV in comparison with the unvaccinated group (Table 2). The above decrease was transient, and no differences in B IgM^+ ACC were observed on day 14 PV.

In Experiment II, B IgM^+ ACC increased significantly in HG of MDA+14/V birds on 7 DPV (Table 2).

In Experiments III and IV, vaccination against TRT induced a highly significant increase in B IgM^+ cell counts in TC on 14 DPV (Table 2). In Experiment IV, the vaccine virus also caused a significant decrease in IgM^+ B cell count in HG of MDA-14/V birds on 14 DPV in comparison with control.

Serology

No statistical differences in the level of specific anti – aMPV antibodies in tracheal washes were observed between vaccinated and not vaccinated birds in any of the experiments (Table 3). In all MDA+ groups on the day of vaccination, in tracheal washes turkeys had detectable maternally derived antibodies (Table 3), and their level decreased with age in large part proportionally to their level in the serum. Only in MDA-14/V group the level of these antibodies increased in tracheal washes on day 14 PV, but this increase was not statistically significant (Table 3).

In Experiment I, high level of anti-aMPV antibodies were reported in the serum and tracheal washes on the day of vaccination. In the MDA+0/V group, mean (S/P)-ratios in the serum and tracheal washes decreased faster

than in unvaccinated birds. In most of cases, the observed decrease was not statistically significant, except on day 3 PV when mean serum antibody level were significantly lower in vaccinated turkeys than in unvaccinated birds (Table 4).

In Experiment II, MDA levels were detectable on vaccination day with the mean (S/P)-ratio (at 500-fold dilution) of 0.41 (data not shown), which is twice the recommended (S/P)-ratio (0.2) cut-off value. In the MDA+14/V group, MDA levels increased significantly on 14 DPV in comparison with unvaccinated birds, but differences were noted only when serum were diluted 100-fold (Table 4), and not 500-fold (data not shown).

In Experiment III and IV, anti-aMPV antibodies were not detected in the serum (at 100-fold dilution) or in tracheal washes on the day of vaccination (Tables 3 and 4). Serum level of anti-aMPV IgY antibodies in MDA-0/V increased gradually after vaccination and peaked significantly on 14 DPV (Table 4). Similar results were observed in Experiment IV, where serum antibody levels in MDA-14/V turkeys began to increase significantly (at 100-fold serum dilution) on 7 DPV, and increased further on 14 DPV (Table 4).

Molecular biology

The effectiveness of aMPV-A vaccine virus detection varied considerably between experiments. Between day 3 and 7 PV in Experiments I and III, aMPV RNA was detected by nested RT-PCR in 100% (5 out of 5) of choanal swabs in both MDA+0/V and MDA-0/V groups. On 14 DPV, aMPV RNA was detected in 40% (2/5) and 100% (5/5) of samples from groups MDA+0/V and MDA-0/V, respectively (Table 5).

In Experiment II, aMPV RNA was barely detectable in the MDA+14/V group. In this group, genetic material of the vaccine virus was identified only on day 3 PV in 40% (2/5) of choanal swabs. aMPV/A RNA was undetectable on days 7 and 14 PV (Table 5).

In Experiment IV, no viral RNA was detected at any stage of the experiment in choanal swabs of MDA-14/V birds (Table 5). The viral genome was not identified in unvaccinated birds in any experiments (data not shown).

Discussion

Different TRT vaccination schedules in parent flocks of turkeys are likely to cause highly variable transfer of specific anti-aMPV maternal antibodies to hatching poults. Although these antibodies do not protect turkey poults against TRT, their impact on the development of vaccine-induced immunity against aMPV infections has been investigated by very few studies. The present situation is problematic because most breeder turkey flocks are kept in areas with endemic prevalence of aMPV [19].

Table 2 Mean x-fold change of IgM^+ B ACC at days post aMPV vaccination[a] in HG and TC

| Experiment | Group | | Mean x-fold change[b] | | | |
			0	3	7	14
I	MDA+0/V	HG	1	0,72	1,33	0,88
		TC	1	0,83	0,75*	0,88
II	MDA+14/V	HG	1	1,23	1,49*	0,76
		TC	1	1,28	1,32	1,08
III	MDA-0/V	HG	1	1,24	0,85	0,89
		TC	1	1,31	0,91	1,66**
IV	MDA-14/V	HG	1	1,18	0,99	0,74*
		TC	1	0,78	1,17	3,31**

[a]In all experiments vaccinated birds were inoculated oculonassaly with 10^4 $TCID_{50}$ of live attenuated aMPV/A vaccine.

[b]x-fold change = mean IgM^+ B ACC of vaccinated group divided by mean IgM^+ B ACC of not vaccinated group.

*/**Significant difference in mean IgM^+ B ACC of vaccinated birds in comparison to the not vaccinated group (T-test, *as p < 0,05 and **as p < 0,01).

Table 3 Tracheal washings anti – aMPV IgY antibody level after aMPV vaccination[a] of turkeys

| Experiment | Group | Mean (S/P)-ratio ± S.D.[b] at days post aMPV/A vaccination | | | |
		0	3	7	14
I	MDA+0/V	1.152 ± 0.995	0.446 ± 0.476	0.117 ± 0.136	0.097 ± 0.102
	MDA+0/NV	1.152 ± 0.995	0.598 ± 0.695	0.123 ± 0.204	0.128 ± 0.097
III	MDA-0/V	0.00 ± 0.00	0.00 ± 0.00	0.00 ± 0.00	0.005 ± 0.011
	MDA-0/NV	0.00 ± 0.00	0.00 ± 0.00	0.00 ± 0.00	0.00 ± 0.00
II	MDA+14/V	0.128 ± 0.097	0.025 ± 0.036	0.022 ± 0.033	0.023 ± 0.025
	MDA+14/NV	0.128 ± 0.097	0.025 ± 0.039	0.031 ± 0.039	0.025 ± 0.042
IV	MDA-14/V	0.00 ± 0.00	0.00 ± 0.00	0.00 ± 0.00	0.029 ± 0.058
	MDA-14/NV	0.00 ± 0.00	0.00 ± 0.00	0.00 ± 0.00	0.00 ± 0.00

[a]In all experiments vaccinated birds were inoculated oculonassaly with 10^4 $TCID_{50}$ of live attenuated aMPV/A vaccine.
[b]10 samples of undiluted tracheal washings per group were analyzed.

Cook et al. [11,12] did not report any differences in the development of post-vaccination immunity between MDA+ and MDA- turkeys immunized with an attenuated aMPV strain (3B (Att.)) on 1 or 7 DOL. However, the attenuated aMPV strain used by the cited authors was characterized by a relatively high virulence index indicated by post-vaccination clinical scoring system. Contemporary TRT vaccines are less pathogenic, and they do not cause such acute side effects [20,21]. Re-evaluating research aiming to compare the development of vaccine-induced immunity to aMPV infections in MDA+ and MDA- birds has not been undertaken to date.

Liman and Rautenschlein [7] demonstrated that the percentage of $CD4^+$ T cells subpopulation (but not $CD8^+$ T cells) increased briefly in HG of turkeys 7–14 DPV after vaccination with aMPV/B or after infection with aMPV/A or B, which corroborates our results for MDA+ vaccinated birds. The cited authors suggested that the short-lived protection against TRT offered by vaccination and the frequency of TRT outbreaks could be explained by the transient character of the observed stimulation. Liman and Rautenschlein [7] analyzed turkeys from a breeder flock

immunized against TRT, and vaccinated the birds at the age of 33 days when specific anti-aMPV IgY antibodies could still be detected in their serum. Their findings corroborate our observations and indicate that the presence of maternal antibodies somehow protects the upper respiratory tract of turkeys against infiltration by $CD8^+$ T cells regardless of the birds' age. In this context, the presence of specific antibodies could contribute to the induction of aMPV/A immunophagocytosis through opsonization of the vaccine virus. The above observation is additionally validated by faster viral clearance in the upper respiratory tract and a significant decrease in MDA levels in MDA+0/V birds after vaccination.

Cha [17] demonstrated that inoculation of two-week old MDA- turkeys with aMPV/C increased the percentage of $CD8^+$ T cells in nasal turbinate mucosa, without inducing any changes in the percentage of $CD4^+$ T cells. Additionally, an increase in absolute counts of $CD4^+$ and $CD8^+$ T cells was reported in HG in MDA- chickens inoculated with aMPV/A or B [9], which is consistent with our results in MDA- vaccinated groups. The observed increase in absolute counts of both T cell

Table 4 Serum anti – aMPV IgY antibody level after aMPV vaccination[a] of turkeys

| Experiment | Group | Mean S/P-ratio ± S.D.[b] at days post aMPV/A vaccination | | | |
		0	3	7	14
I	MDA+0/V (1:500)[c]	2.19 ± 1.87	0.9 ± 0.51*	0.57 ± 0.5	0.23 ± 0.16
	MDA+0/NV (1:500)	2.19 ± 1.87	1.9 ± 1.36	0.6 ± 0.62	0.41 ± 0.36
III	MDA-0/V (1:100)	0.001 ± 0.00	0.006 ± 0.01	0.015 ± 0.017	0.179 ± 0.164**
	MDA-0/NV (1:100)	0.001 ± 0.00	0.005 ± 0.005	0.005 ± 0.008	0.00 ± 0.00
II	MDA+14/V (1:100)	0.598 ± 0.492	0.42 ± 0.361	0.21 ± 0.200	0.307 ± 0.217*
	MDA+14/NV (1:100)	0.598 ± 0.492	0.423 ± 0.345	0.228 ± 0.242	0.140 ± 0.116
IV	MDA-14/V (1:100)	0.00 ± 0.00	0.014 ± 0.038	0.034 ± 0.055*	0.123 ± 0.194*
	MDA-14/NV (1:100)	0.00 ± 0.00	0.00 ± 0.00	0.00 ± 0.00	0.00 ± 0.00

[a]In all experiments vaccinated birds were inoculated oculonassaly with 10^4 $TCID_{50}$ of live attenuated aMPV/A vaccine.
[b]15 samples of serum were analyzed per group.
[c]Sample dilution for ELISA procedure.
*/**Significant difference in mean (S/P)-ratio of vaccinated birds in comparison to the not vaccinated group (U-test, *as p < 0,05 and **as p < 0,01).

Table 5 Detection of aMPV genome in choanal swabs of aMPV vaccinated turkeys by nested RT-PCR

Group	Experiment	Number of aMPV/A positive birds/total[a] at days post vaccination			
		0	3	7	14
MDA+0/V	I	0/5	5/5	5/5	2/5
MDA-0/V	III	0/5	5/5	5/5	5/5
MDA+14/V	II	0/5	2/5	0/5	0/5
MDA-14/V	IV	0/5	0/5	0/5	0/5

[a]In all experiments vaccinated birds were inoculated oculonassaly with 10^4 TCID$_{50}$ of live attenuated aMPV/A vaccine.

subpopulations in HG and CD8$^+$ T lymphocytes in TC could indicate that CD4$^+$ T cells alone are unable to control the vaccine virus replication. Greater stimulation of vaccine-induced humoral immunity in MDA- vaccinated birds could indicate that the CD4$^+$ T cells are unable to maintain such metabolic pressure, which triggers the additional CD8$^+$ T cells infiltration in the upper respiratory tract of vaccinated turkeys.

Studies of other respiratory infections demonstrated that CD8$^+$ T memory cells confer immunity to reinfection by restricting the spread of the virus at the site of its replication [22,23] but in turn, they may be directly responsible for damage to the host's anatomical structures (e.g. mucous membranes) [24]. The question that arises in connection with our results is whether the presence of maternal antibodies interferes with the acquisition of T memory cells after vaccination against TRT. Further research is needed to examine the role of CD4$^+$ and/or CD8$^+$ T memory cells in protection against aMPV infections.

As demonstrated earlier, the TRT virus has immunosuppressive activity [25-28]. In our study a significant decrease in CD4$^+$ and/or CD8$^+$ T ACC in tracheal mucosa was noted in vaccinated birds 3–7 DPV in Experiments II - IV. Although, we can not assume that the above changes are indicative of T cell immunosuppression we may speculate that attenuated aMPV strains could also deliver such effects. Further research is necessary to establish whether aMPV vaccine strains possess immunosuppressive activity and if this activity *in vivo* could depend on specific antibody levels and birds' age on the day of vaccination.

The role of double positive CD4$^+$CD8$^+$ T cells in the host's immune response has not yet been fully elucidated, but in some production lines of hens those cells were found to represent a significant percentage of T lymphocytes in secondary immune structures [29]. Double-positive T cells could also have regulatory functions or could play the role of both T helper cells and cytotoxic T cells [30]. As it turned out in our study, this parameter varied significantly only in MDA- vaccinated turkeys.

Although most of the cited authors concluded their studies based on relative T cell count and not ACC,

these values are highly proportional. Therefore it can be concluded that differences exist in the development and activation of CMI in the upper respiratory tract of turkeys vaccinated against TRT, and that those variations are correlated mainly with the birds' age and maternal antibody level on the day of vaccination. The cited experiments produced similar results despite the use of different aMPV strains, which seems to suggest that differences in TRT immunopathogenesis are not strain-related [6,7,17].

In our study, MDA+0/V was the only group of vaccinated birds that did not produce anti-aMPV IgY antibodies in response to vaccination. On day 3 PV, anti-aMPV antibody level in the serum of MDA+0/V birds was significantly lower in comparison with unvaccinated birds. Those findings are partly consistent with results reported by Cook et al. [12] who did not observe an increase in serum levels of specific anti-aMPV antibodies in most MDA+ chickens vaccinated against TRT on the first day of life. In our experiment, a faster decrease in MDA levels in MDA+0/V birds after vaccination could be attributed to immunophagocytosis.

MDA+14/V and both MDA- vaccinated groups of turkeys responded to vaccination by producing specific IgY anti-aMPV antibodies that were detected in the serum (but not in tracheal washings) at 100-fold dilution on 14 DPV. In MDA-14/V birds, the level of those antibodies were elevated already on day 7 PV. Those results indicate that the level and the time required to induce humoral immunity after TRT vaccination are determined by age and MDA level on the day of vaccination. The above could impair early assessment of vaccine-induced immunity against TRT based on the results of routine serological monitoring which also has other disadvantages [4,31-33].

The absolute count of IgM$^+$ B cells is a general, nonspecific indicator of humoral immunity stimulation after vaccination. In this study, the only group of birds in which this parameter did not change or decreased significantly was MDA+0/V. A significant decrease in IgM$^+$ B ACC in HG was also reported in the MDA-14/V group on day 14 PV, but in this case, it was probably compensated by intensive IgM$^+$ B cell infiltration in tracheal mucosa.

Secretory IgA plays the main role in humoral immunity of upper respiratory tract. IgA$^+$ B cells and specific IgA participates in the local immune response against TRT in the upper respiratory tract [15]. Absolute counts of IgA$^+$ B cells and the levels of specific IgA were not determined in this study, but it could be hypothesized that, similarly to IgM$^+$ B cell infiltration and specific IgY production, the production of specific IgA could also depend on the MDA level and the age of birds on the day of vaccination against TRT. Further research is needed to determine the involvement of IgA$^+$ B cells and the role of IgA in protection against aMPV infections.

The observed differences in aMPV/A replication in nasal choanae between the MDA+0/V and MDA-0/V groups could be associated with high antibody levels in MDA+ birds upon vaccination. High levels of the these immunoglobulins probably facilitated and stimulated (upon immunophagocytosis) viral clearance from the upper respiratory tract, as suggested earlier by Cook et al. [11,12].

In both groups vaccinated on 14 DOL, aMPV/A RNA was practically undetectable in choanal swabs. Despite the above, the upper respiratory tract immune system was strongly stimulated in those groups after vaccination. Those results partially corroborate the findings of Rubbenstroth and Rautenschlein [16] who reported very high levels of vaccine-induced immunity against aMPV infections despite the fact the aMPV/A RNA was not regularly detected in nasal turbinates of turkeys vaccinated against TRT on 13 or 14 DOL. Differences between birds vaccinated at different age suggest that the replication of vaccine aMPV/A is limited during the maturation of the immune and/or respiratory system, but this does not influence the development of vaccine-induced immunity.

This work has some limitations. Given the fact that MDA+ and MDA- turkeys had different origin we were unable to perform statistical analysis of assayed parameters between them. However we could trace the diversity of their development after vaccination in each experiment in comparison to adequate not vaccinated control group. To ensure the reproducibility of the results, in each experiment, before the vaccination the birds were confirmed to be free (with PCR technique) from other common respiratory pathogens *Mycoplasma spp.*, *Ornithobacterium rhinotracheale*, *Bordetella avium* and Newcastle Disease Virus (data not shown). Experiments I and III as well as II and IV were performed simultaneously. Additionally, birds for experiment I and II as well as III and IV were obtained from the hatcheries at the same time.

Conclusion

Previous studies demonstrated that, under laboratory conditions, the live attenuated vaccines are highly efficient in protecting against TRT [7,9,17,21]. On the other hand, despite vaccination, TRT outbreaks are frequently observed in the field [7-9], which may stem not only from aMPV high virulence but, additionally, from differences in post-vaccination immunity development in birds with diversified immunological status and from the impact of other negative environmental and microbiological agents.

From the perspective of our study, at least a few pathomechanisms of this adverse situation may be concluded: (I) possible immunosuppressive activity of aMPV vaccine strains causing disorders in T cells activity or T cells activation, (II) possible disorders in antigen specificity acquisition of B and/or T lymphocytes in MDA+ groups, (III) high infiltration of CD8$^+$ T lymphocytes in TC of MDA- groups, that (most likely) is not neutral to the morphology of tracheal mucosa, as well as (IV) temporary character of CD4$^+$ T lymphocytes increase in the upper respiratory tract of MDA+ birds.

Abbreviations
ACC: Absolute cell count; ALC: Absolute lymphocyte count; aMPV: Avian Metapneumovirus; CMI: Cell mediated immunity; DPV: Days post vaccination; FBS: Fetal bovine serum; HG: Harderian gland; IFN: Interferon; IL: Interleukin; MDA: Maternally derived antibodies; PBS: Phosphate-buffered saline; PV: Post vaccination; RCC: Relative cell count; RT-PCR: Reverse transcriptase polymerase chain reaction; (S/P)-ratio: Sample to positive ratio; TC: Tracheal mucosa; TCID: Tissue culture infectious dose; TRT: Turkey rhinotracheitis.

Competing interests
None of the authors of this paper have a financial or personal relationship with other people or organizations that could inappropriately influence or bias the content of the paper.

Authors' contributions
MS designed the study, conducted the experiments, collected all samples, performed flow cytometry and serological analysis and wrote the manuscript. DP performed molecular biology analysis. BT and TS were responsible for the animals and helped obtain the samples. AK supervised the study and helped to write the manuscript. All authors read and approved the final manuscript.

Acknowledgements
The project has been defrayed with the funds from the National Science Centre granted in terms of decision number DEC-2011/01/N/NZ6/05757.

References
1. Pedersen JC, Reynolds DL, Ali A. The sensitivity and specificity of a reverse transcriptasepolymerase chain reaction assay for the avian pneumovirus (Colorado strain). Avian Dis. 2000;44:681–5.
2. Buys SB, Du Preez JH. A preliminary report on the isolation of a virus causing sinusitis in turkeys in South Africa and attempts to attenuate the virus. Turkeys. 1980;28:36.
3. Collins MS, Gough RE, Alexander DJ. Antigenic differentiation of avian pneumovirus isolates using polyclonal antibody and mouse monoclonal antibodies. Avian Pathol. 1993;22:469–79.
4. Cook JKA, Jones BV, Ellis MM, Li J, Cavanagh D. Antigenic differentiation of strains of Turkey rhinotracheitis virus using monoclonal antibodies. Avian Pathol. 1993;22:257–73.
5. Seal BS. Matrix protein gene nucleotide and predicted amino acid sequence demonstrate that the first US avian pneumovirus isolate is distinct from European strains. Virus Res. 1998;58:45–52.

6. Smialek M, Tykalowski B, Stenzel T, Koncicki A. The perspective of immunoprophylaxis and selected immunological issues in the course of the turkey rhinotracheitis. Pol J Vet Sci. 2012;15:175–80.

7. Liman M, Rautenschlein S. Induction of local and systemic immune reactions following infection of turkeys with avian Metapneumovirus (aMPV) subtypes A and B. Vet Immunol Immunopathol. 2007;115:273–85.

8. Catelli E, Lupini C, Cecchinato M, Ricchizzi E, Brown P, Naylor CJ. Field avian metapneumovirus evolution avoiding vaccine induced immunity. Vaccine. 2010;28:916–21.

9. Rautenschlein S, Aung YH, Haase C. Local and systemic immune responses following infection of broiler-type chickens with avian Metapneumovirus subtypes A and B. Vet Immunol Immunopathol. 2011;140:10–22.

10. Jones RC, Wolliams RA, Baxter-Jones C, Savage CE, Wilding GP. Experimental infection of laying turkeys with rhinotracheitis virus: distribution of virus in the tissues and serological response. Avian Pathol. 1988;17:841–50.

11. Cook JKA, Ellis MM, Dolby CA, Holmes HC, Finney PM, Huggins MB. A live attenuated turkey rhinotracheitis virus vaccine. 1.Stability of the attenuated strain. Avian Pathol. 1989;18:511–22.

12. Cook JKA, Holmes HC, Finney PM, Dolby CA, Ellis MM, Huggins MB. A live attenuated turkey rhinotracheitis virus vaccine. 2. The use of the attenuated strain as an experimental vaccine. Avian Pathol. 1989;18:523–34.

13. Jirjis FF, Noll SL, Halvorson DA, Nagaraja KV, Shaw DP. Pathogenesis of avian pneumovirus infection in turkeys. Vet Pathol. 2002;39:300–10.

14. Jones RC, Naylor CJ, al-Afaleq A, Worthington KJ, Jones R. Effect of cyclophosphamide immunosuppression on the immunity of turkeys to viral rhinotracheitis. Res Vet Sci. 1992;53:38–41.

15. Cha RM, Khatri M, Sharma JM. B-cell infiltration in the respiratory mucosa of turkeys exposed to subtype C avian metapneumovirus. Avian Dis. 2007;51:764–70.

16. Rubbenstroth D, Rautenschlein S. Compromised T-cell immunity in turkeys may lead to an unpredictable avian metapneumovirus vaccine response and variable protection against challenge. Avian Pathol. 2010;39:349–57.

17. Cha RM. Immunopathogenesis of avian Metapnumovirus in the turkeys. PhD thesis. University of Minnesota, United States; 2009.

18. Cavanagh D, Mawditt K, Britton P, Naylor CJ. Longitudinal field studies of infectious bronchitis virus and avian pneumovirus in broilers using type-specific polymerase chain reactions. Avian Pathol. 1999;28:593–605.

19. Gough RE, Jones RC. Avian Metapneumovirus. In: Saif YM, editor. Diseases of poultry. 12th ed. Ames: Blackwell Publishing; 2008. p. 100–10.

20. Wiliams RA, Savage CE, Jones RC. Development of a live attenuated vaccine against turkey rhinotracheitis. Avian Pathol. 1991;20:45–55.

21. Patnayak DP, Sheikh AM, Gulati BR, Goyal SM. Experimental and field evaluation of a live vaccine against avian pneumovirus. Avian Pathol. 2002;31:377–82.

22. Kimpen JL, Rich GA, Mohar CK, Ogra PL. Mucosal T cell distribution during infection with respiratory syncytial virus. J Med Virol. 1992;36:172–9.

23. de Bree GJ, van Leeuwen EM, Out TA, Jansen HM, Jonkers E, van Lier RA. Selective accumulation of differentiated CD8+ T cells specific for respiratory viruses in the human lung. J Exp Med. 2005;202:1433–42.

24. Scott KG, Buret AG. Role of CD8+ and CD4+ T lymphocytes in jejunal mucosal injury during murine giardiasis. Infect Immun. 2004;72:3536–42.

25. Timms LM, Jahans KL, Marshall RN. Evidence of immunosuppression in turkey poults affected by rhinotracheitis. Vet Rec. 1986;119:91–2.

26. Chary P, Rautenschlein S, Njenga MK, Sharma JM. Pathogenic and immunosuppressive effects of avian pneumovirus in turkeys. Avian Dis. 2002;46:153–61.

27. Chary P, Rautenschlein S, Sharma JM. Reduced efficacy of hemorrhagic enteritis virus vaccine in turkeys exposed to avian pneumovirus. Avian Dis. 2002;46:353–9.

28. Marien M, Decostere A, Martel A, Chiers K, Froyman R, Nauwynck H. Synergy between avian pneumovirus and Ornithobacterium rhinotracheale in turkeys. Avian Pathol. 2005;34:204–11.

29. Davidson F, Kaspers B, Schat KA. Avian immunology. 1st ed. Great Britain: Academic Press; 2008.

30. Parel Y, Chizzolini C. CD4+ CD8+ double positive (DP) T cells in health and disease. Autoimmune Rev. 2004;3:215–20.

31. Eterradossi N, Toquin D, Guittet M, Bennejean G. Evaluation of different turkey rhinotracheitis viruses used as antigens for serological testing following live vaccination and challenge. Zentralbl Veterinarmed B. 1995;42:175–86.

32. Mekkes DR, de Wit JJ. Comparison of three commercial ELISA kits for the detection of turkey rhinotracheitis virus antibodies. Avian Pathol. 1998;27:301–5.

33. Cook JKA. Avian rhinotracheitis. Rev Sci Tech. 2000;19:602–13.

21

Seroprevalence and molecular characteristics of hepatitis E virus in household-raised pig population in the Philippines

Xiaofang Liu[1], Mariko Saito[1,2], Yusuke Sayama[1], Ellie Suzuki[1], Fedelino F Malbas Jr[3], Hazel O Galang[3], Yuki Furuse[1], Mayuko Saito[1], Tiancheng Li[4], Akira Suzuki[1] and Hitoshi Oshitani[1,2]*

Abstract

Background: Hepatitis E virus (HEV) infection is a significant public health concern in Asia, and swine is an important source of sporadic HEV infection in human. However, no epidemiological data are available regarding HEV infection among the swine or human population in the Philippines. To assess the HEV infection status among pigs in rural areas, we investigated the molecular characteristics and seroprevalence of HEV among household-raised pigs in San Jose, Tarlac Province, the Philippines.

Result: Serum and rectal swab samples were collected from 299 pigs aged 2–24 months from 155 households in four barangays (villages) between July 2010 and June 2011. Enzyme-linked immunosorbent assay (ELISA) revealed that 50.3% [95% confidence interval (CI) 44.5–56.2%] and 22.9% (95% CI 18.2–28.1%) of pigs tested positive for anti-HEV IgG and IgM, respectively. HEV RNA was detected in the feces of 22 pigs (7.4%, 95% CI 4.7–10.9%). A total of 103 households (66.5%, 95% CI 58.4–73.8%) had at least one pig that tested positive for anti-HEV IgG or IgM or HEV RNA. The prevalence of anti-HEV IgG and IgM in breeding pig (8–24 months) were higher than that in growing pigs (2–4 months) ($p < 0.0001$ and $p = 0.008$, respectively). HEV RNA was more frequently detected in 2–4-month-old pigs (9.2%, 95% CI 5.4–14.6%) than in ≥5-month-old pigs (4.8%, 95% CI 1.1–8.5%) without statistical significance ($p = 0.142$). HEV RNA showed 0–27.6% nucleotide difference at the partial ORF2 gene among the detected viruses, and a majority of them belonged to subtype 3a (20/22, 90.9%).

Conclusion: We found a high prevalence of HEV antibodies in the household-raised pig population in rural areas of the Philippines, which indicates the potential risk of HEV infection among local residents. Only genotype 3 of HEV was observed, and genetically diverse strains of HEV were found to be circulating in pigs in this study.

Keywords: Hepatitis E virus, Household-raised pig, Seroprevalence, Genotype 3, Philippines

Background

Hepatitis E was first documented as a unique clinical entity distinct from hepatitis A and B in water-borne epidemic hepatitis in India in 1978 [1]. Hepatitis E virus (HEV), the sole member of genus *Hepevirus* in the *Hepeviridae* family, is the causative agent of self-limited or fulminant hepatitis [2]. The virion of HEV is spherical, nonenveloped, 27–34 nm in diameter, with a single-stranded, positive sense RNA genome. The RNA is approximately 7300 nucleotides in length and contains three open reading frames (ORFs). ORF1 encodes nonstructural proteins, while ORF2 encodes capsid proteins and ORF3 encodes a small protein of unknown function [3]. Mammalian HEV falls into four major genetically distinct genotypes based on nucleotide differences [4-6]. Genotypes 1 and 2 are the most common causes of epidemic hepatitis in humans in tropical and subtropical countries with poor sanitation and unsafe water supply [1,7]. Genotypes 3 and 4 are considered to be of zoonotic origin and are together recognized as an important cause of sporadic hepatitis cases in humans both in developing and industrialized countries [6,8,9].

* Correspondence: oshitanih@med.tohoku.ac.jp
[1]Department of Virology, Tohoku University Graduate School of Medicine, 2-1 Seiryo-machi, Aoba-ku, Sendai, Miyagi 980-8575, Japan
[2]Tohoku-RITM Collaborating Research Center on Emerging and Reemerging Infectious Diseases, RITM compound, FCC, Alabang, Muntinlupa City 1781, Philippines
Full list of author information is available at the end of the article

Some evidence indicates that pigs are an important source of zoonotic HEV genotypes 3 and 4. Case reports have shown that viruses recovered from clinical patients with hepatitis E and the consumed pork were genetically similar [8,10]. A cluster of human isolates from autochthonous hepatitis E cases were found to be genetically similar to the local swine strains by phylogenetic analysis [11]. Meta-analysis of 10 cross-sectional studies revealed greater chances of HEV seropositivity in people with occupational exposure to pigs than in the general human population [12].

HEV genotype 3, which was first isolated in 1997 [6] from domestic pigs in the United States, has been shown to be widely distributed in pigs in all continents. Genotype 4 was first reported in China [5,9], and it appears to be present in pigs and humans exclusively in Southeast Asia. Recently, however, genotype 4 has been detected in pigs and in human cases with more severe clinical manifestations than those with other HEV genotypes in Europe [13,14]. Genotypes 3 and 4 are quite diverse and can be further classified into 10 (3a–3j) and seven (4a–4 g) subtypes, respectively, on the basis of five different regions of HEV, including 5994–6294 nucleotide positions of ORF 2 (GenBank accession number M73218) [4].

The increasing documentation of zoonotic HEV in Asian countries such as China, Japan, Korea, Indonesia, Cambodia, Thailand, and Laos [15-17] suggests a significant health risk for the people. No epidemiological data are available regarding HEV infection among pigs or humans in the Philippines. However, recently, Li et al. reported that genotype 3 of HEV was found in the river water in Manila [18]. HEV infection

in commercial pig farms were previously reported; however, there are very few reports on HEV infections in family-scale farms (backyard pig farms), where local people could be more frequently exposed to pigs or pig feces because of the open breeding system and poor sanitation of backyard pigs. The seroprevalence of HEV in family-scale pig farms was higher than that in large-scale pig farms as reported from Thailand [19] and China [20]. In rural areas of the Philippines, backyard pig farms are still quite common, and backyard pigs are an important source of income for pig owners. As a part of the project conducted in the Philippines to assess the prevalence of zoonotic pathogens, including Japanese encephalitis virus and Reston Ebola virus [21], we investigated the molecular characteristics and seroprevalence of HEV among household-raised pigs in four barangays (Villa Aglipay, Moriones, Pao, and Lubigan) in San Jose, Tarlac Province, the Philippines. Notably, San Jose is a third-class municipality and comprises mainly of rural areas in the Tarlac Province (Figure 1), where the density of household-raised pigs is quite high.

Results

Detection of anti-HEV IgG and IgM in pig sera and HEV RNA in stool swabs

Serum and rectal swab samples were collected from a total of 299 pigs aged 2–24 months (median age, 4 months) from 155 households in four barangays. The median numbers of pigs raised and numbers of samples per household were 2 [interquartile range 1–5] and 1[interquartile range 1–2], respectively. A majority of pigs were healthy, raised in simple piggeries in backyards,

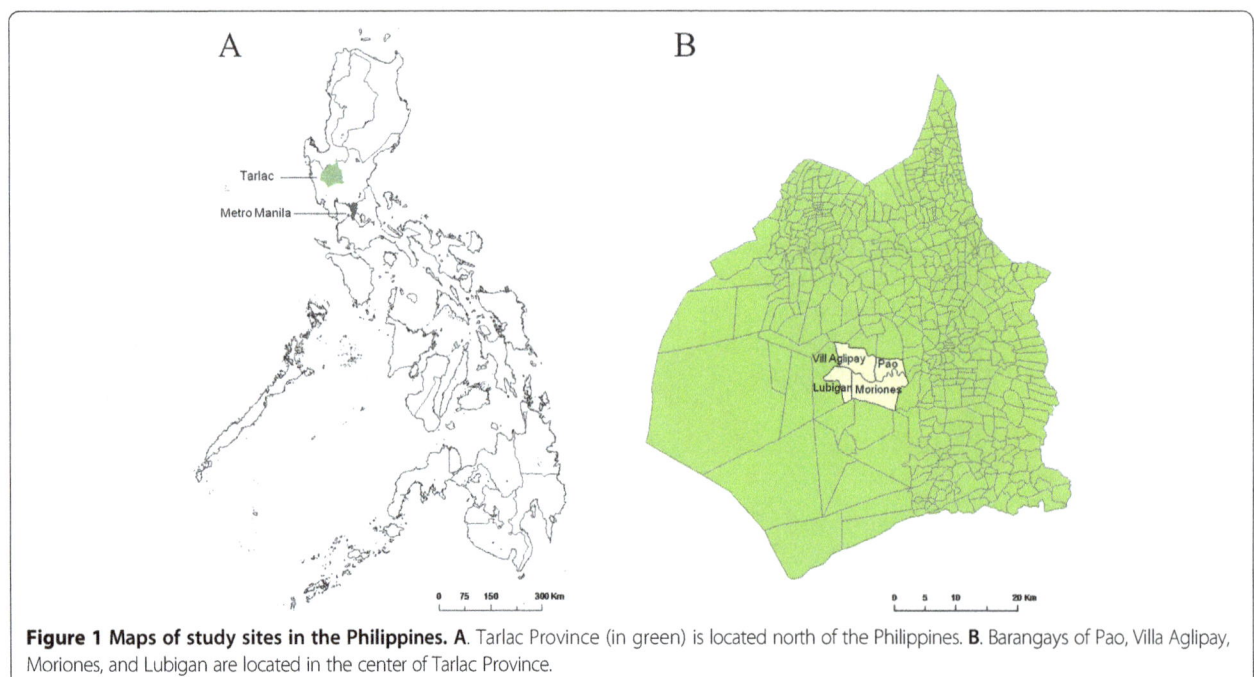

Figure 1 Maps of study sites in the Philippines. A. Tarlac Province (in green) is located north of the Philippines. **B**. Barangays of Pao, Villa Aglipay, Moriones, and Lubigan are located in the center of Tarlac Province.

fed with commercial feeding or kitchen residues, and living with other domestic animals such as chickens and ducks. Anti-HEV IgG was found in 150 serum samples [50.3%, 95% confidence interval (CI) 44.5–56.2%] from 93 households (60.0%), with the similar average prevalence of 43.4–55.1% among four barangays (Table 1). Anti-HEV IgM was detected in 68 serum samples (22.9%, 95% CI 18.2–28.1%) from 52 households (33.5%). On the other hand, a total of 22 rectal swabs (7.4%, 95% CI 4.7–10.9%) from 16 households (10.3%) were positive for HEV RNA (Table 1). The average prevalence (56.2%, 95% CI 50.4–61.9%) of any of the three markers (anti-HEV IgG, IgM, and RNA) in the pig population was observed at similar range between 47.0% and 62.5% among the four barangays. Overall, 66.5% households (103/155, 95% CI 58.4–73.8%) had pigs positive for either anti-HEV IgG, IgM, or viral RNA. Among the 22 RNA positive samples, six samples were positive for both anti-HEV IgM and IgG and 10 samples were only positive for anti-HEV IgG. The remaining six samples were negative for both anti-HEV IgM and IgG.

The presence of anti-HEV IgG, IgM, and HEV RNA in different age groups

The prevalence of anti-HEV IgG (37.6%, 95% CI 30.3–45.2%) was the lowest in growing pigs (P < 0.0001) and then increased in finishing pigs (64.1%, 95% CI 53.6–73.9%) and reached a peak of 78.8% (95% CI 61.1–91.0%) in breeding pigs (Table 2). Also, the prevalence of anti-HEV IgM was the lowest in growing pigs (16.9%, 95% CI 11.6–23.3%), comparing to that in finishing pigs (27.2%, 95% CI 18.4–37.4%) and breeding pigs (42.4%, 95% CI 25.5–60.8%) (p = 0.05 and p = 0.0008, respectively). Growing pigs had the highest prevalence of viral RNA (9.2%, 95% CI 5.4–14.6%), followed by finishing pigs (5.4%, 95% CI 1.8–12.1%), and breeding pigs (3.0%, 95% CI 0.1–15.8%), although it was not statistically significant (p = 0.26 and p = 0.23, respectively).

Genetic analysis of HEV strains from stool swabs

Phylogenetic analysis of 301 nucleotides corresponding to nucleotide positions 5994–6294 of M73218 in ORF2 revealed that 22 HEV strains in the Philippines belonged to genotype 3 (Figure 2). Pairwise comparison of 22

strains over 301 nucleotides revealed a 0–27.6% nucleotide difference. Compared with representative strains from river water in Manila, the strains in this study showed 10.0–24.0% nucleotide difference. With the exception of two strains (HEV_Vil_PHL_2011_Tjs-224_ORF2 and HEV_Vil_PHL_2010_Tjs-078_ORF2), the other 20 strains fell into a unique cluster within subtype 3a with a genetic distance of 0–4.9%. BLAST analysis revealed that these 20 strains shared less than 94% nucleotide similarities with any other sequence in GenBank. HEV_Vil_PHL_2011_Tjs-224_ORF2 shared the highest similarity (91%) with unclassified strains (JSW-Kyo-FH06L, AB291955) and subtype 3b strains (swJA11, AB082567) from Japan [22] and was also clustered with genotype 3b strains in the phylogenetic tree. The remaining strain HEV_Vil_PHL_2010_Tjs-078_ORF2 displayed 15.9–27.6% pairwise distance with other strains in this study. In the phylogenetic tree, it was clustered with unclassified reference strains from pigs (G3-HEV83-2-27 and G3-4531) and humans (HRC-HE200, HEJSB6151, and E088-STM04C) in Japan and shared 94–100% similarity with them. This cluster was genetically distant from other subtypes and may represent a novel subtype. Strains detected from the same household were closely clustered except two strains (HEV_Vil_PHL_2011_Tjs-223_ORF2 and HEV_Vil_PHL_2011_Tjs-224_ORF2). HEV_Vil_PHL_2011_Tjs-223_ORF2 and HEV_Vil_PHL_2011_Tjs-224_ORF2, which were collected in the same batch of pigs raised in the same household, genetically differed from each other by 15.4% and were grouped into subtype 3a and 3b in the phylogenetic tree, respectively.

Discussion

We used the recombinant antigen (112–660 amino acids of ORF2) of one of the prototype strains of genotype 1 (GenBank accession number D10330), which proved to be effective in detecting HEV antibodies in both human and pig serum [23,24]. Notably, numerous commercial or in-house enzyme immunoassays, which were developed to detect antibodies in human sera, were also adapted to detect anti-HEV in pigs since only one serotype has been described [3,6,25]. We found that the

Table 1 The detection of anti-HEV IgG, IgM, and HEV RNA in household-raised pigs in four barangays

Barangay	No. of swine	% RNA (95% CI)	% IgG (95% CI)	% IgM (95% CI)	% one of three markers (95% CI)	No. of household	% household positive for one of three markers (95% CI)
Pao	83	3.6 (0.8–10.2)	43.4(32.5–54.7)	22.0 (13.6–32.5)	47.0 (35.9–58.3)	49	53.1 (38.3–67.5)
Villa Aglipay	70	15.7 (8.1–26.4)	49.3 (37.0–61.6)	24.6 (15.1–36.5)	57.1 (44.7–68.9)	24	70.8 (48.9–87.4)
Moriones	98	7.1 (2.9–14.2)	55.1 (44.7–65.2)	21.4 (13.8–30.9)	60.2 (49.8–70.0)	52	73.1 (59.0–84.4)
Lubigan	48	2.1 (0.5–11.1)	54.2 (39.2–68.6)	25.0 (13.6–39.6)	62.5 (47.4–76.0)	30	73.3 (54.1–87.7)
Total	299	7.4 (4.7–10.9)	50.3 (44.5–56.2)	22.9 (18.2–28.1)	56.2 (50.4–61.9)	155	66.5 (58.4–73.8)

Table 2 The presence of anti-HEV IgG, IgM, and HEV RNA in pigs of different age groups

Age group of pigs	No. of pig	% RNA (95% CI)	% IgG (95% CI)	% IgM (95% CI)
Growing pigs (2–4 months)	173	9.2 (5.4–14.6)	37.6 (30.3–45.2)	16.9 (11.6–23.3)
Finishing pigs (5–7 months)	93	5.4 (1.8–12.1)	64.1 (53.5–73.9)	27.2 (18.4–37.4)
Breeding pigs (8–24 months)	33	3.0 (0.1–15.8)	78.8 (61.1–91.0)	42.4 (25.5–60.8)
Total	299	7.4 (4.7–10.9)	50.3 (44.5–56.2)	22.9 (18.2–28.1)

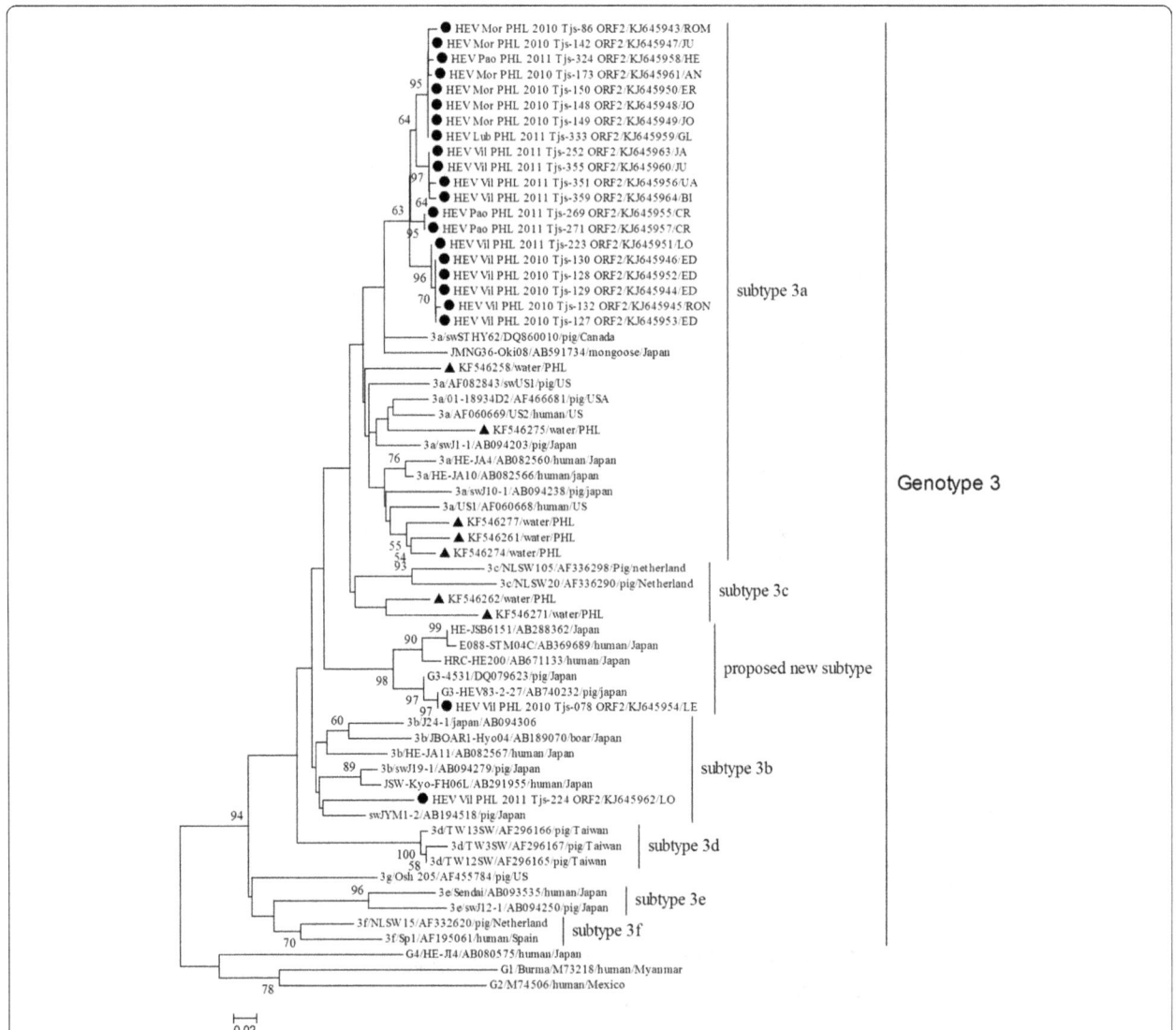

Figure 2 Phylogenetic analysis of HEV strains from pigs in San Jose, Tarlac Province, the Philippines. The phylogenetic tree was constructed using the neighbor-joining method (Kimura 2-parameter model) based on 301 nucleotides of ORF2 of HEV. Strains from this study were labeled with ● and tagged with household name (in capital letters) from where they originated. HEV genotype 3 strains from rivers in Manila, the Philippines, which were labeled with ▲, with GenBank accession numbers of KF546258, 546261, 546262, 546271, 546274, and 546277, were also included. Other reference strains were representatives of genotypes 1, 2, and 4 and subtypes 3a–3 g of genotype 3 in other countries. Reference strains were indicated as genotypes or subtypes, name, country, and GenBank accession number. The numbers on branches were bootstrap values (1,000 replicates; values less than 50% were not shown).

anti-HEV IgG prevalence (50.3%) in pigs from rural communities of the Philippines was much higher than that in a similar study conducted in smallholder-raised pigs in rural villages of Laos (15.3%) [26] and comparable to that in large-scale surveys of pigs of all age groups from commercial pig farms in Japan (56%) [15], Germany (46.9%) [27] and Italy (50.2%) [28]. It is worthwhile to mention that in several other studies, discrepant results have been reported when comparing ELISAs using different antigens of HEV with human or porcine origin for detecting anti-HEV in pigs [29,30]. Compared with the prevalence of anti-HEV IgG, there are limited data on the seroprevalence of anti-HEV IgM in domestic pigs. The seroprevalence of IgM in this study (22.9%) was much higher than that in large-scale surveys in Japan (3%) [15] and similar to that in Spain (28.2%) [31]. Furthermore, 66.5% of households had at least one pig positive for anti-HEV IgG, IgM, or HEV RNA. In the present study, the piggeries of pigs were simple, in poor sanitary conditions and located at the household or near to the household. Such a high level of HEV infection in household-raised pigs, frequent exposure to pigs or pig waste, and poor sanitation in rural areas in the Philippines indicate potential risks of HEV transmission from pigs to local residents. Besides, the local people commonly consume the cooked pig livers, pork and sausages made by local manufactures. Therefore, workers in slaughterhouses and pork handlers in the local area are at potential risk of getting HEV infection. However, there are no available data on viral hepatitis incidence due to HEV in the Philippines. The human health impact of HEV should be properly defined to establish appropriate interventions.

Our data revealed that the seroprevalence of anti-IgG increased with age from 2–4-month-old pigs to 8–24-month-old pigs. A higher seroprevalence of IgG in adult pigs than in young pigs has also been documented in other studies [25,32]. However, according to antibody dynamics studies, there may be two seroprevalence peaks of anti-HEV IgG at less than one month old pigs due to maternal antibody and adult pigs in commercial pig herds [6,33-35]. In the present study, we did not observe the first peak of anti-IgG because the pigs in the present study were ≥2 months old and the maternal anti-IgG could persist up to 8–9 weeks of age in young pigs depending on the titers in breeding pigs [6,34,35]. It has been reported that seroconversion of IgM occurs in pigs aged 2–3 months and its duration varies from 4 to 7 weeks in commercial herds [6,34,35]. However, in some commercial herds, the peak prevalence of IgM was reported in pigs aged 25 weeks, which could be slaughtered, and IgM were also frequently detected in sows (up to 40%) [33]. We observed that the prevalence of IgM increased from 2-4-month-old pigs (16.9%) and reached a peak in 8–24-month-old pigs (42.4%); however,

no infectious RNA was detected in rectal swabs of these breeding pigs except one. All these pigs were raised under poor sanitary condition, and breeding pigs usually lived with young pigs in rural communities. The high seroprevalence of IgM in breeding pigs was probably caused by the secondary immune response to frequent HEV exposure as reported among the vaccinated population exposed to measles virus [36]. This quick secondary immune response could prevent viral proliferation in the early phase; therefore, no RNA was detected. In the current study, we have provided important information about HEV infection status of pigs aged above 6 months while a majority of prevalence studies have been performed among pig aged less than 6 months. Six pigs with age ranging from 2–4 months were found negative for both IgG and IgM antibodies in sera but positive for HEV RNA in feces probably because of a recent infection [37]. On the other hand, in 10 pigs with age ranging from 2 to 8 months, RNA was detected in feces and IgG was found positive, but IgM was found negative. Detected IgG antibody might be due to persistent maternal antibody among 2–3 months old pigs (n = 5) and existed antibody from past infection in other five pigs aged 4–8 months. IgM negative results were probably because of a recent recurrent viral infection which could result in a low IgM immune response to HEV and a false negative result of IgM serological test. Moreover, it is possible that positive HEV in stools might reflect transient exposure to the virus through ingestion of contaminated food or water.

The average RNA-positive rate in rectal swab samples in this study (7.4%) was similar to that in Japan (5%) [15], Laos (11.6%) [16] and Thailand (2.9–7.75%) [19,38]. In this study, the viral RNA-positive rate was higher in 2–4-month-old pigs than in adult pigs, however the difference was not found statistically significant. Our finding is in line with other reports which stated that the highest incidence of HEV infections occurs in young pigs (2–4 months old) [15,39]. In Southeast Asia, both HEV genotypes 3 and 4 are circulating in human and swine; however, the geographical distribution of genotypes of zoonotic HEV in pigs varies. In Cambodia [40] and Thailand [19,38], only HEV genotype 3 has been reported in local pigs, while only genotype 4 of HEV has been reported in pigs from Laos [16]. In China [41], Japan [42], Korea [43], Indonesia [17], and Taiwan [44], both genotypes 3 and 4 were circulating in domestic pigs or wild boars. In the present study, we only detected HEV genotype 3 strains and a majority of them (20/22) were classified into the existing subtype 3a. Subtype 3a was also the most frequently detected subtype in Japan, Korea, and North America [4,45,46] as well as in river water in Manila in 2012 [18]. Subtype 3a strains in San

Jose shared less than 94% nucleotide similarity with strains in GenBank (including strains from river water in Manila), which suggests that area-specific strains of HEV were circulating in the Philippines. HEV_Vil_PHL_2010_Tjs-078_ORF2 shares 100% sequence identity with the strain (G3-HEV83-2-27, AB740232) from a domestic pig in Japan in 2003; thus, HEV_Vil_PHL_2010_Tjs-078_ORF2 may have the same origin as the strain detected in a domestic pig in Japan. However, the exact transmission route of this virus remains unknown. HEV_Vil_PHL_2010_Tjs-078_ORF2 together with G3-HEV83-2-27 and some unclassified strains from Japan formed a distinct cluster from other subtypes. The full sequence of G3-HEV83-2-27 is available in GenBank (accession number AB740232), and it can also form a distinct cluster in a phylogenetic tree based on the full genome sequence (see Additional file 1: Figure S1). Therefore, this cluster, including HEV_Vil_PHL_2010_Tjs-078_ORF2, could represent a new subtype.

Conclusion

The present study is the first report on the seroprevalence and molecular characterization of HEV in pigs in the Philippines. We found a high proportion of IgG and IgM, and three different subtypes of HEV among household-raised pigs suggesting that the risk of HEV transmission to humans in this geographical area was substantial. Hepatitis E is not included as a notifiable disease in the Philippines, and laboratory testing for acute hepatitis is not routinely performed in the country. Since only pig population from a small geographic area were investigated in the present study, further studies are required to define the genotype distribution in other areas, genetic relationship between HEV strains from swine and human and human health impact of HEV in the Philippines.

Methods
Samples

Swine blood and rectal swab samples from previous cross-sectional survey for validation of an ELISA assay [21] were tested for prevalence of HEV at the research institute for tropical medicine in Manila, Philippines. The sample collection was divided in six phases between July 2010 and June 2011. Households known to have pigs in their backyard farms were visited and owners were asked for the participation into the study. Informed consent was obtained from the pig owners. The pigs were stratified by age in months and selected to have all age groups available in each household. Piglets less than two months old were excluded from the sampling. The sampling was not systematic or random. Up to 50 samples were collected per sampling phase. This study was approved by ethics committee of Research Institute for Tropical Medicine and Institutional Animal Care and

Use Committee at the Animal Welfare Division of Bureau of Animal Industry, the Department of Agriculture.

Assessment of HEV infection by serology

To detect anti-HEV IgM and IgG, ELISA was performed. Virus-like particles (VLPs) were expressed by a recombinant HEV Burma strain (genotype 1) ORF2 (112–660 amino acids of D10330) using baculovirus in Tn5 cells, as described previously [47]. Flat-bottom 96-well polystyrene microplates (Becton, Dickinson and Company, NJ, USA) were coated with purified VLPs (1 μg/ml, 100 μl/well) and incubated at 4°C overnight. Unbound VLPs were washed out with 300 μl of 10 mM phosphate-buffered saline containing 0.05% Tween 20 (PBS-T). The wells were blocked for 1 h with 200 μl of 5% skim milk (Becton, Dickinson and Company, NJ, USA) in PBS-T at 37°C. After the plates were washed three times with PBS-T, swine serum samples (100 μl/well) were added in duplicate at a dilution of 1:200 in PBS-T containing 5% skim milk. The plates were then incubated for 1 h at 37°C. The plates were washed three times as described above and were administered 100 μl of horseradish peroxidase-conjugated goat anti-pig IgG (Bethyl, Laboratories, Inc., TX, USA) (1:10,000 dilution) or IgM (Kirkegaard & Perry Laboratories, Inc., MD, USA) (1:2,500 dilution) in PBS-T containing 1% skim milk. The plates were incubated for 1 h at 37°C and washed three times with PBS-T. Subsequently, 100 μl of o-phenylenediamine dihydrochloride (Sigma-Aldrich, Co., MO, USA) was added to each well. The plates were incubated in a dark room for 30 min at room temperature, following which 100 μl of 4 N H_2SO_4 was added to each well. The optical density was measured at 492 nm. Four standard deviation values above the mean OD value of negative controls (n = 4) were applied as the cut-off value for each plate.

Detection and genotyping of HEV infection

Rectal swabs were soaked in a viral transport medium containing Hank's balanced salt solution supplemented with gelatin, streptomycin, penicillin-G, and amphotericin B. RNA was extracted from 140 μl of sample using the QIAamp MinElute Virus Spin Kit (Qiagen, Hilden, Germany). Reverse transcription was performed using SuperScript III reverse transcriptase with a random hexamer (Life technologies, Carlsbad, CA, USA). A previously described nested polymerase chain reaction (PCR) [8] was performed to amplify part of ORF2, which corresponds to the nucleotide positions 5939–6316 of the genotype 1 HEV genome (GenBank accession number M73218). The PCR products were purified using the QIAquick® PCR Purification Kit (Qiagen), sequenced using BigDye Terminator version 1.1 (Life technologies), and analyzed using Applied Biosystems 3700 Genetic Analyzer (Life technologies). HEV genotypes were determined by phylogenetic analysis using MEGA (version 5) [48]. The pairwise distance was calculated by the neighbor-joining method, and the phylogenetic tree was constructed by the Kimura 2-parameter model, neighbor-joining method by MEGA 5. Strains in this study were named as HEV_ Barangay code_PHL _year_ID number of strain_ORF2 and were deposited in the GenBank database under the accession number of KJ645943–KJ645964. The GenBank accession numbers of reference strains are given as follows: DQ860010, AB082566, AB194492, AF060669, AB740232, DQ079632, AB671133, AB369689, AB288362, AB291955, AB094279, AB082567, AF296167, AF296165, AF336298, AF336290, AF336293, AB093535, AF332620, AF455784, AB080575, AF296166, AB094250, AF195061, AB591734, AB291955, AB194518, M73218, and M74506.

Availability of supporting data
The data set supporting the results of this article is included within the article and its additional file.

Statistical Analysis
Pigs in this study were classified into three age groups according to local pig production stage: growing pigs (2–4 months), finishing pig (5–7 months), and breeding pigs (8–24 months). The prevalence of anti-HEV IgG, IgM and HEV RNA between different age groups were compared by using Chi-square test in Stata software, version 12 (StataCorp, College Station, Texas), $p \leq 0.05$ was considered statistically significant.

Additional file

Additional file 1: Figure S1. Phylogenetic analysis of HEV based on complete genome. The phylogenetic tree was constructed by the neighbor-joining method with the Kimura 2-parameter model. The strain G3-HEV83-2-7 (sharing 100% similarity in 301 nucleotides with HEV_Vil_PHL_2010_Tjs-078_ORF2) with ♦ label could represent a new subtype under genotype 3 based on full genome sequence analysis.

Abbreviations
HEV: Hepatitis E virus; ORF: Open reading frame; nt: Nucleotide; ELISA: Enzyme-linked immunosorbent assay; PCR: Polymerase chain reaction; VLP: Virus-like particle; Ig: Immunoglobulin; PBS-T: Phosphate buffered saline containing 0.05% Tween 20.

Competing interests
The authors declare that they have no competing interests.

Authors' contributions
XFL carried out molecular analysis and draft the manuscript. MS participated in the design of the study, carried out the sample collection, immunological assay and involved to drafting the manuscript. YS participated in the design of the study, carried out the sample collection, immunological assay and molecular analysis. ES carried out the molecular analysis. FFM and HOG worked on the coordination with local government unit and carried out the sample collection. YF helped in phylogenetic analysis for the revised manuscript. MS carried out the epidemiological analysis and helped to draft the manuscript. TCL prepared the virus-like particle for immunological assay. AS carried out the sample collection and helped to draft the manuscript. HO

conceived of the study and helped to draft the manuscript. All authors read and approved the final manuscript.

Authors' information
XFL and YS are postgraduate students at Department of Virology, Tohoku University Graduate School of Medicine. ES is an undergraduate student in Medical School of Tohoku University. FFM and HOG are staff at Research Institute for Tropical Medicine. TCL is staff at Department of Virology II, National Institute of Infectious Disease. YF, MS, MS, AS and HO are staff at Department of Virology, Tohoku University Graduate School of Medicine.

Acknowledgement
We are grateful to the Local Government Unit of San Jose Municipality of Tarlac Province, the Philippines for their considerable support. We especially thank Dr. Lorna Baculanta, Provincial Veterinarian of Provincial Veterinary Office in Tarlac and Ms. Cecille Lopez,Epidemiologist of Tarlac Provincial Hospital for their valuable assistance. We thank the staff of RITM, Department of Virology, Tohoku University Graduate School of Medicine, and Tohoku-RITM Collaborating Research Center on Emerging and Re-emerging Infectious Diseases for technical assistance and logistic support. This work received financial support from a grant-in-aid for the Japan Initiative for Global Research Network on Infectious Diseases (J-GRID) from the Ministry of Education, Culture, Sports, Science and Technology of Japan.

Author details
[1]Department of Virology, Tohoku University Graduate School of Medicine, 2-1 Seiryo-machi, Aoba-ku, Sendai, Miyagi 980-8575, Japan. [2]Tohoku-RITM Collaborating Research Center on Emerging and Reemerging Infectious Diseases, RITM compound, FCC, Alabang, Muntinlupa City 1781, Philippines. [3]Research Institute for Tropical Medicine, FCC, Alabang, Muntinlupa City 1781, Philippines. [4]Depatment of Virology II, National Institute of Infectious Diseases, 4-7-1Gakuen, Musashimurayama-shi, Tokyo 208-0011, Japan.

References
1. Khuroo MS. Study of an epidemic of non-A, non-B hepatitis. Possibility of another human hepatitis virus distinct from post-transfusion non-A, non-B type. Am J Med. 1980;68(6):818–24.
2. Emerson SU, Anderson D, Arankalle A, Meng XJ, Purdy M, Schlauder GG, et al. Genus hepevirus. In: Fauquet CM, Mayo MA, Maniloff J, Desselberger U, Ball LA, editors. Virus taxonomy eighth report of the international committee on taxonomy of viruses. London: Elsevier; 2004. p. 853–7.
3. Khudyakov Y, Kamili S. Serological diagnostics of hepatitis E virus infection. Virus Res. 2011;161(1):84–92.
4. Lu L, Li C, Hagedorn CH. Phylogenetic analysis of global hepatitis E virus sequences: genetic diversity. Rev Med Virol. 2006;16(1):5–36.
5. Hsieh SY, Yang PY, Ho YP, Chu CM, Liaw YF. Identification of a novel strain of hepatitis E virus responsible for sporadic acute hepatitis in Taiwan. J Med Virol. 1998;55(4):300–4.
6. Meng XJ, Purcell RH, Halbur PG, Lehman JR, Webb DM, Tsareva TS, et al. A novel virus in swine is closely related to the human hepatitis E virus. Proc Natl Acad Sci U S A. 1997;94(18):9860–5.
7. Panduro A, Escobedo Meléndez G, Fierro NA, Ruiz Madrigal B, Zepeda-Carrillo EA, Román S. Epidemiology of viral hepatitis in Mexico. Salud Publica Mex. 2011;53 Suppl 1:S37–45.
8. Li TC, Chijiwa K, Sera N, Ishibashi T, Etoh Y, Shinohara Y, et al. Hepatitis E virus transmission from wild boar meat. Emerg Infect Dis. 2005;11(12):1958–60.
9. Wang Y, Ling R, Erker JC, Zhang H, Li H, Desai S, et al. A divergent genotype of hepatitis E virus in Chinese patients with acute hapetitis. J Gen Virol. 1999;80(Pt 1):169–77.
10. Yazaki Y, Mizuo H, Takahashi M, Nishizawa T, Sasaki N, Gotanda Y, et al. Sporadic acute or fulminant hepatitis E in Hokkaido, Japan, may be food-borne, as suggested by the presence of hepatitis E virus in pig liver as food. J Gen Virol. 2003;84(Pt 9):2351–7.
11. Bouquet J, Tessé S, Lunazzi A, Eloit M, Rose N, Nicand E, et al. Close similarity between sequences of hepatitis E virus recovered from humans and swine, France, 2008–2009. Emerg Infect Dis. 2011;17(11):2018–25.

12. Wilhelm BJ, Rajić A, Greig J, Waddell L, Trottier G, Houde A, et al. A systematic review/meta-analysis of primary research investigating swine, pork or pork products as a source of zoonotic hepatitis E virus. Epidemiol Infect. 2011;139(8):1127–44.

13. der Honing RW H-v, van Coillie E, Antonis AF, van der Poel WH. First isolation of hepatitis E virus genotype 4 in Europe through swine surveillance in the Netherlands and Belgium. PLoS One. 2011;6(8):e22673.

14. Jeblaoui A, Haim-Boukobza S, Marchadier E, Mokhtari C, Roque-Afonso AM. Genotype 4 hepatitis E virus in France: an autochthonous infection with a more severe presentation. Clin Infect Dis. 2013;57(4):e122–6.

15. Takahashi M, Nishizawa T, Tanaka T, Tsatsralt-Od B, Inoue J, Okamoto H. Correlation between positivity for immunoglobulin A antibodies and viraemia of swine hepatitis E virus observed among farm pigs in Japan. J Gen Virol. 2005;86(Pt 6):1807–13.

16. Conlan JV, Jarman RG, Vongxay K, Chinnawirotpisan P, Melendrez MC, Fenwick S, et al. Hepatitis E virus is prevalent in the pig population of Lao People's Democratic Republic and evidence exists for homogeneity with Chinese Genotype 4 human isolates. Infect Genet Evol. 2011;11(6):1306–11.

17. Widasari DI, Yano Y, Utsumi T, Heriyanto DS, Anggorowati N, Rinonce HT, Utoro T, Lusida MI, Soetjipto, Asmara W, Hotta H, Hayashi Y. Hepatitis E Virus Infection in Two Different Community Settings with Identification of Swine HEV Genotype 3 in Indonesia. Microbiol Immunol. in press.

18. Li TC, Yang T, Shiota T, Yoshizaki S, Yoshida H, Saito M, et al. Molecular detection of hepatitis E virus in rivers in the Philippines. Am J Trop Med Hyg. 2014;90(4):764–6.

19. Hinjoy S, Nelson KE, Gibbons RV, Jarman RG, Chinnawirotpisan P, Fernandez S, et al. A cross-sectional study of hepatitis E virus infection in pigs in different-sized farms in northern Thailand. Foodborne Pathog Dis. 2013;10(8):698–704.

20. Li W, She R, Wei H, Zhao J, Wang Y, Sun Q, et al. Prevalence of hepatitis E virus in swine under different breeding environment and abattoir in Beijing, China. Vet Microbiol. 2009;133(1–2):75–83.

21. Sayama Y, Demetria C, Saito M, Azul RR, Taniguchi S, Fukushi S, et al. A seroepidemiologic study of Reston ebolavirus in swine in the Philippines. BMC Vet Res. 2012;8:82.

22. Takahashi K, Kitajima N, Abe N, Mishiro S. Complete or near-complete nucleotide sequences of hepatitis E virus genome. Virology. 2004;330(2):501–5.

23. Li TC, Zhang J, Shinzawa H, Ishibashi M, Sata M, Mast EE, et al. Empty virus-like particle-based enzyme-linked immunosorbent assay for antibodies of hepatitis E virus. J Med Virol. 2000;62(3):327–33.

24. Kanai Y, Tsujikawa M, Yunoki M, Nishiyama S, Ikuta K, Hagiwara K. Long-term shedding of hepatitis E virus in the feces of pigs infected naturally, born to sows with and without maternal antibodies. J Med Virol. 2010;82(1):69–76.

25. Di Bartolo I, Ponterio E, Castellini L, Ostanello F, Ruggeri FM. Viral and antibody HEV prevalence in swine at slaughterhouse in Italy. Vet Microbiol. 2011;149(3–4):330–8.

26. Blacksell SD, Myint KS, Khounsy S, Phruaravanh M, Mammen Jr MP, Day NP, et al. Prevalence of hepatitis E virus antibodies in pigs: implications for human infections in village-based subsistence pig farming in the Lao PDR. Trans R Soc Trop Med Hyg. 2007;101(3):305–7.

27. Krumbholz A, Joel S, Neubert A, Dremsek P, Durrwald R, Johne R, et al. Age-related and regional differences in the prevalence of hepatitis E virus-specific antibodies in pigs in Germany. Vet Microbiol. 2013;167(3–4):394–402.

28. Martinelli N, Luppi A, Cordioli P, Lombardi G, Lavazza A. Prevalence of hepatitis E virus antibodies in pigs in Northern Italy. Infect Ecol Epidemiol. 2011;1:10.

29. Baechlein C, Schielke A, Johne R, Ulrich RG, Baumgaertner W, Grummer B. Prevalence of Hepatitis E virus-specific antibodies in sera of German domestic pigs estimated by using different assays. Vet Microbiol. 2010;144(1–2):187–91.

30. Peralta B, Casas M, de Deus N, Martin M, Ortuno A, Perez-Martin E, et al. Anti-HEV antibodies in domestic animal species and rodents from Spain using a genotype 3-based ELISA. Vet Microbiol. 2009;137(1–2):66–73.

31. Seminati C, Mateu E, Peralta B, de Deus N, Martin M. Distribution of hepatitis E virus infection and its prevalence in pigs on commercial farms in Spain. Vet J. 2008;175(1):130–2.

32. Jiménez de Oya N, de Blas I, Blázquez AB, Martín-Acebes MA, Halaihel N, Gironés O, et al. Widespread distribution of hepatitis E virus in Spanish pig herds. BMC Res Notes. 2011;4:412.

33. Casas M, Cortés R, Pina S, Peralta B, Allepuz A, Cortey M, et al. Longitudinal study of hepatitis E virus infection in Spanish farrow-to-finish swine herds. Vet Microbiol. 2011;148(1):27–34.

34. de Deus N, Casas M, Peralta B, Nofrarías M, Pina S, Martín M, et al. Hepatitis E virus infection dynamics and organic distribution in naturally infected pigs in a farrow-to-finish farm. Vet Microbiol. 2008;132(1–2):19–28.

35. Feng R, Zhao C, Li M, Harrison TJ, Qiao Z, Feng Y, et al. Infection dynamics of hepatitis E virus in naturally infected pigs in a Chinese farrow-to-finish farm. Infect Genet Evol. 2011;11(7):1727–31.

36. Lievano FA, Papania MJ, Helfand RF, Harpaz R, Walls L, Katz RS, et al. Lack of evidence of measles virus shedding in people with inapparent measles virus infections. J Infect Dis. 2004;189 Suppl 1:S165–70.

37. Bouwknegt M, Rutjes SA, Reusken CB, Stockhofe-Zurwieden N, Frankena K, de Jong MC, et al. The course of hepatitis E virus infection in pigs after contact-infection and intravenous inoculation. BMC Vet Res. 2009;5:7.

38. Keawcharoen J, Thongmee T, Panyathong R, Joiphaeng P, Tuanthap S, Oraveerakul K, et al. Hepatitis E virus genotype 3f sequences from pigs in Thailand, 2011–2012. Virus Genes. 2013;46(2):369–70.

39. Kaba M, Davoust B, Marie JL, Barthet M, Henry M, Tamalet C, et al. Frequent transmission of hepatitis E virus among piglets in farms in Southern France. J Med Virol. 2009;81(10):1750–9.

40. Caron M, Enouf V, Than SC, Dellamonica L, Buisson Y, Nicand E. Identification of genotype 1 hepatitis E virus in samples from swine in Cambodia. J Clin Microbiol. 2006;44(9):3440–2.

41. Liu P, Li L, Wang L, Bu Q, Fu H, Han J, et al. Phylogenetic analysis of 626 hepatitis E virus (HEV) isolates from humans and animals in China (1986–2011) showing genotype diversity and zoonotic transmission. Infect Genet Evol. 2012;12(2):428–34.

42. Sato Y, Sato H, Naka K, Furuya S, Tsukiji H, Kitagawa K, et al. A nationwide survey of hepatitis E virus (HEV) infection in wild boars in Japan: identification of boar HEV strains of genotypes 3 and 4 and unrecognized genotypes. Arch Virol. 2011;156(8):1345–58.

43. Kim YM, Jeong SH, Kim JY, Song JC, Lee JH, Kim JW, et al. The first case of genotype 4 hepatitis E related to wild boar in South Korea. J Clin Virol. 2011;50(3):253–6.

44. Wu JC, Chen CM, Chiang TY, Tsai WH, Jeng WJ, Sheen IJ, et al. Spread of hepatitis E virus among different-aged pigs: two-year survey in Taiwan. J Med Virol. 2002;66(4):488–92.

45. Kim SE, Kim MY, Kim DG, Song YJ, Jeong HJ, Lee SW, et al. Determination of fecal shedding rates and genotypes of swine hepatitis E virus (HEV) in Korea. J Vet Med Sci. 2008;70(12):1367–71.

46. Huang FF, Haqshenas G, Guenette DK, Halbur PG, Schommer SK, Pierson FW, et al. Detection by reverse transcription-PCR and genetic characterization of field isolates of swine hepatitis E virus from pigs in different geographic regions of the United States. J Clin Microbiol. 2002;40(4):1326–32.

47. Li TC, Yamakawa Y, Suzuki K, Tatsumi M, Razak MA, Uchida T, et al. Expression and self-assembly of empty virus-like particles of hepatitis E virus. J Virol. 1997;71(10):7207–13.

48. Tamura K, Peterson D, Peterson N, Stecher G, Nei M, Kumar S. MEGA5: molecular evolutionary genetics analysis using maximum likelihood, evolutionary distance, and maximum parsimony methods. Mol Biol Evol. 2011;28(10):2731–9.

22

Spatial characterization of colonies of the flying fox bat, a carrier of Nipah Virus in Thailand

Weerapong Thanapongtharm[1,2*], Catherine Linard[2,3], Witthawat Wiriyarat[4], Pornpiroon Chinsorn[1], Budsabong Kanchanasaka[5], Xiangming Xiao[6,7], Chandrashekhar Biradar[8], Robert G Wallace[9] and Marius Gilbert[2,3]

Abstract

Background: A major reservoir of Nipah virus is believed to be the flying fox genus *Pteropus*, a fruit bat distributed across many of the world's tropical and sub-tropical areas. The emergence of the virus and its zoonotic transmission to livestock and humans have been linked to losses in the bat's habitat. Nipah has been identified in a number of indigenous flying fox populations in Thailand. While no evidence of infection in domestic pigs or people has been found to date, pig farming is an active agricultural sector in Thailand and therefore could be a potential pathway for zoonotic disease transmission from the bat reservoirs. The disease, then, represents a potential zoonotic risk. To characterize the spatial habitat of flying fox populations along Thailand's Central Plain, and to map potential contact zones between flying fox habitats, pig farms and human settlements, we conducted field observation, remote sensing, and ecological niche modeling to characterize flying fox colonies and their ecological neighborhoods. A Potential Surface Analysis was applied to map contact zones among local epizootic actors.

Results: Flying fox colonies are found mainly on Thailand's Central Plain, particularly in locations surrounded by bodies of water, vegetation, and safe havens such as Buddhist temples. High-risk areas for Nipah zoonosis in pigs include the agricultural ring around the Bangkok metropolitan region where the density of pig farms is high.

Conclusions: Passive and active surveillance programs should be prioritized around Bangkok, particularly on farms with low biosecurity, close to water, and/or on which orchards are concomitantly grown. Integration of human and animal health surveillance should be pursued in these same areas. Such proactive planning would help conserve flying fox colonies and should help prevent zoonotic transmission of Nipah and other pathogens.

Keywords: Flying foxes, Nipah, Species distribution model, Ensemble modeling, Potential surface analysis

Background

Habitat loss is the greatest threat to wildlife and biodiversity. The loss and fragmentation of wildlife habitats can lead to increasing contact among wildlife, domestic animals, and people, potentially leading to the emergence and spread of zoonotic diseases [1]. The Nipah virus (NiV) is one such pathogen. The novel RNA paramyxovirus (genus *Henipavirus*), closely related to Hendra virus, is named after the village Sungai Nipah in the State of Negeri Sembilan, Malaysia from which the virus was first isolated from a human patient in 1998 [2]. In humans, NiV causes Nipah virus infection, presenting a range of clinical outcomes, from asymptomatic infection to acute respiratory syndrome and fatal encephalitis [3].

Investigations of the origins of NiV identified the flying fox genus *Pteropus* to be a major reservoir [4,5]. Subclinical infections have been found in flying fox populations in Malaysia, Cambodia, Thailand and Madagascar [4-8]. Flying foxes are mammals, members of the *Pteropididae* or fruit bat family, and are the largest of all bats [9]. They are found throughout tropical and sub-tropical Asia and Australia and on islands of the Indian Ocean and the western Pacific [9]. *Pteropididae* play a crucial role in rainforest ecosystems [10]. They pollinate flowers and disperse seeds as they forage on the nectar and pollen of plants and on the fruits of rainforest trees and vines [10]. In Thailand, flying foxes are protected by the Wildlife Preservation and Protection Act, B.E. 2535 (1992), which forbids hunting protected wild animals and protects wildlife

---

* Correspondence: weeraden@yahoo.com
[1]Department of Livestock Development (DLD), Bangkok, Thailand
[2]Lutte biologique et Ecologie spatiale (LUBIES), Université Libre de Bruxelles, Brussels, Belgium
Full list of author information is available at the end of the article

sanctuaries. A better understanding of the flying fox and its habitat preferences and dispersal would be a useful contribution to its conservation in Thailand. In addition, such an investigation should help efforts in better preventing potential disease transmission.

Work outside Thailand shows that in response to losses in its natural foraging areas, the adaptive *Pteropus* have turned to foraging in orchards, including those grown on pig farms where the NiV it carries are intermittently passed to pigs via urine or the contamination of partially-eaten fruit [4,5,11]. Investigation showed the virus to subsequently spill over from pigs to other animals and humans via respiratory droplets or close contact [2,12]. Pig farmers and workers exposed to respiratory illness and encephalitis in pigs were the first group of humans infected with the virus [13]. In 1999, abattoir workers in Singapore developed Nipah virus encephalitis [14]. Investigation showed direct contact with live pigs imported from Malaysia appeared to be the most important risk factor for those infections [15]. In contrast, a retrospective study of human cases in Bangladesh in 1999, the consumption of raw date palm sap proved one of the main risk factors of infection [16-18]. The result suggests NiV may have passed directly from bats to humans without an amplification host, as was apparently the case in Malaysia [11,12]. Human-to-human transmission was observed in several outbreaks in Bangladesh and India [18-20].

The situation of Nipah virus infection in Thailand showed that there has been no evidence of the viruses in domestic animals but they have been found in wildlife. Thailand's National Institute of Animal Health (NIAH), the Department of Livestock Development (DLD)'s central laboratory, conducted a retrospective study of all specimens of swine interstitial pneumonia submitted during 1998 to 2001 using immunohisto-chemistry (IHC) technique [21]. All samples reported negative for NiV. Since 2002, The DLD has conducted a sero-surveillance of 4,000 – 5,000 samples of pig per year by using Modified ELISA technique. The pig blood samples have been collected in high pig density areas and bordering area of Thailand and Malaysia (south). Simultaneously, the veterinarians of the DLD have conducted clinical surveillance by investigating any suspected cases of NiV, they can consider to collect samples submitting for laboratory confirmation [22] but NiV has never been found so far [23]. On the other hand, the Molecular Biology Laboratory for Neurological Diseases, Chulalongkorn University Hospital conducted surveillance for NiV antibody by using enzyme immunoassay and for NiV by using the duplex reverse transcription–polymerase chain reaction (RT-PCR) in Thailand's bat population during 2002–2004. The results showed 82 of 1,304 positives to NiV antibody and the tests for NiV presence in the urine and saliva of 12 bat species

produced positives for 3 species of fruit bats (*P. hypomelanus, P. vampyrus,* and *P. lylei*) and 1 species of insect-eating bat (*Hipposideros larvatus*) with being a probable accidental case [7]. In only one species of flying fox (*P. lylei*) was NiV found in both saliva and urine. A longitudinal study subsequently conducted on *P. lylei* populations between 2005 to 2007 in Thailand showed that 2 NiV strains previously identified circulating in Malaysia and Bangladesh were found in the bat's urine [24]. The study also highlighted a seasonal pattern with peaks between April and June, when viral RNA could be detected in urine. This seasonal pattern was associated with the observed fluctuation of population numbers, as May corresponds to the time of the year when young bats fledge [24].

The objectives of the present study were threefold. First, we aimed to describe the characteristics of the flying fox colonies and their neighborhoods in the central plain of Thailand (including central and eastern Thailand) from field observations, remote sensing (RS), and geographic information systems (GIS) data. Second, we aimed to predict the potential distribution of flying foxes in the study area using species distribution models (SDM). Finally, we aimed to map the areas where the three key elements of NiV ecology coincide, specifically flying fox habitat, human population, and pig farms, with the aim of informing NiV surveillance on the central plain of Thailand.

Methods
Characteristics of bat colonies and their vicinities
Field observations

The study area covered 23 provinces of western, central and eastern Thailand of a total area of 93,826 km^2 (Figure 1). The distribution of flying foxes in central and eastern Thailand was studied in 2004 and 2011. Boonkird and Wanghongsa [25] surveyed the colony of flying foxes in central and eastern Thailand 2001–2004 and reported 16 sites in 10 provinces with 2 species of flying foxes: the Lyle's flying fox (*P. lylei*) living in central Thailand and the Large flying fox or Greater flying fox (*P. vampyrus*) living along the coast of eastern Thailand. Sedsawai *et al.* [26] conducted a study of the distribution of flying foxes in central Thailand 2010–2011 and found 14 roosting sites within 10 provinces, including 10 previously reported and 4 newly discovered sites. Locations of bat colonies located in this area were obtained from these previous studies complemented by locations from field surveys by the Department of National Parks, Wildlife and Plant Conservation (DNP) conducted from March to August 2013. We surveyed each of those 22 bat colonies from June 2013 to January 2014 to verify the presence of flying foxes and to collect information on site characteristics for the roosting trees and

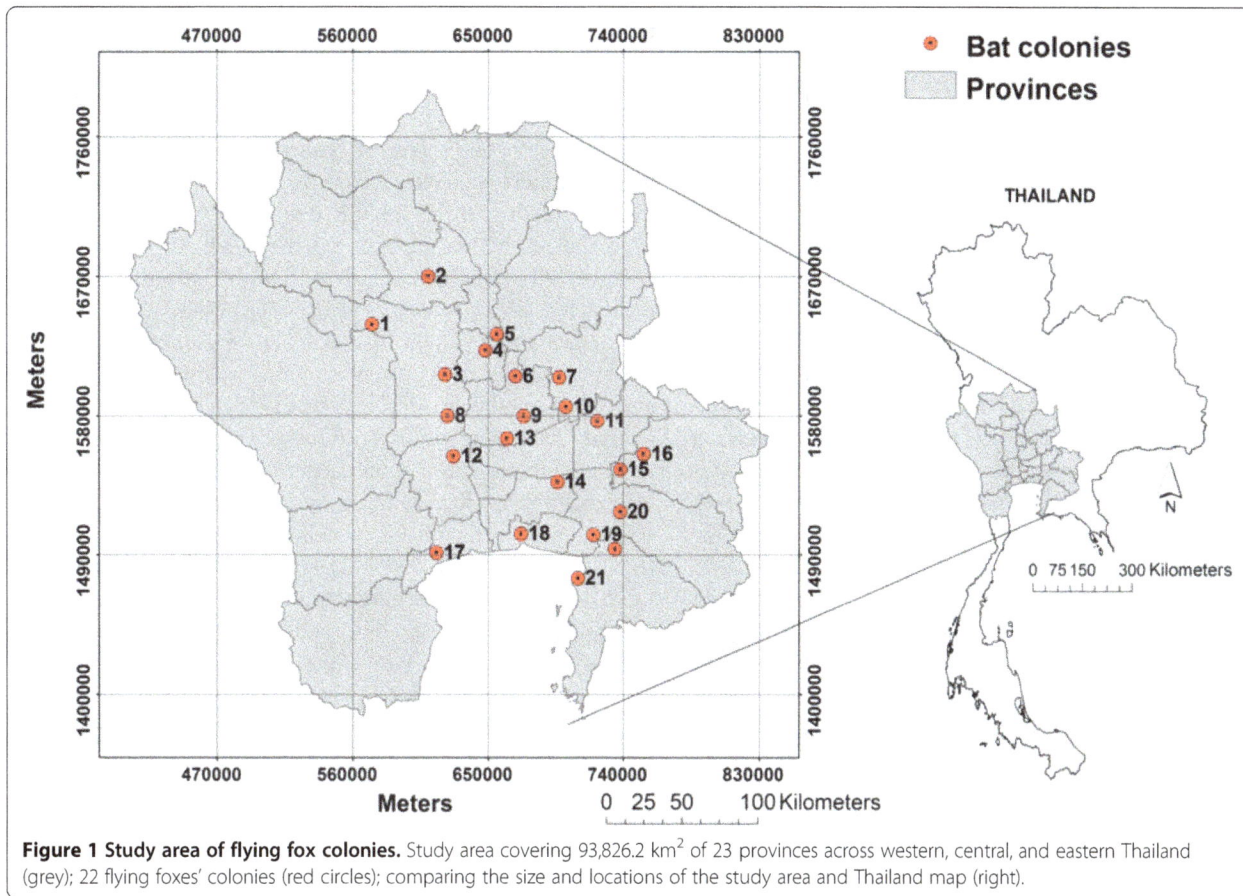

Figure 1 Study area of flying fox colonies. Study area covering 93,826.2 km² of 23 provinces across western, central, and eastern Thailand (grey); 22 flying foxes' colonies (red circles); comparing the size and locations of the study area and Thailand map (right).

their vicinities. We also estimated the margins of each colony with a hand-held GPS in order to delineate their spatial extent polygons.

Descriptive analyses

The GIS layer of the colonies was overlaid on other layers, including of bodies of water, human population density, elevation, and land cover. The vector map of permanent bodies of water was provided by the Ministry of Transportation. A human population density raster map at 100 m resolution was obtained from the World-pop project [27]. We used the SRTM elevation database with 90 m spatial resolution produced by NASA [28].

A land cover map was developed using LANDSAT images with the Exelis VIS ENVI image processing software. Eleven scenes of the LANDSAT 7 Enhanced Thematic Mapper Plus (LANDSAT 7-ETM+) were used to cover the 23 provinces of the study area (path/row = 131/49-50, 130/49-51,129/49-51,128/49-51). The LANDSAT 7 ETM+ sensor has six optical spectral bands at 30 m spatial resolution and one panchromatic band at 15 m spatial resolution and a 16 day revisit cycle. We searched the LANDSAT image archive at the United States Geological Survey EROS Data Center (http://glovis.usgs.gov) and downloaded images with low cloud cover acquired in

January 2014. All images were mosaicked and the minimum distance technique supervised classification method [29] was used to classify images into 4 land cover types most-related to flying fox habitat, including forest, irrigated vegetation, settlement/rainfed vegetation, and bodies of water. The regions of interest (ROIs) were built as classification training sets using ground truth data, 2D scatter plots, visible composition images, and spectral profiles. We evaluated the accuracy of the classes with 100 points per class of additional ground truth data and high-resolution data from Google Earth images for accuracy. Overall accuracy was 93%, with 98% accuracy for forest, 95% for irrigated vegetation, 91% for settlement/rainfed vegetation, and 86% for bodies of water, results considered acceptable and sufficient for the analysis.

For each bat colony polygon, we estimated summary descriptive statistics on the environment, geography, and anthropogenic variables. Specifically, we estimated the area of each colony, the distance from each colony to its nearest neighbor (another colony), the distance from each colony to the nearest body of water, the distance from each colony to the nearest temple, the average elevation within the colony, the average human population density, the proportion of irrigated vegetation land cover in a 10 km buffer around the colony, and the mean normalized difference vegetation index (NDVI) within the colony acquired from LANDSAT images. The vector map of Buddhist temples was provided by the Ministry of Transportation.

Species distribution models

In this study, we used ensemble modeling (EM) (or consensus methods or ensemble forecasting) with the 'dismo' and 'raster' packages in R, which combines the predictions from several different statistical modeling techniques into a single prediction. Species distribution models (SDM) were initially used to map the ecological suitability for flying fox colonies across the study area. SDM can be used to predict the geographical distribution of species as a function of a series of spatial variables, as they relate species distribution data (occurrence or abundance in known locations) to information on the environmental and/or spatial characteristics of those locations [30]. They have been widely used both for describing patterns and making predictions across terrestrial, freshwater and marine ecosystems [30,31]. Flying fox colonies can occasionally move, and such modeling should allow inferring other areas to which colonies might move, even those from which they are presently absent. The variables used to build the models were selected according to field observations and the results of the descriptive analysis. This would allow, for example, to map areas where colonies are not present at the time of the study, but where the colonies may move in the future if they are too disturbed, or if their current habitat became degraded. The seven different SDM methods used in analyses include: Bioclim, Domain, generalized linear model (GLM), generalized additive model (GAM), maximum entropy model (Maxent), boosted regression tree (BRT), and random forests (RF). The Bioclim and Domain are presence-only modeling methods. Bioclim characterizes the occurrences that are located within the environmental hyper-space occupied by a species, whereas Domain is a distance-based method that assesses new locations in terms of their environmental similarity to locations of presence [32]. The GLM and GAM are presence-absence models based on the regression framework. The GLM is a generalization of ordinary least squares regression using maximum likelihood allowing the linear model to be related to the response variable via a logit link function. The GAM is an extension of the GLM, where the linear predictor is the sum of smoothing functions. It is more flexible and much as machine learning methods can fit very complex functions [33].

Maxent, BRT, and RF are machine learning methods using presence-absence data. Maxent, sometimes misleadingly referred to as presence-only methods, actually does require the use of background data [33]. It estimates species' distributions by finding the distribution of maximum entropy (i.e. closest to uniform) subject to the constraint that the expected value of each environmental variable (or its transform and/or interactions) under the distribution matches its empirical average [34]. BRT combines the strengths of two algorithms, regression trees and boosting, creating a single best model from a large numbers of relatively simple models, each formed by a regression tree [35]. RF combines tree predictors such that each tree depends on the values of a random vector sampled independently and with the same distribution for all trees in the forest [36]. When compared with other methods, RF shows a very high accuracy, an ability to model complex interactions among predictors, and the flexibility to perform several types of statistical analysis [37]. The predictions of the seven SDM were then combined into a single ensemble model prediction by weighting each prediction by the performance of its source model, a procedure called ensemble modeling (EM) recognized as producing significantly more robust predictions than all the single models alone [38-42].

For three reasons, all our models were subject to 10 bootstraps. First, there was a very low proportion of positive samples in our data set, which can introduce bias into the logistic regression analysis framework. So for each trial we bootstrapped a different set of pseudo-absences [33,43]. Second, the bootstrapping also aims at preventing overfitting. That is, we aim at avoiding modeling the noise rather than the main pattern in the data by assembling across a population of models trained with different subsets of data. Third, the pseudo-absences were distributed within a given distance of the presence sites. We wanted to bootstrap through different distance values. The 10 sets of absence data were randomly selected from the background and from 6–15 kilometers beyond the presence sites. Then each set was randomly selected again and divided into two parts equally: a model set used to train the model and a test set used to evaluate the models. These were then used as weights in combining the methods. Nine times the number of positives was randomly selected at each bootstrap to maintain 10% of the positive values of the outcome variable. This 10% ratio was chosen because previous studies compared the various prevalences across models and reported that GAM was not influenced by prevalence, whereas the accuracy increased up to an asymptote when the number of presences reached one tenth of the number of absences for GLM, BRT, and RF [33]. All predictor variables were simultaneously tested in the models.

The performance of the models was evaluated using the area under the curve (AUC) of the receiver operating characteristics (ROC) plots. AUC is a quantitative measure of the overall fit of models that varies from 0.5 (chance event) to 1.0 (perfect fit) [44]. Although AUC was recently criticized as an absolute measure of goodness of fit by many authors, it remains valuable in comparing the performances of several models tested on the same data set [32].

Mapping the risk area of NiV

A Potential Surface Analysis (PSA) was applied to map the risk area of NiV by measuring the extent of the overlay between the factors that influence the risk of NiV infection, including potential flying fox habitats, and pig farm and human population densities. The PSA approach is somewhat simpler than other more complex knowledge-based approaches such as a Multi-Criteria Decision Analysis (MCDA) that can be employed to spatialize areas at risk [45]. However, MCDA methods require an extensive collection of knowledge on the important risk factors by experts, and at the present time, the knowledge of important cofactors that may be applicable to Thailand remains limited. In previous studies, the PSA method was used in similar conditions, where the knowledge of a particular outcome was limited. For instances; Ano *et al.* [46] estimated the drought risk area in the northeastern Thailand and used the result for managing water supply and Udomsap and Iamtrakul [47] studied the factors influencing the diversity of activities on Rachadamnoen Klang Avenue, Bangkok, which aimed to use the result in a planning process for maximizing efficiency of space usage and bringing economic enhancement to the local people and tourism. The PSA method ranks the spatial factors according to their importance using different weightings [48],

$$S = W_1R_1 + W_2R_2 + (W_nR_n)$$

Where S represents a summation of scores, $W_1 - W_n$, the weight of each factor according to its importance, and $R_1 - Rn$ the rating score of each variable, which corresponds to its scaling into bins. For these maps we assumed two potential scenarios for *human infection:* 1) humans are directly infected by the virus from the bats, and 2) humans are infected through a pig intermediate host. The overlay corresponding to the first scenario was

hence based on three factors: the flying fox distribution map, the distance to the flying fox colonies, and the house density in the sub-district. For the second scenario, the pig farm density map was added to the first three factors. For mapping the overlay of factors important to *pig infection,* we used three factors: the flying fox distribution map, distance to the flying fox colonies, and the pig farm density at the sub-district level.

The flying fox distribution map was obtained from the ensemble model described above, whose predicted values were divided into four bins according to their standard deviation (<0.5, 0.5-1.5, 1.5-2.5, and >2.5 of σ). The distance to the flying fox colonies was divided into bins corresponding to 5, 10, 20, 30, 50, 100, and 200 km. The pig farm density in the sub-district level was obtained from the 2010 surveys of the Department of Livestock Development (DLD), with the density values divided into 6 bins according to σ. The house density in the sub-district level was obtained from the Department of Provincial Administration, and the density values were divided into four bins according to their σ. We assigned initial rating and weighting scores to factors with values ranging from 0 to 9 (no risk to highest risk) based on literature and expert opinions [46-48] (Table 1). The layers were overlaid and analyzed by using the intersect tool. In each unit (intersected polygon), the summation score for each layer was summed. The mean and standard deviation were calculated from the summation scores of all units. The risk level was interpreted based on the summation score and the difference of mean ($\bar{x}$) and standard deviation (σ). Risk was low if the summation score was less than $\bar{x}-\sigma$, moderate if the summation score ranged between $\bar{x}-\sigma$ and $\bar{x}-\sigma$, and high if the summation score was more than $\bar{x}-\sigma$.

Ethical considerations

This study was approved by the Research Committee of the Bureau of Disease Control and Veterinary Services, Department of Livestock Development (Permit Number: 0601/1325).

Table 1 Scores given for a Potential Surface Analysis (PSA)

Flying fox distribution zones (probability during 0 to1)				Distance to the flying foxes colonies (km)				Pig farm density (farm per km^2)				House density (house per km^2)			
Scale	R	W	R*W	Scale	R	W	R*W	Scale	R	W	R*W	Scale	R	W	R*W
0.83x10^{-3} - 0.83x10^{-2}	1	2	2	<5	9	1	9	0	0	3	0	0.13 – 907	2	3	6
0.84x10^{-2} - 0.14	2	2	4	5-10	8	1	9	0.9x10^{-3} -0.035	1	3	3	908-1968	4	3	12
0.15 - 0.27	3	2	6	10-20	7	1	7	0.036-0.88	2	3	6	1969-3028	3	3	9
0.28 - 0.87	4	2	8	20-30	5	1	5	0.89-1.72	3	3	9	3029-12510	1	3	3
				30-50	3	1	3	1.73-2.56	4	3	12				
				>50	1	1	7	2.57-16.55	5	3	15				

R = rating score W = weighting score.
Weighting and rating scores of 4 factors used to map the overlay between NiV hosts on the central plain of Thailand.

Results

During field observation we observed flying foxes roosted on several types of trees: tamarind, coconut tree, bamboo (grass family), mangrove forests, and others (mostly members of evergreen forests) (Table 2). The colonies occupied a median area of 6,562 m² (ranging 1,463-30,751 m²), and the median distance to the nearest neighbor colony was 23.2 km (ranging 12.5-57.7 km) (Table 3). Almost all colonies were located on the central plain (Figure 2A), with a median elevation of 9 m (ranging 5–65 m). The colonies clustered into 4 groups according to the type of roosting trees: 1) bamboo only; 2) mangrove forests only; 3) rubber trees only; and 4) various types of trees. We observed that while some trees failed to protect against sunlight, some colonies remained. Most colonies were located nearby Buddhist temples (median nearest distance 262 m, range 42–2704 m), with 13 of the 22 colonies roosting on trees located within the temple area (no. 3–7, 9–11, 13, 15, 16, 20 and 22). When overlaid over the land cover maps (Figure 2B), the majority of colonies were surrounded by irrigated vegetation covering 96% of the landscape within 10 km², followed by settlement/rainfed vegetation (2.3%), bodies of water (1.5%), and forest (0.1%). Colonies were found on an island (no. 18) and riverside (no. 19), accessible to humans by boat alone. One colony was protected by the Wildlife Conservation Park (no. 1) and others located on private lands (no. 2, 8, 12, 14, 17, and 21). All colonies were located nearby bodies of water such as rivers, canals, ponds, and the sea (Figure 2C, median distance 120 m, range 30–4815 m). Some colonies were located in places with relatively high human population densities (Figure 2D), usually within Buddhist temples, where the number of tourists can be high (median population density of 232 people km⁻², range 0–1307 people km⁻²), while one bat colony was located on an island uninhabited by humans. We observed that some colonies had moved away from their previously known sites. Colony no. 21 moved away from its old site to a new isolated site along the sea and colony no. 17 moved away from a site with numerous destroyed mangrove forest trees to an adjacent area.

The predicted values obtained from the seven SDMs were combined as an ensemble model (EM) weighted by the predictive performance of each source model (Figure 3). All models captured the strong structuring effects of distance to rivers. The presence-only models (BC and DM) showed higher predicted values (more than 0.6) than that of the others in high-suitability areas. The model with the greatest AUC for evaluation was RF followed by BRT, Maxent, GAM, GLM, Domain, and Bioclim, respectively (Figure 4). The mean AUC of EM was 0.980 for model sets (ranged from 0.969-0.989) and 0.981 for test sets (ranged from 0.971-0.991). The effect of the predictive variable on predicted response (the fitted function) of the BRT model showed that the distance to temple, the distance to water, and elevation had a negative association and the area of vegetation within 10 km had a positive association with the presence of a colony (Figure 5). The human population density showed a positive association with the fitted function when human density was greater than 100 people per square kilometer and turned negative when the density was higher than 500 people per a square kilometer. The association remained steady when

Table 2 Characteristics of the trees roosted by flying foxes

Group	Colony	Botanic description
Group 1 Bamboo	8 and 12	Bamboo is generally found interspersed in many other types of forest and as a pioneer species. It is a fast growing species that easily colonizes disturbed forest sites, both natural and man-made. As such, and due to the logging excesses in Thailand in the past, many bamboo forests have become established in man-made disturbed sites [72].
Group 2 Mangrove forest	17,18, 19, and 21	Trees in mangrove forest are evergreen species with a very dense forest floor. The roots of the trees are both for anchoring it in the soil and for breathing. This type of forest is found close to the seat of the mouth of major rivers where the sea washes ashore. The important tree species include the Kongklang (*Rhizophora* spp.), Prasak. The plants grow on the forest floor include the various types of sea grasses [73,74].
Group 3 Rubber	2,5, and 11	The rubber (*Dipterocarpus alatus*) is a tropical forest tree, of dense evergreen or mixed dense forests, common in Thailand, Cambodia, Laos and Vietnam. It is a medium-sized to fairly large tree of up to 40 m tall (sometimes more), bole tall, straight, cylindrical, branchless up to 20 m, up to 150 cm in diameter. Leaves narrowly ovate to ovate to elliptical-oblong, 9–25 cm x 3.5-15 cm, base cuneate to rounded, apex acute or shortly indistinctly acuminate [75].
Group 4 Various trees	1,3,4,6,7,9,10,13,14, 15,16, 20 and 22	The various type of trees (mostly are in the Buddhist temple) composed of rubber (*Dipterocarpus spp*), ficus tree (*Ficus spp*), bohhi tree (*Ficus religiosa* L.), bengal almond (*Terminalia catappa* L.), rain tree (*Samanea saman*), neem plant (*Azadirachta indica*), tamarind (Tamarindus indica Linn), sal tree (*Shorea robusta* Roxb.), bamboo (*Bambusa sp.*), coconut (*Cocos nucifera Linn.*), and others [75]. Most of trees are a medium-sized to fairly large tree of up to 40 m tall, which mostly found in the tropical evergreen forest which is distributed in all areas of Thailand. They are concentrated in pockets of high moisture such as valleys and close to water sources such as rivers, streams and mountains. A common characteristic of tropical evergreen forest is the appearance of a lush green vegetation all year round.

Characteristics of bat roosting trees of 22 flying fox colonies in the central plain of Thailand grouped by type of trees.

Table 3 Descriptive statistics of the flying foxes' colonies and vicinity

Statistics	Size (m²)	Distance from each colony			Elevation (m)	Human density (people/km²)	Land cover in 10 km. of radius (m²)				**NDVI
		To nearest neighbor (km)	To nearest water (m)	To nearest temple (m)			Forest	Irrigated vegetation	Settlement/ rainfed vegetation	Bodies of water	
Median	6562	23.2	120	262	9	232.07	259	246700	55840	3805	0.0119
*SD	8595	12.5	1442	683	13	339.39	4493	61194	47550	10017	0.0686
Minimum	1463	13.0	30	42	5	0	0	88680	14510	437	−0.1061
Maximum	30751	57.7	4815	2704	65	1307.15	16450	331800	158600	40470	0.1429

*Standard deviation **Normalized difference vegetation index.
Descriptive statistics of environmental, geographical, and anthropogenic factors of 22 colonies of flying fox on the central plain of Thailand.

the density was higher than 800 people per square kilometer. The average relative contributions were 46% (35-62%) for the distance to a temple, 43% (31-55%) for the distance to the nearest body of water, 5.0% (2.6-8.7%) for the human density, 3.3% (0.6-6.5%) for vegetation area within 10 km of radius, and 3.2% (1.4-5.0%) for elevation.

The overlay of potential surface maps corresponding to the first scenario under which *humans* are directly infected with NiV by bats show the higher-risk areas cover 6,199 km² of 1,003 sub-districts, 159 districts, and 23 provinces and are mainly located to the north, northeast and east of Bangkok (Figures 6 and 7A). For the second scenario in which humans are infected via a pig reservoir, higher-risk areas cover 5,629 km² of 653 sub-districts, 143 districts, and 23 provinces (Figure 7B). The higher-risk area of NiV in *pigs* cover 5,417 km² of 607 sub-districts, 125 districts, and 23 provinces (Figure 7C). The two risk maps factoring in pig density looked very similar (Figure 7B & C). The higher-risk areas on both maps are located around the Bangkok metropolitan area, with environs to the west and north most affected. A slight difference in NiV risk levels between humans and pigs was observed in Bangkok, with greater risk for humans (Figure 7B) than for pigs (Figure 7C).

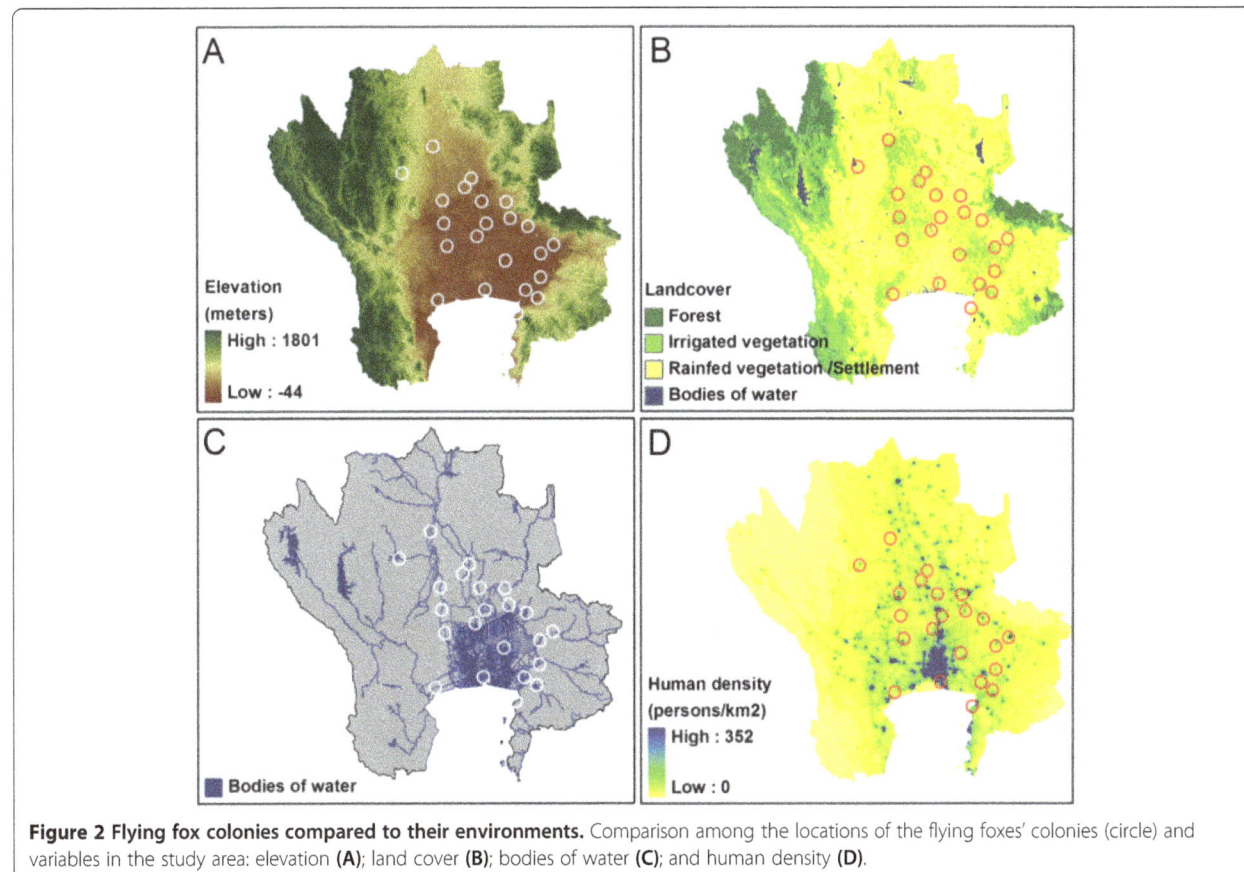

Figure 2 Flying fox colonies compared to their environments. Comparison among the locations of the flying foxes' colonies (circle) and variables in the study area: elevation **(A)**; land cover **(B)**; bodies of water **(C)**; and human density **(D)**.

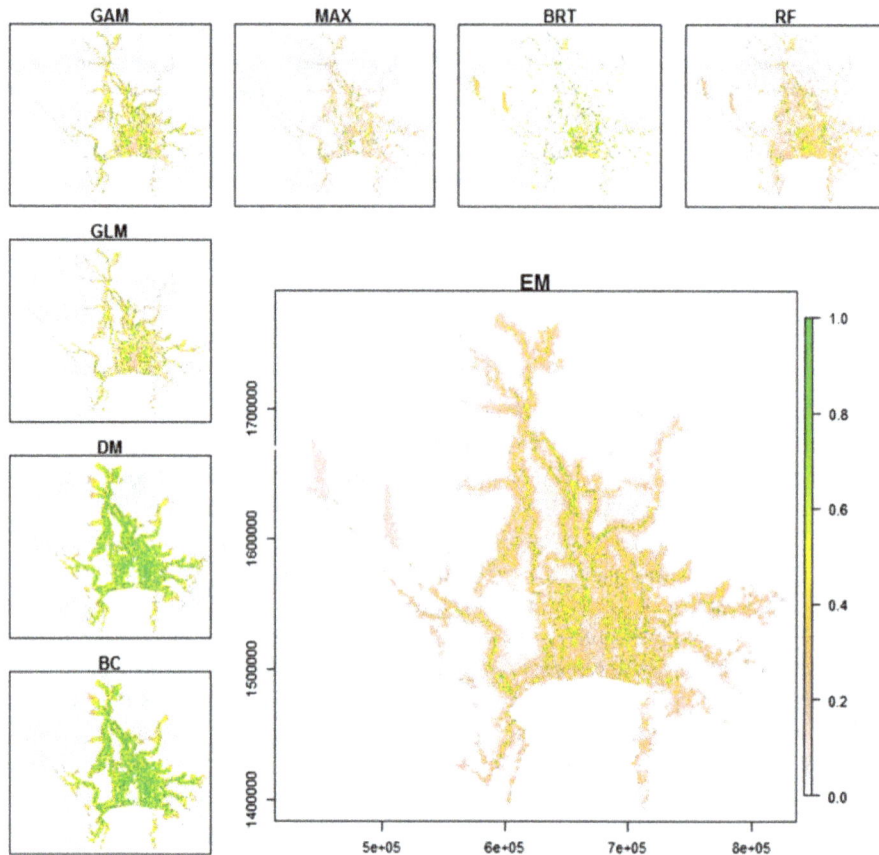

Figure 3 Predicted suitability maps for flying fox colonies on the central plain of Thailand. The maps explained by Bioclim (BC), Domain (DM), Generalized Linear Model (GLM), Generalized Additive Model (GAM), Maximum Entropy Model (MAX), Boosted Regression Tree (BRT), and Random Forest (RF). The large map shows the Ensemble model (EM) output obtained by combining the 7 SDMs weighted by their respective predictive performance.

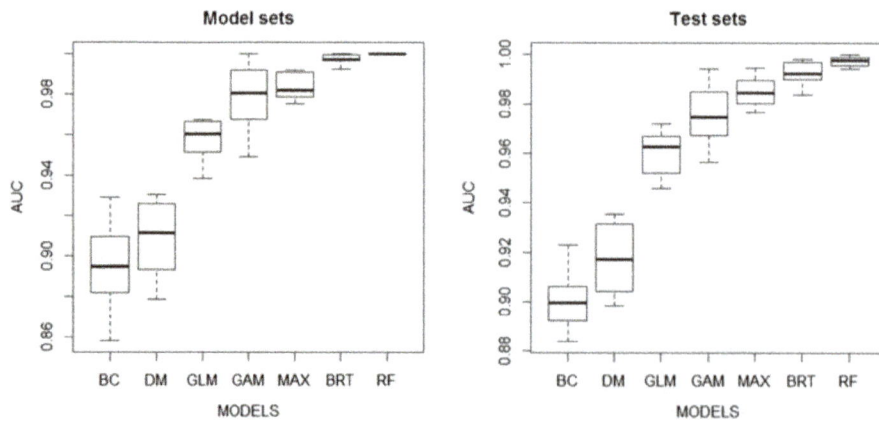

Figure 4 The predictive performance of 7 species distribution models. Box plots showing the predictive performance of 7 SDMs evaluated using the area under the curve (AUC) of ROC plots for the model sets (left) and test sets (right).

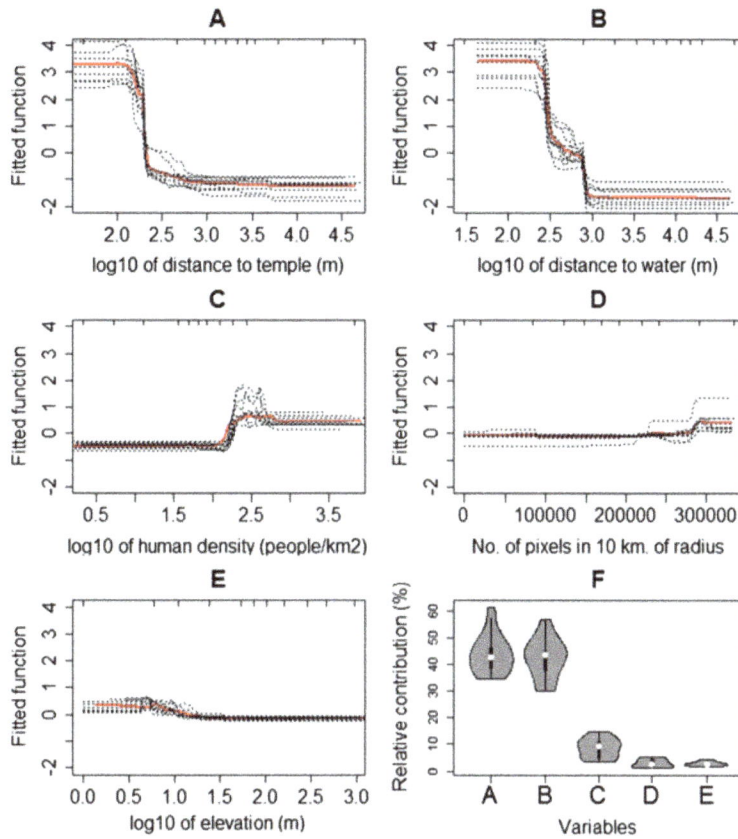

Figure 5 Fitted functions and relative contributions of variables predicted by the BRT. Partial dependence plots show the effect of a predictive variable on the response after accounting for the average effects of all other variables in the model: distance to water **(A)**; distance to temple **(B)**; human density **(C)**; amount of vegetation area within 10 km radius **(D)**; and elevation **(E)**. The relative contributions of each variable from the BRT is shown in **(F)**.

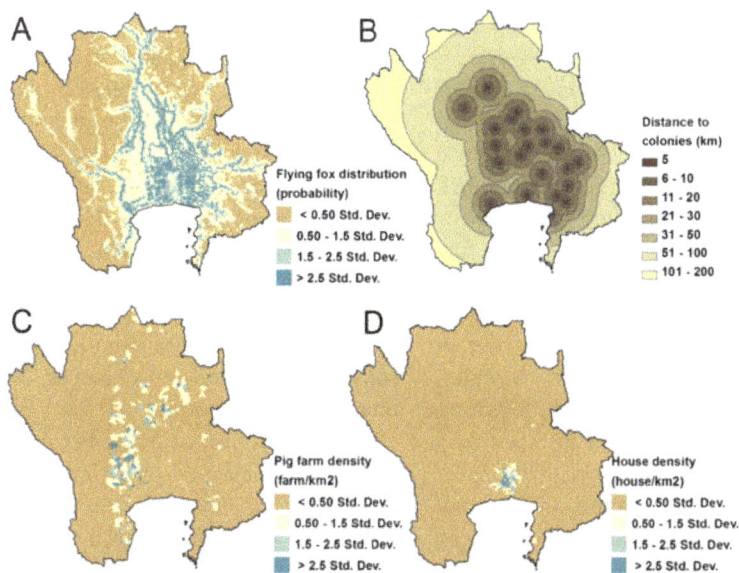

Figure 6 Factors used in mapping NiV risk. Maps of 4 factors used for analyzing the risk map of NiV in the central plain of Thailand: flying fox distribution map **(A)**; distance to the flying foxes colonies **(B)**; pig farm density at the sub-district level **(C)**; house density at the sub-district level **(D)**.

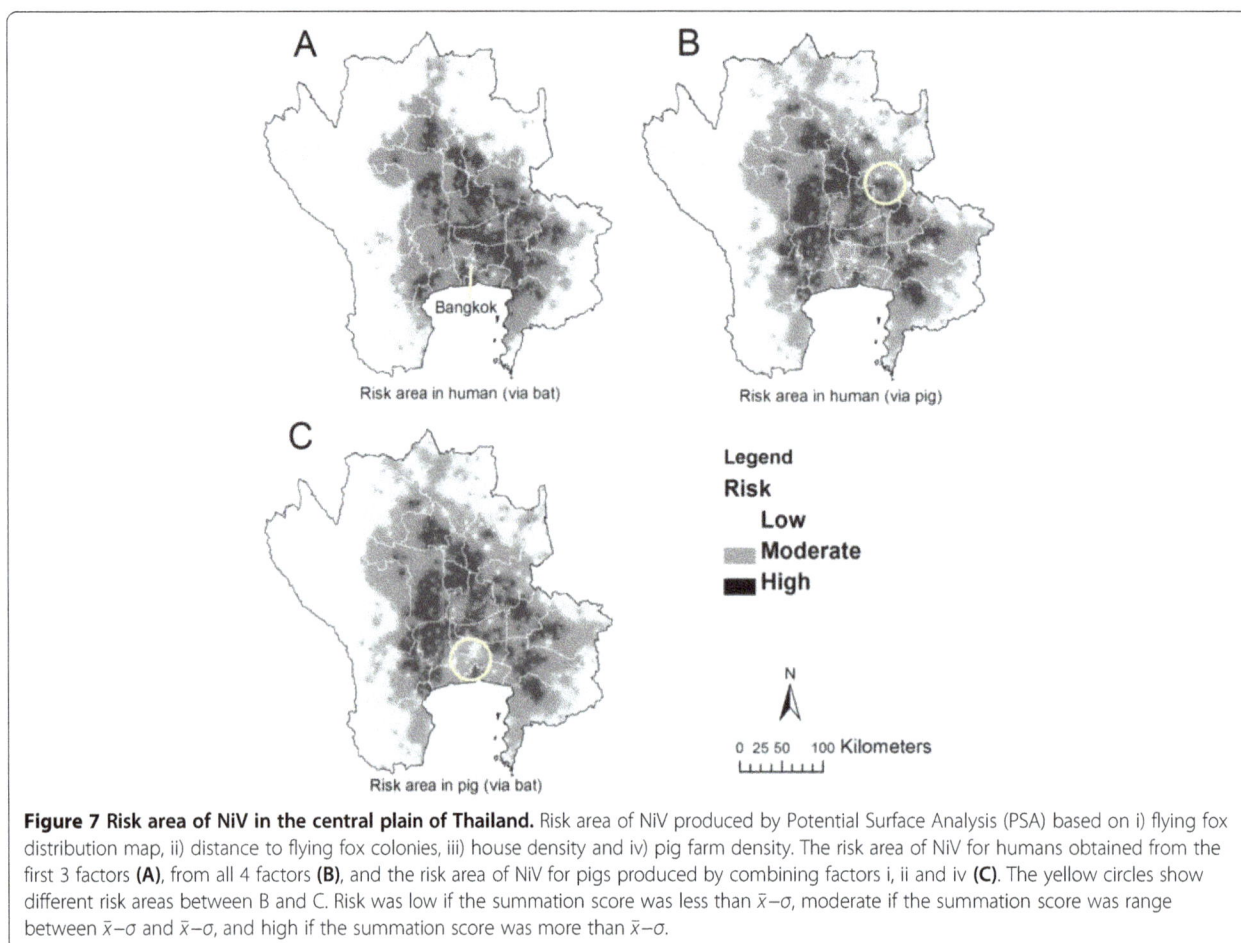

Figure 7 Risk area of NiV in the central plain of Thailand. Risk area of NiV produced by Potential Surface Analysis (PSA) based on i) flying fox distribution map, ii) distance to flying fox colonies, iii) house density and iv) pig farm density. The risk area of NiV for humans obtained from the first 3 factors (**A**), from all 4 factors (**B**), and the risk area of NiV for pigs produced by combining factors i, ii and iv (**C**). The yellow circles show different risk areas between B and C. Risk was low if the summation score was less than $\bar{x}-\sigma$, moderate if the summation score was range between $\bar{x}-\sigma$ and $\bar{x}-\sigma$, and high if the summation score was more than $\bar{x}-\sigma$.

Discussion

Our field observations indicated that flying foxes choose a variety of tree types, especially members of evergreen forests, for roosting, even if the trees no longer protect the bats from sunlight. The observations are supported by remote sensing, showing a normalized difference vegetation index acquired from January 2014 LANDSAT imagery with relatively low values at some of the roosting sites. This suggests flying foxes prefer evergreen forests to protect themselves from the sunlight while roosting, but also show a tolerance to trees damaged by bat urine and roosting [25]. We found roosting sites in relatively safe places, including Buddhist temples, islands, the Wildlife Conservation Park, and private lands, as marked by SDMs that included distance to a temple as an important predictor. Even as flying foxes are protected by the Wildlife Preservation and Protection Act, B.E. 2535 (1992), they are still threatened by human hunting, efforts to protect fruit orchards, and informal efforts at disease prevention. Most of the population is Buddhist (>90%) and would largely refrain from threatening animals in the vicinity of temples. Human

density appears to correspond positively with roosting sites for temple communities but is negatively associated for the greatest densities in and around urban areas. Some bat colonies are located in private lands and study informants indicated landlords and/or the people in the local community around these sites had tried to protect the bats against hunters. Finally, the other colonies were located in isolated areas such as islands, riverside, and at seaside that are hard to reach by hunters. The Wildlife Conservation Park is closed off as a unit of wildlife conservation. Therefore, all bat colonies, across a variety of locales, were protected from hunters for an array of reasons, including cultural practices, ownership, local sentiment, and remoteness.

The distribution of flying fox colonies is dynamic and changes are observed over time. In 2004–2014, new colonies were observed and a few colonies moved away from their previously known sites [26]. Apart from disturbances caused by hunters, other factors may trigger colony migration. Disturbance by visitors or tourists is assumed to have caused colony no. 21 to move away from its old site to a new isolated site seaside. The roosting trees may have been damaged or killed by the flying foxes themselves by way of their urine and/or roosting [25]. Colony no. 17 moved away from a site with numerous destroyed mangrove forest trees to an adjacent area. Competition with other species using the same habitat could also play an important role as former bat colonies sites were observed colonized by large bird populations. Finally, colonies may move if their sizes increase beyond the capacity of a roosting site, if the foraging areas are reduced or too impacted by urban development, or in relation to the mating season [49]. Colony mobility supports the concept of mapping potentially suitable sites. Even should these sites be presently empty, they may be occupied in the near future.

The distance to bodies of water was found to be an important factor, both in the field and through statistical analysis. Rainho and Palmeirim [50] made similar observations in two cave-dwelling species (*Rhinolophus mehelyi* and *Miniopterus schreibersii*), for which proximity to a source of drinking water was an important factor. The Department of Environment of the Australian government also reported that flying foxes sites were usually found close to water [10]. Several studies indicated that bats lose a significant amount of water while they are roosting, especially under conditions of low relative humidity and high temperature [51-53]. Furthermore, lactating females need more frequent drinking than non-reproductive females [54]. Flying foxes may also need water for cooling down. Welbergen *et al.* [55] reported temperatures exceeding 42°C in January 2002 in New South Wales, Australia, causing the deaths of thousands of flying foxes from hyperthermia. The high temperature may lead flying foxes to dip their bellies into water to cool down [56]. The maximum temperatures in central Thailand in most months are above 30°C, with temperatures of 40°C commonly recorded in April [57]. As some roosting trees fail to protect bats from sunlight, the availability of nearby water may help those populations to resist the worst of the heat during the hottest months. Informants living nearby bat colonies suggested flying foxes may use bodies of water as landmarks for foraging. They reported flying foxes frequently flying along the river when they depart their roosting sites in the evening and when flying back along the river in the morning. Using water bodies as foraging landmarks was reported in insect-eating bats. For example, in the little brown bat, water bodies have been shown to be used as landmarks to help foraging on patches of insects found in abundance above rivers, streams, ponds, or lakes [58]. The association that we found between flying foxes and areas located in the lowland central plain, which is surrounded by vegetation, may also simply correspond to the extensive irrigation that allows greater vegetation than elsewhere, as observed in Australia [9].

Further studies, focusing on the distribution, ecology, behaviors, and disease status of flying foxes should be conducted in Thailand in the central region but also elsewhere. Although the foraging plants and some of the environmental factors associated with flying fox colonies have been reported in other countries, a follow-up should be pursued in Thailand and for its singular ecologies [9,59]. Such data would be useful for conserving flying fox populations and in disease prevention and surveillance. Flying fox movements, heat relief, water usage, and other behaviors should be more fully characterized as they are likely to have impacts upon transmission patterns. For instance, during the mating season, large aggregations of individuals migrating from different sites are observed, and, as documented in Arctic waterfowl, could potentially contribute to the spread of pathogens across bat and other populations [49,60].

The SDM maps converged with the observations discussed above, showing highly suitable areas for flying foxes mainly located along riversides, in river basins in the central plain, and in areas of moderate human population density. The number of known occurrences in our study was low (*n* = 22) and many studies note that small sample sizes can significantly reduce the predictive potential of models [31,61-63]. Several methods have been proposed to deal with the problem [33,64-66]. While some methods are more effective at predicting species' distributions than others, no modeling method has proven to be the best in all situations. The ensemble modeling approach used in this study appears as a way to limit the potential influence of one particular modeling method, which was found to provide good results in previous studies [38,67,68]. However, we recognize that one of the limitations of our study may be the low sample size. One option for improvement might be to pool locations from wider areas and across countries, to have a larger sample size and sets of environmental conditions.

Even more challenging than mapping the suitability for a colony is to map the suitability for NiV infection. Generally, identifying risk factors associated with the spatial distribution of disease relies on disease distribution data that are used to quantify the effect of a set of explanatory variables on the spatial distribution of a particular disease outcome [69]. The outcome variable can be a count of disease events in a unit area or more simply a binary response indicating the presence or absence of disease at a given location. Each outcome can be used to map other areas sharing similar risk factors [69]. However, such an approach was not possible for NiV in Thailand since no case of NiV infection in human or pig has yet been found [23]. What we do have outside an etiological agent, in this case NiV, are susceptible hosts (bats, pigs and humans) and environments that connect hosts and the potential agent. By PSA we mapped areas where the virus's documented reservoirs potentially coincide. The approach has not been used in epidemiological study but may be useful in the absence of disease data, as a way to spatialize disease surveillance and regionally plan livestock production. Even though it has not been used in epidemiological study and is not based on a formal statistical model, it remained useful in the present case of a disease that is absent (and hence provides no data to train a model) as a way to integrate different factors in a risk map that can inform further planning and disease surveillance in a context of very limited knowledge. A limitation of the approach is, however, the somewhat arbitrary choices on weights that are made along the process, that are defined in a more explicit and thorough way in using MCDA approaches. Ultimately, the spatial validity of both approaches could only be formally evaluated in retrospect, if NiV infection were eventually identified in the country.

Conclusions

Broad-scale delineation of areas where three potential host types—bat, pig and human—are present could improve NiV surveillance strategy [70]. Indeed, in a context of limited financial support for animal disease surveillance systems, a more optimal use of resources could be implemented if active surveillance is targeted at higher-risk farms or areas [70]. One approach could circle around developing passive and active surveillance programs on pig farms of predicted risk, for example, with particular focus on farms of low biosecurity, nearby bodies of water, and/or hosting orchards as additional risk factors [11]. The surveillance program should be integrated with those for other diseases to reduce cost and manpower. Simultaneously, such surveillance efforts could be reinforced with enhanced communication on good farm management practices and public awareness campaigns.

In addition, preventing direct transmission of NiV from bats to humans could be adapted to the characteristic habitats identified in this study. For instance, it is apparent that flying foxes on the central plain of Thailand are found in particular conditions in spatial (e.g., distance to water, vegetation) and social terms (e.g., undisturbed environment and community). An active surveillance program could be conducted on the people who live closely to flying fox colonies. A new colony detected in 2011 (no. 17) is surrounded by commercial orchards, in particular coconut trees [26]. Testing NiV in a fresh coconut-palm sugar, usually produced by leaving a container on the trees overnight, may be useful for a focal study. In Bangladesh, sap harvesters were encouraged to use bamboo skirts on their trees to prevent contacts between fruit bats and raw date palm sap. Authorities educated locals to avoid drinking raw date palm sap or eat partially eaten fruit, and these

efforts could be adapted for Thailand [71]. Finally, the central plain of Thailand is an area with intense farming activities, including pig husbandry, reflecting strongly the convergence across multiple risk models here. Surveillance programs in pigs and humans should be integrated to mutually increase their effectiveness.

Competing interests
The authors declare that they have no competing interests.

Authors' contributions
WT and MG conceived and designed the study. WT generated the raw data and performed statistical analysis with contributions from MG, CL, XX, and CB. WT drafted the paper, which MG, CL and RW critically reviewed. PC, WW, and BK provided raw data. All authors read and approved the final manuscript.

Acknowledgements
Part of this work was supported through the NIH NIAID grant (1R01AI101028-01A1). We thank the staff of the Department of Livestock Development (DLD) for conducting the surveillance on the animals; National Institute of Animal Health (NIAH) and Regional Veterinary Research and Development Centers for evaluating the NiV; Ministry of Transportation for geodata; Department of Provincial Administration, Ministry of Interior for population data; and Department of National Parks, Wildlife and Plant Conservation, Ministry of Resources and Environment for location data for the fruit bats. We also thank colleagues at Lutte biologique et Ecologie spatiale (LUBIES), ULB, Belgium, for assistance and suggestions.

Author details
[1]Department of Livestock Development (DLD), Bangkok, Thailand. [2]Lutte biologique et Ecologie spatiale (LUBIES), Université Libre de Bruxelles, Brussels, Belgium. [3]Fonds National de la Recherche Scientifique (FNRS), Brussels, Belgium. [4]The Monitoring and Surveillance Center for Zoonotic Diseases in Wildlife and Exotic Animals (MOZWE), Mahidol University, Nakhonpatom, Thailand. [5]Department of National Parks, Wildlife, and Plant Conservation, Bangkok, Thailand. [6]Department of Microbiology and Plant Biology, Center for Spatial Analysis, University of Oklahoma, Norman, OK 73019, USA. [7]Institute of Biodiversity Science, Fudan University, Shanghai 200433, China. [8]International Center for Agricultural Research in Dry Areas (ICARDA), Amman, Jordan. [9]Institute for Global Studies, University of Minnesota, Minneapolis, USA.

References
1. Suzán G, Marcé E, Giermakowski JT, Armién B, Pascale J, Mills J, et al. The effect of habitat fragmentation and species diversity loss on hantavirus Prevalence in Panama. Ann N Y Acad Sci. 2008;1149:80–3.
2. Mohd Nor MN, Gan CH, Ong BL. Nipah virus infection of pigs in peninsular Malaysia. Rev Sci Tech Int Off Epizoot. 2000;19:160–5.
3. WHO | Nipah Virus (NiV) Infection [http://www.who.int/csr/disease/nipah/en/]
4. Chua KB, Lek Koh C, Hooi PS, Wee KF, Khong JH, Chua BH, et al. Isolation of Nipah virus from Malaysian Island flying-foxes. Microbes Infect. 2002;4:145–51.
5. Mohd Yob J, Hume F, Azmin Mohd R, Christopher M, Van Der Heide B, Paul R, et al. Nipah virus infection in bats (order Chiroptera) in peninsular Malaysia. Emergin Infect Dis. 2001;7:439–41.
6. Reynes J-M, Counor D, Ong S, Faure C, Seng V, Molia S, et al. Nipah virus in Lyle's flying foxes, Cambodia. Emerg Infect Dis. 2005;11:1042–7.
7. Wacharapluesadee S, Lumlertdacha B, Boongird K, Wanghongsa S, Chanhome L, Rollin P, et al. Bat Nipah Virus, Thailand. Emerg Infect Dis. 2005;11:1949–51.
8. Iehlé C, Razafitrimo G, Razainirina J, Andriaholinirina N, Goodman SM, Faure C, et al. Henipavirus and tioman virus antibodies in pteropodid bats, Madagascar. Emerg Infect Dis. 2007;13:159–61.
9. DEPI - Flying-foxes [http://www.depi.vic.gov.au/environment-and-wildlife/wildlife/flying-foxes]
10. Flying-foxes and national environmental law [http://www.environment.gov.au/node/16394]

11. Chua K, Chua B, Wang C. Anthropogenic deforestation, El Niño and the emergence of Nipah virus in Malaysia. Malays J Pathol. 2001;24(1):15–21.

12. Tan K-S, Tan C-T, Goh K-J. Epidemiological aspects of Nipah virus infection. Neurol J Southeast Asia. 1999;4:77–81.

13. Chua KB, Goh KJ, Wong KT, Kamarulzaman A, Tan PSK, Ksiazek TG, et al. Fatal encephalitis due to Nipah virus among pig-farmers in Malaysia. Lancet. 1999;354:1257–9.

14. Paton NI, Leo YS, Zaki SR, Auchus AP, Lee KE, Ling AE, et al. Outbreak of Nipah-virus infection among abattoir workers in Singapore. Lancet. 1999;354:1253–6.

15. Chew MHL, Arguin PM, Shay DK, Goh K-T, Rollin PE, Shieh W-J, et al. Risk factors for Nipah virus infection among abattoir workers in Singapore. J Infect Dis. 2000;181:1760–3.

16. Hsu VP, Hossain MJ, Parashar UD, Ali MM, Ksiazek TG, Kuzmin I, et al. Nipah virus encephalitis reemergence, Bangladesh. Emerg Infect Dis. 2004;10:2082–7.

17. Luby S, Rahman M, Hossain M, Blum L, Husain M, Gurley E, et al. Foodborne transmission of Nipah virus, Bangladesh. Emerg Infect Dis. 2006;12:1888–94.

18. Luby SP, Gurley ES, Hossain MJ. Transmission of human infection with Nipah virus. Clin Infect Dis. 2009;49:1743–8.

19. Luby SP, Hossain MJ, Gurley ES, Ahmed B-N, Banu S, Khan SU, et al. Recurrent zoonotic transmission of Nipah virus into humans, Bangladesh, 2001–2007. Emerg Infect Dis. 2009;15:1229–35.

20. Chadha MS, Comer JA, Lowe L, Rota PA, Rollin PE, Bellini WJ, et al. Nipah virus-associated encephalitis outbreak, Siliguri, India. Emerg Infect Dis. 2006;12:235–40.

21. Pathchimasiri T, Kalpravidh W, Damrongwatanapokin S, Chantamaneechote T, Daniels P, Buranathai C: Immunohistochemistry Investigation of Nipah Virus : A Retrospective study in Thailand. In *The 11th International Symposium of the World Association of Veterinary Laboratory Diagnosticials and OIE Seminar on Biotechnology*. Thai Association of Veterinary Laboratory Diagnosticians; 2003:44–45.

22. Department of Livestock Development. Animal health in Thailand 2011. Bangkok, Thailand: Department of Livestock Development; 2012.

23. OIE World Animal Health Information System [http://www.oie.int/wahis_2/public/wahid.php/Countryinformation/Animalsituation]

24. Wacharapluesadee S, Boongird K, Wanghongsa S, Ratanasetyuth N, Supavonwong P, Saengsen D, et al. A longitudinal study of the prevalence of Nipah virus in *Pteropus lylei* bats in Thailand: evidence for seasonal preference in disease transmission. Vector-Borne Zoonotic Dis. 2010;10:183–90.

25. Boonkird K, Wanghongsa S. On the population number and distribution fo flying foxes (Pteropus lylei) in central plain. Wildl Yearb. 2004;5:89–100.

26. Sedwisai P, Changbunjong T, Chamsai T, Yongyuttawichai P, Sangkachai N, Weluwanarak T, et al. The distribution of flying fox (Pteropus spp.) in the central region of Thailand. J Appl Anim Sci. 2011;4:21–9.

27. Gaughan AE, Stevens FR, Linard C, Jia P, Tatem AJ. High resolution population distribution maps for Southeast Asia in 2010 and 2015. PLoS One. 2013;8:e55882.

28. CGIAR-CSI SRTM 90 m DEM Digital Elevation Database [http://srtm.csi.cgiar.org/]

29. Classification References (Using ENVI) | Exelis VIS Docs Center [http://www.exelisvis.com/docs/ClassificationReferences.html]

30. Elith J, Leathwick JR. Species distribution models: ecological explanation and prediction across space and time. Annu Rev Ecol Evol Syst. 2009;40:677–97.

31. McPherson JM, Jetz W, Rogers DJ. The effects of species' range sizes on the accuracy of distribution models: ecological phenomenon or statistical artefact?: Species' range and distribution model accuracy. J Appl Ecol. 2004;41:811–23.

32. Elith J, Graham CH, Anderson RP, Dudík M, Ferrier S, Guisan A, et al. Novel methods improve prediction of species' distributions from occurrence data. Ecography. 2006;29:129–51.

33. Barbet-Massin M, Jiguet F, Albert CH, Thuiller W. Selecting pseudo-absences for species distribution models: how, where and how many? Methods Ecol Evol. 2012;3:327–38.

34. Phillips SJ, Anderson RP, Schapire RE. Maximum entropy modeling of species geographic distributions. Ecol Model. 2006;190:231–59.

35. Elith J, Leathwick JR, Hastie T. A working guide to boosted regression trees. J Anim Ecol. 2008;77:802–13.

36. Breiman L. Random forests. In: Machine learning, vol. 45. The Netherlands: Kluwer Academic Publishers; 2001. p. 5–32.

37. Cutler DR, Edwards TC, Beard KH, Cutler A, Hess KT, Gibson J, et al. Random forests for classificaiton in ecology. Ecology. 2007;88:2783–92.

38. Marmion M, Parviainen M, Luoto M, Heikkinen RK, Thuiller W. Evaluation of consensus methods in predictive species distribution modelling. Divers Distrib. 2009;15:59–69.

39. Araujo M, New M. Ensemble forecasting of species distributions. Trends Ecol Evol. 2007;22:42–7.

40. Robert J. Hijmans, Jane Elith: Species distribution modeling with R. 2013.

41. Engler R, Waser LT, Zimmermann NE, Schaub M, Berdos S, Ginzler C, et al. Combining ensemble modeling and remote sensing for mapping individual tree species at high spatial resolution. For Ecol Manag. 2013;310:64–73.

42. Thuiller W, Lafourcade B, Engler R, Araújo MB. BIOMOD - a platform for ensemble forecasting of species distributions. Ecography. 2009;32:369–73.

43. Augustin NH, Mugglestone MA, Buckland ST. An autologistic model for the spatial distribution of wildlife. J Appl Ecol. 1996;33:339–47.

44. Fielding AH, Bell JF. A review of methods for the assessment of prediction errors in conservation presence/absence models. Environ Conserv. 1997;24:38–49.

45. Stevens KB, Gilbert M, Pfeiffer DU. Modeling habitat suitability for occurrence of highly pathogenic avian influenza virus H5N1 in domestic poultry in Asia: a spatial multicriteria decision analysis approach. Spat Spatio-Temporal Epidemiol. 2013;4:1–14.

46. Ano T, Hormwichian R, Jitrapinate N, Compliew S, Kangrang A. The estimation of drought risk area using potential surface analysis technique. UBU Eng J. 2013;6:13–21.

47. Udomsap I, Iamtrakul P. Accessibility improvement for district's urban diversity: case study of Rachadamnoen klong avenue, Bangkok. J Soc Transp Traffic Stud JSTS. 2011;2:1–17.

48. Nakya S, Leopairojna SK, Rangsiraksa L. Use of satellite data and potential surface analysis for Urban expansion of Hua Hin Municipality, Prachuap Khiri Khan Province, Thailand. In: 31st Asian conference on remote sensing 2010. Volume 1. Hanoi, Vietnam: Asian Association on Remote Sensing; 2010. p. 293–302.

49. Eby P. Seasonal movements of grey-headed flying-foxes, Pteropus poliocephalus (Chiroptera : Pteropodidae), from two maternity camps in northern New South Wales. Wildl Res. 1991;18:547.

50. Rainho A, Palmeirim JM. The importance of distance to resources in the spatial modelling of bat foraging habitat. PLoS One. 2011;6:e19227.

51. Webb PI. The comparative ecophysiology of water balance in microchiropteran. 67;1995:203–218

52. Webb PI, Speakman JR, Racey PA. Evaporative water loss in two sympatric species of vespertilionid bat, Plecotus auritus and Myotis daubentoni: relation to foraging mode and implications for roost site selection. J Zool. 2009;235:269–78.

53. Studier EH, O'Farrell MJ. Biology of Myotis thysanodes and M. lucifugus (Chiroptera: Vespertilionidae)—III. Metabolism, heart rate, breathing rate, evaporative water loss and general energetics. Comp Biochem Physiol A Physiol. 1976;54:423–32.

54. Adams RA, Hayes MA. Water availability and successful lactation by bats as related to climate change in arid regions of western North America. J Anim Ecol. 2008;77:1115–21.

55. Welbergen JA, Klose SM, Markus N, Eby P. Climate change and the effects of temperature extremes on Australian flying-foxes. Proc R Soc B Biol Sci. 2008;275:419–25.

56. Killer climate: tens of thousands of flying foxes dead in a day [http://www.brisbanetimes.com.au/queensland/killer-climate-tens-of-thousands-of-flying-foxes-dead-in-a-day-20140225-33drr.html]

57. Thai Meteorological Department [http://www.tmd.go.th/en/]

58. Clare EL, Barber BR, Sweeney BW, Hebert PDN, Fenton MB. Eating local: influences of habitat on the diet of little brown bats (Myotis lucifugus): molecular detection of variation in diet. Mol Ecol. 2011;20:1772–80.

59. Flying foxes | NSW Environment & Heritage [http://www.environment.nsw.gov.au/animals/flyingfoxes.htm]

60. Olsen B. Global patterns of influenza A virus in wild birds. Science. 2006;312:384–8.

61. Stockwell DR, Peterson AT. Effects of sample size on accuracy of species distribution models. Ecol Model. 2002;148:1–13.

62. Chen H, Wood MD, Linstead C, Maltby E. Uncertainty analysis in a GIS-based multi-criteria analysis tool for river catchment management. Environ Model Softw. 2011;26:395–405.

63. Hirzel A, Guisan A. Which is the optimal sampling strategy for habitat suitability modelling. Ecol Model. 2002;157:331–41.

64. Segurado P, Araújo MB. An evaluation of methods for modelling species distributions: methods for modelling species distributions. J Biogeogr. 2004;31:1555–68.

65. Engler R, Guisan A, Rechsteiner L. An improved approach for predicting the distribution of rare and endangered species from occurrence and pseudo-absence data. J Appl Ecol. 2004;41:263–74.

66. Hanberry BB, He HS, Palik BJ. Pseudoabsence generation strategies for species distribution models. PLoS One. 2012;7:e44486.

67. Lauzeral C, Grenouillet G, Brosse S. Dealing with noisy absences to optimize species distribution models: an iterative ensemble modelling approach. PLoS One. 2012;7:e49508.

68. Grenouillet G, Buisson L, Casajus N, Lek S. Ensemble modelling of species distribution: the effects of geographical and environmental ranges. Ecography. 2011;34:9–17.

69. Graham A, Atkinson P, Danson F. Spatial analysis for epidemiology. Acta Trop. 2004;91:219–25.

70. Katharina DS, Regula G, Hernandez J, Knopf L, Fuchs K, Morris RS, et al. Concepts for risk-based surveillance in the field of veterinary medicine and veterinary public health: Review of current approaches. BMC Health Serv Res 2006:6–20

71. Khan SU, Gurley ES, Hossain MJ, Nahar N, Sharker MAY, Luby SP. A randomized controlled trial of interventions to impede date palm sap contamination by bats to prevent Nipah virus transmission in Bangladesh. PLoS One. 2012;7:e42689.

72. Forest Types in Thailand [http://wildlifethailand.com]

73. Mangrove Forest Habitat in Tropical Thailand [http://www.kohphrathong.com/thailand_mangrove.html]

74. Asia-Pacific Forestry Sector Outlook Study: Country Report - Thailand [http://www.fao.org/docrep/003/x2649e/X2649E03.htm]

75. Biodiversity & Expert Database [http://www.bedo.or.th/lcdb/default.aspx]

Permissions

List of Contributors

Mehdi Rasoli
Institute of Bioscience, Universiti Putra Malaysia, Serdang 43400, Selangor, Malaysia

Swee Keong Yeap
Institute of Bioscience, Universiti Putra Malaysia, Serdang 43400, Selangor, Malaysia

Sheau Wei Tan
Institute of Bioscience, Universiti Putra Malaysia, Serdang 43400, Selangor, Malaysia

Kiarash Roohani
Institute of Bioscience, Universiti Putra Malaysia, Serdang 43400, Selangor, Malaysia

Ye Wen Kristeen-Teo
Faculty of Biotechnology and Biomolecular Sciences, Universiti Putra Malaysia, Serdang 43400, Selangor, Malaysia

Noorjahan Banu Alitheen
Institute of Bioscience, Universiti Putra Malaysia, Serdang 43400, Selangor, Malaysia
Faculty of Biotechnology and Biomolecular Sciences, Universiti Putra Malaysia, Serdang 43400, Selangor, Malaysia

Yasmin Abd Rahaman
Institute of Bioscience, Universiti Putra Malaysia, Serdang 43400, Selangor, Malaysia
Faculty of Veterinary Medicine, Universiti Putra Malaysia, Serdang 43400, Selangor, Malaysia

Ideris Aini
Institute of Bioscience, Universiti Putra Malaysia, Serdang 43400, Selangor, Malaysia
Faculty of Veterinary Medicine, Universiti Putra Malaysia, Serdang 43400, Selangor, Malaysia

Mohd Hair Bejo
Institute of Bioscience, Universiti Putra Malaysia, Serdang 43400, Selangor, Malaysia
Faculty of Veterinary Medicine, Universiti Putra Malaysia, Serdang 43400, Selangor, Malaysia

Pete Kaiser
The Roslin Institute and R(D)SVS, University of Edinburgh, Easter Bush, Midlothian EH25 9RG, UK

Abdul Rahman Omar
Institute of Bioscience, Universiti Putra Malaysia, Serdang 43400, Selangor, Malaysia
Faculty of Veterinary Medicine, Universiti Putra Malaysia, Serdang 43400, Selangor, Malaysia

Manuel F Chamorro
Department of Clinical Sciences, College of Veterinary Medicine, Auburn University, Auburn, AL, USA

Paul H Walz
Department of Pathobiology, College of Veterinary Medicine, Auburn University, Auburn, AL, USA

Thomas Passler
Department of Clinical Sciences, College of Veterinary Medicine, Auburn University, Auburn, AL, USA

Edzard van Santen
Department of Crop, Soils, and Environmental Sciences, College of Agriculture and Alabama Agricultural Experiment Station, Auburn University, Auburn, AL, USA

Julie Gard
Department of Clinical Sciences, College of Veterinary Medicine, Auburn University, Auburn, AL, USA

Soren P Rodning
Department of Animal Sciences, College of Agriculture, Auburn University, Auburn, AL, USA

Kay P Riddell
Department of Pathobiology, College of Veterinary Medicine, Auburn University, Auburn, AL, USA

Patricia K Galik
Department of Pathobiology, College of Veterinary Medicine, Auburn University, Auburn, AL, USA

Yijing Zhang
Department of Pathobiology, College of Veterinary Medicine, Auburn University, Auburn, AL, USA

Hai-ling Zhang
Division of Infectious Diseases of Special Economic Animal, Institute of Special Animal and Plant Sciences, Chinese Academy of Agricultural Sciences, 4899 Juye Street, Changchun 130112, China

Jian-jun Zhao
Division of Infectious Diseases of Special Economic Animal, Institute of Special Animal and Plant Sciences, Chinese Academy of Agricultural Sciences, 4899 Juye Street, Changchun 130112, China

Xiu-li Chai
Division of Infectious Diseases of Special Economic Animal, Institute of Special Animal and Plant Sciences, Chinese Academy of Agricultural Sciences, 4899 Juye Street, Changchun 130112, China

Lei Zhang
Division of Infectious Diseases of Special Economic Animal, Institute of Special Animal and Plant Sciences, Chinese Academy of Agricultural Sciences, 4899 Juye Street, Changchun 130112, China

Xue Bai
Division of Infectious Diseases of Special Economic Animal, Institute of Special Animal and Plant Sciences, Chinese Academy of Agricultural Sciences, 4899 Juye Street, Changchun 130112, China

Bo Hu
Division of Infectious Diseases of Special Economic Animal, Institute of Special Animal and Plant Sciences, Chinese Academy of Agricultural Sciences, 4899 Juye Street, Changchun 130112, China

Hao Liu
Division of Infectious Diseases of Special Economic Animal, Institute of Special Animal and Plant Sciences, Chinese Academy of Agricultural Sciences, 4899 Juye Street, Changchun 130112, China

Dong-liang Zhang
Jilin Teyan Biotechnological Co. Ltd, 388 Liuying West Road, Changchun 130122, China

Ming Ye
Jilin Teyan Biotechnological Co. Ltd, 388 Liuying West Road, Changchun 130122, China

Wei Wu
Jilin Teyan Biotechnological Co. Ltd, 388 Liuying West Road, Changchun 130122, China

Xi-jun Yan
Division of Infectious Diseases of Special Economic Animal, Institute of Special Animal and Plant Sciences, Chinese Academy of Agricultural Sciences, 4899 Juye Street, Changchun 130112, China

Consuelo Rubio-Guerri
VISAVET Center and Animal Health Department, Veterinary School, Complutense University of Madrid, Av Puerta del Hierro s/n, 28040 Madrid, Spain

Daniel García-Párraga
Veterinary Services, Oceanographic Aquarium of the Ciudad de las Artes y las Ciencias, C/ Junta de Murs i Valls s/n, 46023 Valencia, Spain

Elvira Nieto-Pelegrín
VISAVET Center and Animal Health Department, Veterinary School, Complutense University of Madrid, Av Puerta del Hierro s/n, 28040 Madrid, Spain

Mar Melero
VISAVET Center and Animal Health Department, Veterinary School, Complutense University of Madrid, Av Puerta del Hierro s/n, 28040 Madrid, Spain

Teresa Álvaro
Veterinary Services, Oceanographic Aquarium of the Ciudad de las Artes y las Ciencias, C/ Junta de Murs i Valls s/n, 46023 Valencia, Spain

Mónica Valls
Veterinary Services, Oceanographic Aquarium of the Ciudad de las Artes y las Ciencias, C/ Junta de Murs i Valls s/n, 46023 Valencia, Spain

Jose Luis Crespo
Veterinary Services, Oceanographic Aquarium of the Ciudad de las Artes y las Ciencias, C/ Junta de Murs i Valls s/n, 46023 Valencia, Spain

Jose Manuel Sánchez-Vizcaíno
VISAVET Center and Animal Health Department, Veterinary School, Complutense University of Madrid, Av Puerta del Hierro s/n, 28040 Madrid, Spain

Jianke Wang
State Key Laboratory for Molecular Biology of Special Economic Animals, Institute of Special Animal and Plant Sciences, Chinese Academy of Agricultural Sciences, Changchun 130112, China

Yuening Cheng
Jilin Teyan Biological Technology Company, Changchun 130122, China

Miao Zhang
Jilin Teyan Biological Technology Company, Changchun 130122, China

Hang Zhao
State Key Laboratory for Molecular Biology of Special Economic Animals, Institute of Special Animal and Plant Sciences, Chinese Academy of Agricultural Sciences, Changchun 130112, China

Peng Lin
State Key Laboratory for Molecular Biology of Special Economic Animals, Institute of Special Animal and Plant Sciences, Chinese Academy of Agricultural Sciences, Changchun 130112, China

Li Yi
State Key Laboratory for Molecular Biology of Special Economic Animals, Institute of Special Animal and Plant Sciences, Chinese Academy of Agricultural Sciences, Changchun 130112, China

Mingwei Tong
State Key Laboratory for Molecular Biology of Special Economic Animals, Institute of Special Animal and Plant Sciences, Chinese Academy of Agricultural Sciences, Changchun 130112, China

Shipeng Cheng
State Key Laboratory for Molecular Biology of Special Economic Animals, Institute of Special Animal and Plant Sciences, Chinese Academy of Agricultural Sciences, Changchun 130112, China

Moses Y Otiende
Veterinary Services Department, Forensic and Genetics Laboratory Kenya Wildlife Service, P.O Box 40241–00100, Nairobi, Kenya

Mary W Kivata
Department of Biochemistry and Biotechnology, Kenyatta University, P.O Box 43844–00100, Nairobi, Kenya

Joseph N Makumi
Department of Biochemistry and Biotechnology, Kenyatta University, P.O Box 43844–00100, Nairobi, Kenya

Mathew N Mutinda
Veterinary Services Department, Forensic and Genetics Laboratory Kenya Wildlife Service, P.O Box 40241–00100, Nairobi, Kenya

Daniel Okun
Department of Biochemistry and Biotechnology, Kenyatta University, P.O Box 43844–00100, Nairobi, Kenya

Linus Kariuki
Veterinary Services Department, Forensic and Genetics Laboratory Kenya Wildlife Service, P.O Box 40241–00100, Nairobi, Kenya

Vincent Obanda
Veterinary Services Department, Forensic and Genetics Laboratory Kenya Wildlife Service, P.O Box 40241–00100, Nairobi, Kenya

Francis Gakuya
Veterinary Services Department, Forensic and Genetics Laboratory Kenya Wildlife Service, P.O Box 40241–00100, Nairobi, Kenya

Dominic Mijele
Veterinary Services Department, Forensic and Genetics Laboratory Kenya Wildlife Service, P.O Box 40241–00100, Nairobi, Kenya

Ramón C Soriguer
Estación Biológica de Doñana, Consejo Superior de Investigaciones Científicas (CSIC), Avda. Américo Vespucio s/n 41092, Sevilla, Spain

Samer Alasaad
Estación Biológica de Doñana, Consejo Superior de Investigaciones Científicas (CSIC), Avda. Américo Vespucio s/n 41092, Sevilla, Spain
Institute of Evolutionary Biology and Environmental Studies (IEU), University of Zürich, Winterthurerstrasse 190, 8057 Zürich, Switzerland

Ueli Braun
Department of Farm Animals, Vetsuisse-Faculty, University of Zurich, Winterthurerstrasse 260, CH-8057 Zurich, Switzerland

Monika Hilbe
Institute of Veterinary Pathology, Vetsuisse-Faculty, University of Zurich, Winterthurerstrasse 260, CH-8057 Zurich, Switzerland

Fredi Janett
Department of Farm Animals, Vetsuisse-Faculty, University of Zurich, Winterthurerstrasse 260, CH-8057 Zurich, Switzerland

Michael Hässig
Department of Farm Animals, Vetsuisse-Faculty, University of Zurich, Winterthurerstrasse 260, CH-8057 Zurich, Switzerland

Reto Zanoni
Institute of Veterinary Virology, Vetsuisse-Faculty, University of Bern, Länggass-Strasse 122, 3001 Bern, Switzerland
New Name: Institute of Virology and Immunology, Federal Food Safety and Veterinary Office, University of Bern, Länggass-Strasse 122, CH-3001 Bern, Switzerland

Sandra Frei
Department of Farm Animals, Vetsuisse-Faculty, University of Zurich, Winterthurerstrasse 260, CH-8057 Zurich, Switzerland

Matthias Schweizer
Institute of Veterinary Virology, Vetsuisse-Faculty, University of Bern, Länggass-Strasse 122, 3001 Bern, Switzerland
New Name: Institute of Virology and Immunology, Federal Food Safety and Veterinary Office, University of Bern, Länggass-Strasse 122, CH-3001 Bern, Switzerland

Sabenzia Nabalayo Wekesa
Foot-and-Mouth Disease Laboratory, Embakasi, P. O. Box 18021 00500 Nairobi, Kenya Department of Environmental Management, College of Agricultural and Environmental Sciences, Makerere University, P. O. Box 7062/ 7298, Kampala, Uganda

Abraham Kiprotich Sangula
Foot-and-Mouth Disease Laboratory, Embakasi, P. O. Box 18021 00500 Nairobi, Kenya

Graham J Belsham
National Veterinary Institute, Technical University of Denmark, Lindholm DK-4771 Kalvehave, Denmark

Kirsten Tjornehoj
National Veterinary Institute, Technical University of Denmark, Lindholm DK-4771 Kalvehave, Denmark

Vincent B Muwanika
Department of Environmental Management, College of Agricultural and Environmental Sciences, Makerere University, P. O. Box 7062/ 7298, Kampala, Uganda

Francis Gakuya
Kenya Wildlife Service, Veterinary Services Department, P.O Box 40241 (00100), Nairobi, Kenya

Dominic Mijele
Kenya Wildlife Service, Veterinary Services Department, P.O Box 40241 (00100), Nairobi, Kenya

Hans Redlef Siegismund
Department of Biology, University of Copenhagen, Ole Maaløes Vej 5, DK-2200 Copenhagen, Denmark

Amina Khatun
College of Veterinary Medicine, Chonbuk National University Jeonju, Korea, 664-14 Deokjin-Dong 1 Ga, Jeonju, Jeonbuk 561-756, Republic of Korea

Nadeem Shabir
College of Veterinary Medicine, Chonbuk National University Jeonju, Korea, 664-14 Deokjin-Dong 1 Ga, Jeonju, Jeonbuk 561-756, Republic of Korea

Kyoung-Jin Yoon
Department of Veterinary Diagnostic and Production Animal Medicine, College of Veterinary Medicine, Iowa State University, Ames, IA, USA

Won-Il Kim
College of Veterinary Medicine, Chonbuk National University Jeonju, Korea, 664-14 Deokjin-Dong 1 Ga, Jeonju, Jeonbuk 561-756, Republic of Korea

Emily A Collin
Newport Laboratories Inc., Worthington, MN, USA
Department of Veterinary and Biomedical Sciences, South Dakota State University, Brookings, SD, USA
Veterinary Diagnostic Laboratory, Kansas State University, Manhattan, KS, USA

Srivishnupriya Anbalagan
Newport Laboratories Inc., Worthington, MN, USA

Faten Okda
Department of Veterinary and Biomedical Sciences, South Dakota State University, Brookings, SD, USA
National Research Center, Giza, Egypt

Ron Batman
Newport Laboratories Inc., Worthington, MN, USA

Eric Nelson
Department of Veterinary and Biomedical Sciences, South Dakota State University, Brookings, SD, USA

Ben M Hause
Newport Laboratories Inc., Worthington, MN, USA
Veterinary Diagnostic Laboratory, Kansas State University, Manhattan, KS, USA

Guangjun Chang
College of Veterinary Medicine, Nanjing Agricultural University, Nanjing 210095, PR, China

Kai Zhang
College of Veterinary Medicine, Nanjing Agricultural University, Nanjing 210095, PR, China

Tianle Xu
College of Veterinary Medicine, Nanjing Agricultural University, Nanjing 210095, PR, China

Di Jin
College of Veterinary Medicine, Nanjing Agricultural University, Nanjing 210095, PR, China

Hans-Martin Seyfert
Leibniz Institute for Farm Animal Biology, Wilhelm-Stahl-Allee 2, 18196 Dummerstorf, Germany

Xiangzhen Shen
College of Veterinary Medicine, Nanjing Agricultural University, Nanjing 210095, PR, China

Su Zhuang
College of Animal Science and Technology, Nanjing Agricultural University, Nanjing 210095, PR, China

Xiaoliang Hu Jr
College of Resources and Environment, Northeast Agricultural University, Harbin 150030, People's Republic of China
College of Life Sciences, Northeast Agricultural University, Harbin, Harbin 150030, People's Republic of China

Nannan Li Jr
College of Resources and Environment, Northeast Agricultural University, Harbin 150030, People's Republic of China

Zhige Tian Jr
College of Wildlife Resources, Northeast Forestry University, Harbin 150040, People's Republic of China

Xin Yin Jr
College of Life Sciences, Northeast Agricultural University, Harbin, Harbin 150030, People's Republic of China

Liandong Qu
National Key Laboratory of Veterinary Biotechnology, Harbin Veterinary Research Institute, Chinese Academy of Agricultural Sciences, Harbin 150001, People's Republic of China

Juanjuan Qu
College of Resources and Environment, Northeast Agricultural University, Harbin 150030, People's Republic of China

Han Lei
School of Medicine, Southwest Jiaotong University, Chengdu, 6111756, China
Department of Biomedical Engineering, State University of New York, Binghamton 13902, USA Department of Biotechnology, College of Life Science, Nanchang University, Jiangxi 330031, China

Xiaojue Peng
Department of Biotechnology, College of Life Science, Nanchang University, Jiangxi 330031, China

Jiexiu Ouyang
Department of Biotechnology, College of Life Science, Nanchang University, Jiangxi 330031, China

Daxian Zhao
Department of Biotechnology, College of Life Science, Nanchang University, Jiangxi 330031, China

Huifeng Jiao
Department of Biotechnology, College of Life Science, Nanchang University, Jiangxi 330031, China

Handing Shu
Department of Biotechnology, College of Life Science, Nanchang University, Jiangxi 330031, China

Xinqi Ge
Department of Biotechnology, College of Life Science, Nanchang University, Jiangxi 330031, China

Simon M Kihu
Faculty of Veterinary Medicine, University of Nairobi, PO Box 29053-00625, Uthiru, Kenya Vetworks Eastern Africa, PO Box 10431-00200, Nairobi, Kenya

John M Gachohi
Kenya Agricultural Research Institute -Trypanosomiasis Research Institute, PO Box 362-00902, Kikuyu, Kenya
International Livestock Research Institute (ILRI), PO Box 30709-00100, Nairobi, Kenya

Eunice K Ndungu
Kenya Agricultural Research Institute -Veterinary Research Centre, PO Box 32-00902, Kikuyu, Kenya

George C Gitao
Faculty of Veterinary Medicine, University of Nairobi, PO Box 29053-00625, Uthiru, Kenya

Lily C Bebora
Faculty of Veterinary Medicine, University of Nairobi, PO Box 29053-00625, Uthiru, Kenya

Njenga M John
Faculty of Veterinary Medicine, University of Nairobi, PO Box 29053-00625, Uthiru, Kenya

Gidraph G Wairire
Faculty of Arts, University of Nairobi, PO Box 30197-00100, Nairobi, Kenya

Ndichu Maingi
Faculty of Veterinary Medicine, University of Nairobi, PO Box 29053-00625, Uthiru, Kenya

Raphael G Wahome
Faculty of Veterinary Medicine, University of Nairobi, PO Box 29053-00625, Uthiru, Kenya

Ricky Ireri
Kenya Agricultural Research Institute -Veterinary Research Centre, PO Box 32-00902, Kikuyu, Kenya

Andrea Trovato
Parco Tecnologico Padano, via Einstein, Lodi 26900, Italy

Simona Panelli
Istituto Sperimentale Italiano Lazzaro Spallanzani, Loc. La Quercia, 26027 Rivolta d'Adda, Italy

Francesco Strozzi
Parco Tecnologico Padano, via Einstein, Lodi 26900, Italy

Caterina Cambulli
Istituto Sperimentale Italiano Lazzaro Spallanzani, Loc. La Quercia, 26027 Rivolta d'Adda, Italy

Ilaria Barbieri
Istituto Zooprofilattico Sperimentale della Lombardia e dell'Emilia Romagna, via Bianchi 9, 25124 Brescia, Italy

Nicola Martinelli
Istituto Zooprofilattico Sperimentale della Lombardia e dell'Emilia Romagna, via Bianchi 9, 25124 Brescia, Italy

Guerino Lombardi
Istituto Zooprofilattico Sperimentale della Lombardia e dell'Emilia Romagna, via Bianchi 9, 25124 Brescia, Italy

Rossana Capoferri
Istituto Sperimentale Italiano Lazzaro Spallanzani, Loc. La Quercia, 26027 Rivolta d'Adda, Italy

John L Williams
Parco Tecnologico Padano, via Einstein, Lodi 26900, Italy
School of Animal and Veterinary Sciences, University of Adelaide, Roseworthy, SA 5371, Australia

Ping-Yuan Lin
Department of Biological Science and Technology, Pingtung 91201, Taiwan

Ching-Dong Chang
Veterinary Medicine, National Pingtung University of Science and Technology, Pingtung, Taiwan

Yo-Chia Chen
Department of Biological Science and Technology, Pingtung 91201, Taiwan

Wen-Ling Shih
Department of Biological Science and Technology, Pingtung 91201, Taiwan
Graduate Institute of Biotechnology, National Pingtung University of Science and Technology, 1, Shuefu Rd., Neipu, Pingtung 91201, Taiwan

Jorgen Ravoet
Laboratory of Molecular Entomology and Bee Pathology, Ghent University, Krijgslaan 281 S2, B-9000 Ghent, Belgium

Lina De Smet
Laboratory of Molecular Entomology and Bee Pathology, Ghent University, Krijgslaan 281 S2, B-9000 Ghent, Belgium

Tom Wenseleers
Laboratory of Socioecology and Social Evolution, KU Leuven, Naamsestraat 59, B-3000 Leuven, Belgium

Dirk C de Graaf
Laboratory of Molecular Entomology and Bee Pathology, Ghent University, Krijgslaan 281 S2, B-9000 Ghent, Belgium

Verena Jung-Schroers
Fish Disease Research Unit, University of Veterinary Medicine, Hannover, Germany

Mikolaj Adamek
Fish Disease Research Unit, University of Veterinary Medicine, Hannover, Germany

Felix Teitge
Fish Disease Research Unit, University of Veterinary Medicine, Hannover, Germany

John Hellmann
Fish Disease Research Unit, University of Veterinary Medicine, Hannover, Germany

Sven Michael Bergmann
Friedrich-Loeffler-Institut, Federal Research Institute for Animal Health, Institute of Infectology, Greifswald, Germany

Heike Schütze
Friedrich-Loeffler-Institut, Federal Research Institute for Animal Health, Institute of Infectology, Greifswald, Germany

Dirk Willem Kleingeld
Lower Saxony State Office for Consumer Protection and Food Safety, Veterinary Task-Force, Hannover, Germany

Keith Way
Centre for Environment, Fisheries, and Aquaculture Science (CEFAS), Weymouth, Dorset, UK

David Stone
Centre for Environment, Fisheries, and Aquaculture Science (CEFAS), Weymouth, Dorset, UK

Martin Runge
Lower Saxony State Office for Consumer Protection and Food Safety, Food and Veterinary Institute Braunschweig/Hannover, Hannover, Germany

Barbara Keller
Lower Saxony State Office for Consumer Protection and Food Safety, Food and Veterinary Institute Braunschweig/Hannover, Hannover, Germany

Shohreh Hesami
Department of Infectious Diseases and Pathology, University of Florida, College of Veterinary Medicine, Gainesville, FL, USA

Thomas Waltzek
Department of Infectious Diseases and Pathology, University of Florida, College of Veterinary Medicine, Gainesville, FL, USA

Dieter Steinhagen
Fish Disease Research Unit, University of Veterinary Medicine, Hannover, Germany

Hai-Qiong Yu
Technical Center, Guangdong Entry-Exit Inspection and Quarantine Bureau, Guangzhou, Guangdong Province 510630, PR China

Xian-Quan Cai
Technical Center, Zhongshan Entry-Exit Inspection and Quarantine Bureau, Zhongshan, Guangdong Province 528403, PR China

Zhi-Xiong Lin
Technical Center, Guangdong Entry-Exit Inspection and Quarantine Bureau, Guangzhou, Guangdong Province 510630, PR China

Xiang-Li Li
Zhongshan Torch Polytechnic College, Zhongshan, Guangdong Province 528403, PR China

Qiao-Yun Yue
Technical Center, Zhongshan Entry-Exit Inspection and Quarantine Bureau, Zhongshan, Guangdong Province 528403, PR China

Rong Li
Technical Center, Zhongshan Entry-Exit Inspection and Quarantine Bureau, Zhongshan, Guangdong Province 528403, PR China

Xing-Quan Zhu
State Key Laboratory of Veterinary Etiological Biology, Lanzhou Veterinary Research Institute, Chinese Academy of Agricultural Sciences, Lanzhou, Gansu Province 730046, PR China

Marcin Smialek
Department of Poultry Diseases, Faculty of Veterinary Medicine, University of Warmia and Mazury, Oczapowskiego 13/14, 10-719 Olsztyn, Poland

Daria Pestka
Department of Poultry Diseases, Faculty of Veterinary Medicine, University of Warmia and Mazury, Oczapowskiego 13/14, 10-719 Olsztyn, Poland

Bartlomiej Tykalowski
Department of Poultry Diseases, Faculty of Veterinary Medicine, University of Warmia and Mazury, Oczapowskiego 13/14, 10-719 Olsztyn, Poland

Tomasz Stenzel
Department of Poultry Diseases, Faculty of Veterinary Medicine, University of Warmia and Mazury, Oczapowskiego 13/14, 10-719 Olsztyn, Poland

Andrzej Koncicki
Department of Poultry Diseases, Faculty of Veterinary Medicine, University of Warmia and Mazury, Oczapowskiego 13/14, 10-719 Olsztyn, Poland

Xiaofang Liu
Department of Virology, Tohoku University Graduate School of Medicine, 2-1 Seiryo-machi, Aoba-ku, Sendai, Miyagi 980-8575, Japan

Mariko Saito
Department of Virology, Tohoku University Graduate School of Medicine, 2-1 Seiryo-machi, Aoba-ku, Sendai, Miyagi 980-8575, Japan
Tohoku-RITM Collaborating Research Center on Emerging and Reemerging Infectious Diseases, RITM compound, FCC, Alabang, Muntinlupa City 1781, Philippines

Yusuke Sayama
Department of Virology, Tohoku University Graduate School of Medicine, 2-1 Seiryo-machi, Aoba-ku, Sendai, Miyagi 980-8575, Japan

Ellie Suzuki
Department of Virology, Tohoku University Graduate School of Medicine, 2-1 Seiryo-machi, Aoba-ku, Sendai, Miyagi 980-8575, Japan

Fedelino F Malbas Jr
Research Institute for Tropical Medicine, FCC, Alabang, Muntinlupa City 1781, Philippines

Hazel O Galang
Research Institute for Tropical Medicine, FCC, Alabang, Muntinlupa City 1781, Philippines

Yuki Furuse
Department of Virology, Tohoku University Graduate School of Medicine, 2-1 Seiryo-machi, Aoba-ku, Sendai, Miyagi 980-8575, Japan

Mayuko Saito
Department of Virology, Tohoku University Graduate School of Medicine, 2-1 Seiryo-machi, Aoba-ku, Sendai, Miyagi 980-8575, Japan

Tiancheng Li
Depatment of Virology II, National Institute of Infectious Diseases, 4-7-1Gakuen, Musashimurayama-shi, Tokyo 208-0011, Japan

Akira Suzuki
Department of Virology, Tohoku University Graduate School of Medicine, 2-1 Seiryo-machi, Aoba-ku, Sendai, Miyagi 980-8575, Japan

Hitoshi Oshitani
Department of Virology, Tohoku University Graduate School of Medicine, 2-1 Seiryo-machi, Aoba-ku, Sendai, Miyagi 980-8575, Japan
Tohoku-RITM Collaborating Research Center on Emerging and Reemerging Infectious Diseases, RITM compound, FCC, Alabang, Muntinlupa City 1781, Philippines

Weerapong Thanapongtharm
Department of Livestock Development (DLD), Bangkok, Thailand
Lutte biologique et Ecologie spatiale (LUBIES), Université Libre de Bruxelles, Brussels, Belgium

Catherine Linard
Lutte biologique et Ecologie spatiale (LUBIES), Université Libre de Bruxelles, Brussels, Belgium Fonds National de la Recherche Scientifique (FNRS), Brussels, Belgium

Witthawat Wiriyarat
The Monitoring and Surveillance Center for Zoonotic Diseases in Wildlife and Exotic Animals (MOZWE), Mahidol University, Nakhonpatom, Thailand

Pornpiroon Chinsorn
Department of Livestock Development (DLD), Bangkok, Thailand

Budsabong Kanchanasaka
Department of National Parks, Wildlife, and Plant Conservation, Bangkok, Thailand

Xiangming Xiao
Department of Microbiology and Plant Biology, Center for Spatial Analysis, University of Oklahoma, Norman, OK 73019, USA
Institute of Biodiversity Science, Fudan University, Shanghai 200433, China

Chandrashekhar Biradar
International Center for Agricultural Research in Dry Areas (ICARDA), Amman, Jordan

Robert G Wallace
Institute for Global Studies, University of Minnesota, Minneapolis, USA

Marius Gilbert
Lutte biologique et Ecologie spatiale (LUBIES), Université Libre de Bruxelles, Brussels, Belgium Fonds National de la Recherche Scientifique (FNRS), Brussels, Belgium

www.ingramcontent.com/pod-product-compliance
Lightning Source LLC
Chambersburg PA
CBHW080650200326
41458CB00013B/4806